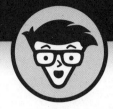

Gut Health

by Kristina Campbell, MSc

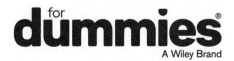

Gut Health For Dummies®

Published by: **John Wiley & Sons, Inc.,** 111 River Street, Hoboken, NJ 07030-5774, www.wiley.com

Copyright © 2024 by John Wiley & Sons, Inc., Hoboken, New Jersey

Published simultaneously in Canada

For general information on our other products and services, please contact our Customer Care Department within the U.S. at 877-762-2974, outside the U.S. at 317-572-3993, or fax 317-572-4002. For technical support, please visit https://hub.wiley.com/community/support/dummies.

Wiley publishes in a variety of print and electronic formats and by print-on-demand. Some material included with standard print versions of this book may not be included in e-books or in print-on-demand. For more information about Wiley products, visit www.wiley.com.

Library of Congress Control Number: 2024931600

ISBN: 978-1-394-22658-0 (pbk); ISBN 978-1-394-22660-3 (ebk); ISBN 978-1-394-22659-7 (ebk)

SKY10066641_021224

Contents at a Glance

Recipes at a Glance

Desserts

Table of Contents

Introduction

I can't convey how exciting it's been to watch gut health gradually emerge into the mainstream. Over a decade ago when I was experiencing debilitating gut symptoms every day, digestion was kept very hush-hush. The science was just starting to emerge, and useful science-based resources were almost nonexistent. When I started writing about gut health and the microbiome, most people who knew me were perplexed. More than once I took an editor's call in a coffee shop and the people at the next table — overhearing me talk about digestion — discreetly moved to another location.

But somewhere along the line, gut health went big. Maybe it was the incredible advancements in gut microbiome science or the publication of popular books on the digestive system, such as Giulia Enders' *Gut*. Maybe it was the fact that fecal matter became established as a lifesaving cure for recurrent *Clostridioides difficile* infection. Now gut health is everywhere — in popular books, on social media, in blogs, in newspapers and online articles, and in documentary films — and now in this book, *Gut Health For Dummies*.

Whether you're here out of desperation to rid yourself of symptoms or you're a fan of GutTok or other gut health content on social media, you've come to the right place. This book gives a solid scientific grounding in everything related to the gut — and this exciting journey shines a light on some dark and twisty corners of your body, with lots of surprising facts along the way. If you become squeamish at any time during this journey, just put down the book, pour yourself a tall glass of water, and remind yourself that what goes in must come out in one way or another. Appreciate that the gut is an incredible, complex system that enables you to be who you are as a human.

Gut health is getting more exposure at just the right time — because more and more people are experiencing digestive health problems that affect their lives. According to the American Gastroenterological Association, up to 70 million people in the United States have a gastrointestinal disease that interferes with their quality of life. And digestive problems have gotten in the way of desired activities for 40 percent of people at some point. In Canada, the incidence of digestive disease is even higher than in the United States — more than 50 percent of people are affected by symptoms. Despite these high numbers, many people delay seeking medical advice for gut-related issues. I hope this book brings clarity about your gut health experiences so you feel confident seeking the care you need — and take proactive steps to avoid gut health problems for many years into the future.

About This Book

Gut Health For Dummies isn't like the other gut health books on bookshelves. Most books about gut health purport to have the one-and-only solution to fix your gut health, whether it's a six-step plan, a restrictive diet, or an expensive array of supplements. The problem with those approaches is that they don't have adequate scientific support: They may have worked well for some person at a particular time, but they're not shown to work reliably. And they're often short-sighted, treating diet as the only thing that matters for gut health. (Spoiler alert: This book identifies many different aspects of your lifestyle that converge to shape your gut health.)

I suffered through years of digestive symptoms without a diagnosis and eventually found relief by changing multiple aspects of my lifestyle, which I share throughout this book. Now, I'm passionate about understanding the science and knowing how to apply it in real life, so everything I report in these pages is based on genuine scientific findings and expert opinion, without hyping any individual findings. Because I make a living working with scientists in this field, I take great care to ensure that everything I say is appropriate and evidence-based according to what they'd expect.

Here I give you the knowledge to tell what claims and information are scientifically backed — so you can understand which products are likely to work versus which ones are relying on more of a wish and a prayer. When you're able to evaluate products with a critical eye, you're not at the mercy of whichever company has the biggest marketing budget. I aim to create the resource that I never had when I suffered from my own gut health issues and felt bombarded by all kinds of confusing and expensive products, all claiming to cure what ailed me. Now with the increased popularity of gut health, the market is even more saturated with products purporting to fix your gut. However, I understand that daily decisions are complex, so if you end up deciding, because of a friend's recommendation or a social media influencer, that you want to try consuming a product with no scientific proof that it works, that's your choice. I only hope you'll be able to navigate your way through the world of gut health with awareness and better confidence.

In true *Dummies* style, the information in this book is presented in a clear, concise format with practical tips throughout. I capture the latest scientific thinking and translate it into everyday actions that represent the best-known ways to take care of your gut throughout your life.

This book extensively covers the microbiome of your gut. Your digestive tract microbiome is really several different microbiomes in different locations. Yet the microbiome of the colon is by far the most frequently studied because of the ease of collecting samples. (I mean, everyone deposits samples of this microbiome regularly into the toilet.) So, the term "gut microbiome" in scientific papers most often refers to the colonic, or fecal, microbiome. Throughout this book, therefore, gut microbiome refers to the colonic microbiome unless otherwise specified.

Sources of information about gut health often use dysbiosis to refer to a disrupted or abnormal gut microbiome. Dysbiosis can look a million different ways, even for a single disease. It can't even be defined as an imbalance between good and bad bacteria in the microbial ecosystem because the concepts of "good" and "bad" simply don't apply to microorganisms. For these reasons, dysbiosis has fallen out of favor in the scientific community, and I avoid it as well in this book. I tend to use the general terms "difference" or "disturbance" when talking about gut microbiome alterations associated with poorer health, lest people think dysbiosis is something that can be specifically defined and diagnosed.

The recipes in this book are complete, but they may not spell out every detail of prepping and cooking the food. For example, certain steps and techniques in cooking are standard no matter what you're preparing. In addition, I require specific types of ingredients and also want to make sure that you adhere to a few of my other cooking preferences. Take a quick look at the following list for points that apply to all the recipes:

>> Fruits and vegetables are washed under cold running water before using.

>> Pepper is freshly ground pepper. Invest in a pepper mill and give it a few cranks when you want pepper bursting with flavor.

>> Fresh herbs are specified in many of the recipes for their bright, authentic flavor. But you can still make a recipe if you don't plan to use these by substituting dry herbs, using one-third the amount of fresh.

>> Dairy products are low-fat.

>> Eggs are large unless otherwise indicated.

>> Olive oil is extra-virgin unless otherwise indicated.

>> All onions are sweet unless otherwise indicated.

>> Water is filtered water.

>> All temperatures are Fahrenheit.

>> Keep pots uncovered unless I tell you to put on the lid.

>> 🍅 This tomato icon indicates that the recipe is vegetarian.

Foolish Assumptions

When writing this book, I make the following assumptions about you:

- » You've heard about gut health but may not be familiar with the scientific jargon, so I define new terms as they're introduced.
- » You're suffering from digestive symptoms and you're open to seeking medical help and taking advantage of the interventions that have the best scientific support.
- » Even if you don't have regular digestive symptoms, you're also interested in leveraging the best science to maintain your gut health and overall wellness.

Icons Used in This Book

Throughout this book you'll see the following icons to draw your attention to certain paragraphs.

When you see this icon, it flags practical advice for putting gut health science into practice.

This icon highlights key points that help you gain a better understanding of gut health in general.

This icon indicates more detailed (nonessential) information for people who want to level up their knowledge.

This icon alerts you about what to watch out for if you want to avoid gut health problems.

This icon shows where a leading scientist weighs in specially for this book to bring you the latest knowledge in the field.

Beyond the Book

I hope you continue your gut health journey even after you read the last page of this book. For more information, you can check out the book's accompanying Cheat Sheet — go to `www.dummies.com` and search for "Gut Health For Dummies Cheat Sheet."

This book is also available as an audiobook — check it out on your favorite audiobook platform.

If you want to share any feedback with me, contact me through my website: `www.bykriscampbell.com`.

Where to Go from Here

This book is designed so you can jump in and start reading anywhere you want. If you prefer a refresher on the digestive tract and how it works, Chapter 2 is the ideal place to start. But if you have a clear memory of those eighth-grade lessons on the digestive tract and need to get up to speed on the microbes living there, start at Chapter 3.

For symptom SOS, jump right in at Chapter 6, or if you're lucky enough not to suffer from major digestive symptoms, you can skip to Chapter 10, which covers how to optimize your diet for gut health. Chapters 13 to 16 have some recipes to try out for supporting your gut if you're a generally healthy person.

If you're not sure where to begin, flip through the table of contents or index and find a topic that piques your interest.

1
Understanding Why Gut Health Is Important

Explore the emerging meaning of gut health and how it's different from digestive health.

Delve into the workings of the digestive system and how it achieves a fine balance between letting in what nourishes you and keeping out harmful substances.

Get a handle on the microorganisms that make their home in the digestive tract and examine what their surprisingly important roles are in maintaining your health.

Find out about the factors in your lifestyle that influence the gut microorganisms and gut health overall.

Discover the connections that scientists are making between your gut health and various diseases — not only digestive diseases, but also metabolic conditions, brain conditions, and more.

Chapter **1**

No Healthy Gut, No Health Glory

I f your body is a temple, your gut is its grand, elaborate foyer. The gut serves as a point of entry for food, medicines, and other substances — and that's where the action begins, but not everything makes it past this entrance hall. Some substances get sent out another door promptly, and others discard layers or become transformed before gaining access to other parts of the body through the gut barrier. The digestive system is your body's primary interface with the outside environment, so it's an area that's not outside you, and not fully inside you either.

Just as managing visitors through the foyer helps keep order in the rest of the building, keeping your gut in good working order is essential for your body's overall health. This chapter dives into what gut health is, then gives an overview of what the digestive tract looks like and how it functions. Finally, this chapter covers the essentials of managing your gut health if you have symptoms or if you want to optimize an already healthy gut.

Defining Gut Health

Decades ago, the term "gut health" didn't even exist. And 10 years ago when I was starting to write about this field, people I interviewed told me the first thing that came to mind when they heard the word "gut" was a protruding belly (as in the phrase "beer gut"). But starting around 2014 I began to hear about gut health more and more, and now, gut health is a term people use all the time — in blogs, in the media, in ads, and elsewhere.

Gut health, however, is often used without necessarily having a clear definition. This section clarifies what gut health is so you can use this definition as you navigate this book.

Discovering the meaning of gut health

So far, scientists haven't agreed on a definition of gut health. Some proposals for the meaning of this term are as follows:

>> Absence of a diagnosed digestive disease

>> Lack of any digestive symptoms

>> Optimal gut structure and function (including the configuration of the gut microbes)

None of these proposals, however, seem to capture the connotations of gut health today and why it's such a popular topic. Clearly many people (myself included, at one time) who are free of diagnosed digestive disease still don't have a healthy gut. And as for using digestive symptoms as the gold standard: Some signs of an unhealthy gut, such as gut barrier permeability or mild inflammation, may not result in symptoms but are nonetheless undesired and linked with health problems later on. Even optimal gut structure and function isn't a definition of gut health that adequately accounts for why the concept is suddenly resonating with millions around the world.

REMEMBER

Because of the general public's growing awareness of the latest science on the gut microbiome and how digestive health relates to other body systems, gut health has come to mean something more like a state of well-being, both mental and physical, that's enabled by what happens in the gut. Whereas the term "digestive health" narrowly refers to the digestive tract and how it functions, *gut health* extends to general wellness from the inside out. Because the gut is the body's crossroads of digestion, immunity, and metabolic health, overall health and well-being can't be achieved without a healthy gut. In other words, without gut health there's no (overall) health glory.

Dietary intake is an important concept intertwined with gut health. The popular conceptualization of gut health appears to signal a new awareness about how people's diets lead to measurable and direct consequences for physical and mental health. Diet, exercise, and other lifestyle factors were previously seen as having vague and long-term health benefits. But now scientists have found that these factors have almost immediate effects on your gut microbes, which are part of the mechanisms for broader health effects throughout the body. Clearly eating a single donut isn't going to shorten a person's lifespan, but donuts (with their high fat and sugar content) pressure the gut microbes in a certain way so that a habit of eating donuts maintains undesirable changes in the gut, which may take years to become visible through the rest of the body and have negative health consequences.

The current meaning of gut health, then, encompasses the optimal structure and function of the gut — with the acknowledgement that it may have the capacity to promote wellness or prevent illness, especially through what you eat.

Identifying components of gut health

Unfortunately, no hard and fast measures exist to confirm you have a healthy gut — and in fact the medical community is much more skilled at defining an unhealthy gut than a healthy gut. However, a healthy gut is generally associated with some specific outcomes:

>> Having fewer sick days

>> Not requiring a restrictive diet

>> Not needing medications for digestive health or other conditions

REMEMBER

As for assessing gut health more precisely, five parameters may be relevant:

>> **Digestive function:** Whether nutrients are broken down and absorbed properly

>> **Digestive tract structure:** Whether the parts of the digestive tract are structurally intact, with no observable damage from inflammation or other injury

>> **Motility:** If materials are moving through the digestive tract appropriately and at the right speed

>> **Gut microbiota characteristics:** Whether the gut microbial composition and function is appropriate (even though a normal gut microbiota hasn't yet been defined)

>> **Gut-brain axis function:** Whether the communication channels between the gut and the brain support both gut and brain health

Scientists may one day come up with a precise list of how to measure each of these parameters to set a standard for a healthy gut, but until then, gut health is more of a judgment call. It includes conscious efforts to maintain health by using knowledge about what affects the digestive tract and its resident microorganisms, as discussed in Chapter 4 as well as Part 5.

Why gut health matters more than ever

Chronic (also called *noncommunicable*) diseases such as heart disease, cancer, respiratory disease, and diabetes, have become a global health emergency. The World Health Organization (WHO) says chronic diseases are responsible for 74 percent of deaths each year. A recent analysis estimated that, in U.S. adults older than 50, the number with a chronic disease will nearly double between 2020 and 2050 — and healthcare systems are poorly prepared to handle the increasing burden of these diseases.

But an opportunity exists to prove these predictions wrong and reverse the chronic disease trend. Importantly, the following preventable factors contribute to the risk of dying from a chronic disease:

>> Smoking

>> Physical inactivity

>> Harmful use of alcohol

>> Unbalanced diets

>> Air pollution

At least three of these factors — inactivity, alcohol, and dietary intake — are now known to have direct connections to health through the gut. Not to mention, scientists are uncovering connections between gut health and chronic diseases themselves as I explain in Chapter 5. Gut health can provide powerful day-to-day motivation to improve habits that have a direct effect on how likely you are to die from a chronic disease — and can perhaps even prevent chronic disease from occurring in the first place. Thus, gut health is at the center of a prevention revolution, empowering people to take charge of their health through diet and other aspects of their lifestyle.

REMEMBER

From this perspective, gut health is one the keys to unlocking better health and longer, healthier lives. The current popularity of gut health is a positive sign that chronic diseases in your families and communities don't have to match up with the latest bleak projections.

Picturing Your Gut

The digestive system includes all the organs and processes in your body that transform your food into energy and eliminate solid waste. A prerequisite for understanding gut health is knowing what the parts of your digestive system look like and how they function; these sections give you a preview.

Understanding how your gut works

The digestive tract is made up of the parts your food moves through — the mouth, esophagus, stomach, small intestine, large intestine, and anus — along with the accessory organs (liver, pancreas, and gallbladder) that produce the substances required to successfully digest your food.

REMEMBER

The digestive system's jobs are to break down food using different mechanical, chemical, and microbial processes, to absorb nutrients, and to send off the waste for elimination. Chapter 2 gives details on how these complex processes work.

Meeting the microbes

The 38 trillion microorganisms you harbor are critical to your body's healthy functioning — and most of them reside in your digestive tract. Chapter 3 introduces you to these microorganisms: bacteria, archaea, fungi, and viruses. Scientists have techniques for not only identifying the composition of these microorganisms in your gut, but also figuring out their functions, or what their genes allow them to do.

Working from home in the gut, the microorganisms have incredibly important jobs that affect distant parts of the body. They strengthen your gut barrier, keep your immune system in check, make vitamins, transform and break down food and medicines, help control metabolism, and even guide your development from a young age.

One of the most exciting areas of science in the past 20 years (in my admittedly biased opinion) has been the study of gut microbes and their effects on overall health. So far the best-known way to get your microbial community to support your health is to keep it diverse and resilient in the face of perturbations.

REMEMBER

Several main things are shown to influence your gut microbes and overall gut health as Chapter 4 details:

>> Medications you take

>> What you eat

>> Other aspects of your lifestyle

Your gut microbiome is particularly sensitive to your everyday choices and habits, which may impact your gut health and perhaps trigger digestive symptoms.

Linking gut health to how you feel

A lot happens in the dark depths of your gut, so you may wonder how much it affects how you feel, physically and mentally. Chapter 5 goes over the known connections between the gut and other organ systems in the body: the skin, respiratory system, liver, kidney, and central nervous system. By studying these communication channels, scientists are linking many specific diseases to gut health — and especially to alterations in the complex ecosystem of intestinal microbes.

In the industrialized world, many aspects of lifestyle have the inadvertent effect of destroying gut microbes, leading some scientists to wonder if missing microbes in people's guts are responsible for the current epidemic of chronic diseases. On the bright side, evidence increasingly suggests that nurturing your gut health and keeping the microbial community diverse may have a positive impact on health, empowering you to prevent chronic disease to the extent it's possible, rather than passively waiting for it to happen.

Managing Your Gut Health

Regardless of the state of your gut health at present, strategies exist for actively managing it. If you experience regular gut symptoms, the first step is accurately describing them to a medical professional who can determine whether or not they fit the pattern of a digestive disease. Then you can take further steps, either through medical management or lifestyle changes, that can help you gain more control over your overall health and wellness as I discuss in these sections.

Identifying symptoms

Everyone experiences unwanted gut health symptoms at some time. Chapter 6 gets to the bottom of your gut symptoms and helps you know how to describe them accurately, including which symptoms are your cue to seek medical advice.

Recognizing possible diagnoses

Some gut-related symptoms signal the presence of digestive disease. Chapter 7 goes through what to expect if you're exploring a digestive disease diagnosis, including what crucial information to tell your doctor and some of the medical tests that may be necessary. That chapter also goes over some of the most common digestive diseases that doctors diagnose and the first steps to take post-diagnosis to make sure you have the most reliable information for your decision-making. I also outline the main categories of treatments for digestive diseases, the details of which should be guided by your healthcare practitioner.

Making dietary and other lifestyle changes

If you have gut symptoms without a digestive disease diagnosis, you can still follow a path of scientific evidence to lead you to appropriate *interventions* (actions you take with the intention to modify your health) that may bring you relief. Chapter 8 focuses on what to do if you don't have an official digestive diagnosis and helps you know how to progress toward better health while navigating the safety and effectiveness of different gut health products and services.

Chapter 9 delves right into the practicalities of managing gut health symptoms in different places, including at home, in public, when visiting others, at work, and while travelling. The chapter is packed with pro tips on lessening the impact of symptoms on your life, including how to leverage apps and other technology, and how to seek social supports.

REMEMBER

Diet is the controllable factor with the biggest impact on your gut health. Chapter 10 starts with the basics of nutrition and the dietary patterns that lead to better health through the actions of the gut microbes, and then covers the surprisingly simple science-backed principles for a diet that supports your gut health:

>> Every week, consume 30 or more varied plant sources of fiber.

>> Consume fermented foods every day.

>> Consume high quantities of live microorganisms — one billion or more — every day.

>> Consume low amounts of omega-6 fats and higher amounts of olive oil and other monounsaturated fats.

>> Avoid emulsifiers and noncaloric sweeteners in your diet.

For delicious inspiration on how to achieve gut-friendly dietary habits, Chapters 13–16 feature a wide array of recipes that support your gut microbes and gut health. Chapter 20 features ten gut-friendly foods to include in your diet each week.

Look to Chapter 10 to give you the lowdown on the biotics — that is, probiotics, prebiotics, synbiotics, and postbiotics — as well as on fermented foods. There I explain how to interpret these products' marketing messages and sort out fact from fiction.

REMEMBER

Diet isn't the only way to adjust your lifestyle for better gut health with the aim of optimizing overall health. Additional powerful factors (see Chapter 11) include the following:

>> Sleep habits

>> Exercise

>> Stress management

>> Outdoor time

Small steps forward in these areas can have compounding effects on your overall health over time.

Staying proactive about gut health throughout life

Certain times of life are especially important for protecting gut health:

>> **Pregnancy:** During this time, even though the fetus is sealed off from direct contact with gut microbes, the microbes of the mother-to-be may have indirect influences. Her microbes may be influenced by a range of factors, including:

- Dietary choices

- Probiotics

- Stress

- Antibiotics

- Infections during pregnancy

>> **Birth and the first three months of life:** Birth is the first exposure of the baby to the vast microbial world, with vaginal birth setting up the infant with a different collection of microbes than Caesarean section birth. Antibiotics and gestational age at birth strongly influence the baby's first microbial

collection, too. Subsequently in the first three months of life, diet (whether breastmilk or formula) has the biggest impact on the gut health of the infant. Various biotics may be added to formula to approximate important components of breastmilk.

>> **The first year of life:** Throughout the first year of a child's life, the factors that specially influence gut health are the transition to solid foods, antibiotics, and exposure to diverse (outdoor) microbes. The farm effect, whereby children who grow up on farms are protected from some chronic diseases later in life, is especially apparent during year one.

>> **Childhood:** From the ages of 1 to 12 years, gut health is primarily supported by the following:

  - Good dietary habits

  - Outdoor microbe exposure

  - Reduction of stress or adverse childhood experiences

>> **Adolescence:** By the time a person reaches adolescence, the gut is less dynamic and potentially less sensitive to external factors. However, a balanced diet and outdoor microbe exposure during adolescence can go a long way to supporting overall health from the gut outward.

>> **Older age:** A gut health transition happens in older age — partly because of the normal process of aging and partly because of age-related diseases as well as lifestyle changes. Diet and biotics, as well as medication management, are the primary ways to support gut health to extend health span in older age.

Science progresses over time, so you'll inevitably encounter new options for improving your gut health in the years to come — not to mention new sources of information that you'll need to evaluate. Chapter 12 empowers you to think critically about gut health products and find out which ones have been scientifically tested and shown to work. You'll be extra savvy about the science if you check out the top ten myths about gut health in Chapter 21.

Chapter **2**

Grasping How the Digestive System Works

What works hard while you're working and works even harder when you take a coffee break? The answer: Your digestive system.

Constantly laboring to transform your food into energy and clear away the substances you no longer need, your digestive system is made up of your digestive tract plus the accessory organs (liver, pancreas, and gallbladder), which produce all the substances needed for digestion. The digestive tract (also known as the gastrointestinal tract, or gut) is essentially a long and winding tube going from your mouth all the way down to your bottom (anus). Every new influx of food — or coffee, for that matter — gives your digestive system something to contend with. But even when you don't ingest food or liquid, this body system keeps working at a steady pace to replenish intestinal tissues and clear out residues.

The main functions of the digestive system are

>> Breaking down food through mechanical, chemical, and microbial processes

>> Absorbing nutrients

>> Eliminating waste products

This chapter gives you the grand tour of your digestive tract, orienting you to all the different parts and how they work — and presenting you with some surprising facts along the way.

Keeping the Outside from Coming Inside

The human digestive tract is a special zone that, strictly speaking, isn't inside your body. Even when your lunch has disappeared from your plate and appears to be inside of you, it's still on the outside — that is, the food is sequestered inside the central shaft of the digestive tract and kept there by the gut barrier. Only when some of the food components are broken down and allowed past the gut barrier are they considered truly inside your body because they then reach blood circulation and travel to where they're needed. Everything that remains trapped in the digestive tract is swept through to the bottom end and eliminated completely through defecation.

REMEMBER

How does the digestive tract keep substances outside from coming inside? It has a sophisticated gut barrier that includes two main parts as follows:

>> **Epithelial cells:** Facing the intestinal *lumen* (the space inside the digestive tract) is a layer of intestinal epithelial cells that's only one cell thick. These cells that line the inside of the intestines are connected by tight junctions — protein structures that open and close like Venetian blinds to let in nutrients while keeping out harmful substances.

>> **The mucus layer:** On top of the epithelial cells is a layer of mucus, gel-like proteins that form a squishy surface. The mucus layer in the gut protects the sensitive epithelial cells and provides stability in the chemical environment, separating the epithelial cells from digestive juices, bacteria, or toxins within the lumen. Chapter 3 discusses the microbes that sit atop the mucus layer.

THE LOWDOWN ON LEAKY GUT

In previous decades, a trendy condition called *leaky gut* was blamed for a huge range of ailments, from skin irritation to brain fog. The way leaky gut was used in alternative health, it served as a diagnosis even though scientists had little evidence for its existence. However, more recently the concept of intestinal permeability is being observed in scientific investigations and is also coming to be known as leaky gut — a state in which more space exists between the tight junctions of the gut, allowing some harmful substances to cross the gut barrier. Today, despite increased acknowledgment of this phenomenon in scientific circles, leaky gut is better characterized as a mechanism of how symptoms occur, rather than a diagnosis. Find more details in Chapter 6.

Immune cells underneath these layers also provide fortification against any harmful substances that could potentially reach the rest of the body. Figure 2-1 illustrates the gut barrier.

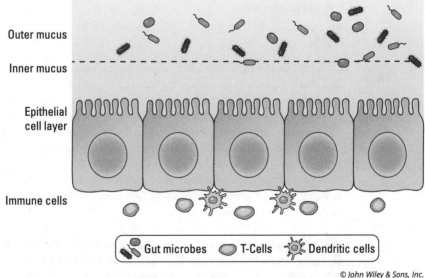

FIGURE 2-1: The parts of the gut barrier.

Outer mucus

Inner mucus

Epithelial cell layer

Immune cells

Gut microbes   T-Cells   Dendritic cells

Reviewing the Parts of the Digestive Tract and How They Work

As a living organism you need energy, and your digestive system creates that energy from things out in the world that contain what you need. For example, a plum or a piece of rye bread has plenty of components for you to digest and nourish your body. But if you happened to eat a piece of paper or some candle wax, they'd move through your digestive system without giving you nourishment.

Figure 2-2 shows the digestive tract. Food moves from top to bottom, through the following parts:

>> Oral cavity (mouth) and oropharynx

>> Esophagus

>> Stomach

>> Small intestine

>> Large intestine

>> Anus

REMEMBER

Each part of the digestive tract either moves food and liquid, or it helps break it into smaller parts — some of which can be absorbed and shipped around the body to where they're needed. *Enzymes* (substances assisting chemical reactions) are essential to the food breakdown. Nerves as well as various hormones help control the digestive processes. (Refer to the section "Recognizing the Essentials about Gut Function" later in this chapter for more information.)

Each part of the digestive tract also harbors live microorganisms that participate in digestion and other critical body functions. Chapter 3 covers these microbial contributors in greater detail.

Many components of your food are absorbed as they make their way through the digestive tract. But some go through, from end to end. Take, for example, the outer covering of a kernel of corn, called the pericarp. You may see evidence of this fibrous food component in your stool after it completes the entire digestive tract journey. The following paragraphs trace the basic journey of a corn kernel on its winding path from the mouth to the stomach and all the way to the toilet.

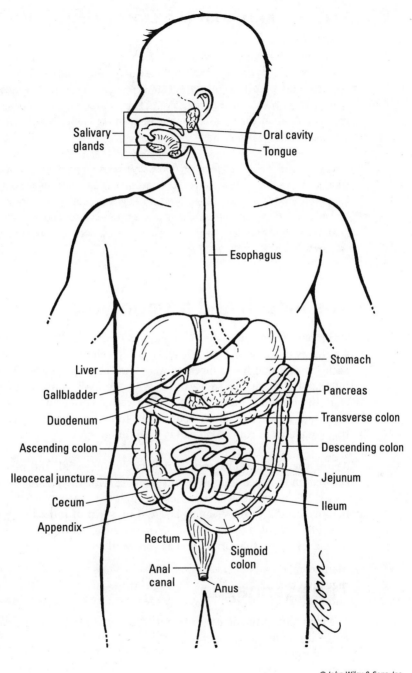

Salivary glands

Oral cavity

Tongue

Esophagus

Liver

Stomach

Gallbladder

Pancreas

Duodenum

Transverse colon

Ascending colon

Descending colon

Ileocecal juncture

Jejunum

Cecum

Ileum

Appendix

Rectum

Anal canal

Sigmoid colon

Anus

K. Born

© John Wiley & Sons, Inc.

FIGURE 2-2:
The parts of the
digestive tract.

THE MAN WHO ATE BICYCLES

You probably have a good idea of what's food and what's not — a pear is perfectly fine to eat, but a pair of boots isn't. Yet there once was a man who ate all manner of unusual items. Michel Lotito, born in 1950 in France, developed a method for eating non-nutritious meals consisting of bicycles, television sets, and shopping carts. He'd disassemble them, cut them into small pieces, and consume the pieces systematically with mineral oil and lots of water.

Doctors determined that he had an unusually thick stomach lining and extra powerful stomach juices that allowed him to consume these objects. From the age of 16, Lotito consumed objects on stage as an entertainer, acquiring the nickname Monsieur Mangetout (Mr. Eat-All). The list of items he consumed throughout his life included 18 bicycles, six chandeliers, two beds, and a *Guinness Book of Records* plaque that he was awarded for the strangest diet.

The mouth and oropharynx

The mouth (also called the *oral cavity*) kicks off the digestion process as soon as you ingest a piece of food. Chewing is typically the first digestive activity that occurs in the mouth — a mechanical process of physically breaking down the food into smaller pieces. As saliva mixes with the food, some of its components also start the chemical digestion of certain carbohydrates and fats — for example, some enzymes called *lingual lipases* start to break down *triglycerides* (a type of fat that circulates in your blood and is used for energy).

As for the hypothetical corn kernel you've ingested, the mouth is where it's chewed and pushed around by the tongue, with the fibrous pericarp remaining intact. When swallowed, it passes through the *oropharynx* (the back part of the mouth, leading to the esophagus). And in a feat of muscular gymnastics, a flap called the *epiglottis* closes off the airway at the exact right moment to prevent you from choking on the corn kernel as you swallow.

The esophagus

The next part of the digestive tract is the *esophagus*, the tube connecting the back of the throat to the stomach.

Muscular contractions called *peristalsis* push the corn kernel down through the esophagus. Peristalsis, a major process that keeps the food moving, occurs when the layer of muscle in the walls of the gastrointestinal tract squeeze in a pattern that propels the food and liquid through the digestive tract. In peristalsis, one part of the muscle contracts while the part directly in front of it relaxes, facilitating the forward movement of the intestinal contents.

Each end of the esophagus has a circular muscle that opens and closes like a drawstring — and at the bottom of the esophagus this muscle (called the *lower esophageal sphincter*) closes tightly so the corn stays in the stomach. For the corn kernel, it's a one-way trip with no return ticket.

The stomach

The stomach has a kind of rockstar status when it comes to digestion — that is, it often stands for the whole of the digestive tract. In everyday language, you may say you have a "stomachache" even though your problem could be at a number of different sites in the digestive tract.

True, important digestive work does happen in the stomach. Food that enters the stomach gets aggressively mixed and broken down, with acid and enzymes added to speed up the digestion process. The stomach walls squeeze the food as the gastric juices continue to break down carbohydrates and fats, and they also start breaking down proteins. Your stomach absorbs some fat-soluble substances, such as aspirin and certain types of alcohol.

The corn kernel gets tossed around in the stomach's acid bath, but even though conditions are harsh, the tough pericarp remains intact. Finally, the kernel is eased out of the stomach when the lower stomach muscle loosens, bringing it to the next part of its journey.

The small intestine

The small intestine is a long and windy tube whose main job is to extract nutrients from your food. It has a velvety lining on the inside with many folds, containing tiny hairlike microvilli that create a huge absorptive area. The small intestine gets first dibs on absorbing most of the food components that nourish the body. Water is also absorbed throughout the length of this part of the digestive tract.

The small intestine has three parts that the corn kernel visits as it moves along:

>> **Duodenum:** The first part of the small intestine immediately below the stomach. This part is where food substances are mixed with different digestive secretions.

>> **Jejunum:** The middle part of the small intestine, making up about two-fifths of its length, where a lot of the nutrient absorption happens.

>> **Ileum:** The bottom part of the small intestine, which is connected to the beginning of the large intestine.

Your pancreas makes digestive enzymes to further break down carbohydrates, fats, and proteins, and delivers them to the duodenum through small tubes called ducts. Furthermore, your liver makes bile and ships it to the gallbladder where it's stored and concentrated. The bile is released into the small intestine when needed to finish the chemical digestion of fats.

After many of the food components are absorbed (that is, they get the all-clear to pass through the gut barrier), your circulatory system delivers them to other parts of your body for immediate use or storage. For example, your blood carries some sugars, amino acids, glycerol, and some vitamins and salts to the liver. The liver processes some of these items and stores them until they're needed at other body sites.

Peristalsis moves the corn kernel down through the small intestine's entire length and onward to the large intestine.

The large intestine and anus

The large intestine (with the colon as its main part) is a beautiful thing. I say this figuratively rather than literally — unless fleshy, squishy, and odorous is your aesthetic. (No judgment.) But the colon really does have its fan club: Neil Pasricha named the colon one of the most awesome things in the original 2010 *Book of Awesome* (Amy Einhorn Books), for example. And Giulia Enders waxed lyrical about the colon in her popular 2014 book *Gut: The Inside Story of Our Body's Most Underrated Organ* (Greystone Books).

The colon is anything but a place for leftovers from the digestive journey. It's a place of transformation and renewal. Its huge population of microorganisms (refer to Chapter 3) turn undigested fiber into substances that maintain health.

REMEMBER

The large intestine is shorter than the small intestine, but it has a bigger diameter. The main parts of the large intestine are as follows:

>> **Cecum:** A pouch located at the junction of the small and large intestines

>> **Ascending colon:** The first tubelike section of the large intestine, which is usually located on the right side of the body and extends upward

>> **Transverse colon:** The middle section of the large intestine, which extends horizontally across the body from right to left

>> **Descending colon:** The section of the colon that extends down from the transverse colon on the left side of the body

>> **Sigmoid colon:** A shorter S-shaped part of the colon, which connects the descending colon to the rectum

>> **Rectum:** The last part of the large intestine, which is a short vertical tube that is the final stop for waste before it passes out of the body through the anus

The appendix is a thin pouch attached to the cecum at the beginning of the large intestine. Even though for many years the appendix was considered to have no special function, more recent investigations show it holds a sample of the gut microbiota that may be useful for repopulating the colon after disturbance by illness or antibiotics.

The intestinal contents continue to move along through peristalsis. Extra water is absorbed into the body through the walls of the large intestine, creating solid waste.

The corn kernel, nearing the end of its journey, moves through all of the parts of the large intestine. Then it exits through the anus, which is an opening surrounded by muscles that relax during the process of defecation. The corn kernel ends up in the toilet, ready to be flushed away and forgotten.

LOOKING CLOSER AT WHAT'S IN YOUR POOP

You produce it every day, but what is your poop made of? Typically, fecal matter is around 75 percent water and 25 percent solids. The solids are a mixture of living and dead microbes as well as undigested carbohydrate, fiber, protein, and fat — and a few inorganic substances such as calcium phosphate and iron phosphate. The bacteria give poop its most distinctive qualities. The brown color comes from bacteria acting on *bilirubin*, which is an end product from the breakdown of old red blood cells. The odor is caused by chemicals produced by bacteria, including indole and hydrogen sulfide.

What you eat is an important determinant of how your waste appears. If you eat lots of dietary fibers, your poop may appear bigger and softer. Specific things you ingest may also affect its appearance; for example, black licorice, blueberries, Pepto Bismol, or an iron supplement can all make your stool appear black. Chapter 6 explains the difference between normal and abnormal bowel movements.

Recognizing the Essentials about Gut Function

Several important processes help digestion proceed normally: the gut's nervous system, proper movement of the intestinal contents, and chemical reactions in the gut. Digestive–immune system interactions also occur. This section covers these complex factors that are necessary for producing smooth digestion.

Getting to know your gut's nervous system

Your central nervous system (CNS) — the brain and spinal cord — gets a lot of attention, but your gut has its own distributed system of nerves called the *enteric nervous system* (ENS).

The ENS consists of nerves within the walls of your gastrointestinal tract, which control various aspects of digestion. The nerves sense food and have the power to influence how fast the food moves as well as the digestive juices that are produced. The nerves also send signals to influence the actions of your gut muscles as they participate in peristalsis.

The ENS nerves relay many signals to the brain through connections to the CNS, mainly the vagus nerve, allowing signals to flow back and forth. Most of the signals between the gut and brain go in the upward direction, so the brain keeps close track of activities in the gut as sensed by the ENS. Chapter 5 has more information on the gut–brain axis.

Understanding gut motility

Digestion can't be rushed. Just think about the figurative meaning of the word "digestion" — when you say you're digesting a piece of information, you're taking the time to understand it and realize its implications. Time is important for literal digestion too. Even though you can eat quickly, the food takes its own sweet time getting through your digestive tract. If the gut contents move too fast or too slow, digestion goes wrong.

Motility encompasses the mechanisms by which food moves through your digestive tract after the moment of ingestion, including through peristalsis.

One way to measure motility is by observing your *gut transit time:* the amount of time it takes for a food item to go all the way through your digestive tract. Here are a couple of possible ways to measure gut transit time:

>> **Blue poop challenge:** A 2021 article in the scientific journal *Gut* outlined a new method for measuring gut transit time, which involved baking muffins with a special blue dye, eating one, and timing how long it took to see blue poop in the toilet. The study found the normal range to be anywhere between 14 and 58 hours to see the blue go through your system. After publication of this article, a gut microbiome testing company chimed in with the #bluepoopchallenge and invited individuals to test their gut transit time. Soon the challenge was all over social media, bringing gut health into the spotlight for a fleeting moment.

>> **Bristol Stool Scale:** Another rough way to measure motility is to look at the quality or appearance of the stool. A fast gut transit time tends to result in looser stool because the material doesn't sit in the colon long enough to have the water absorbed. A slow gut transit time tends to result in constipation because the material sits in the colon too long and has so much water extracted that it becomes a hard mass. A chart referred to as the Bristol Stool Scale (refer to Figure 2-3), is used clinically to indicate an individual's stool shape, with seven categories from hardest to softest, as part of assessing digestive health.

Different disorders can arise when motility goes wrong in different parts of the digestive tract. Chapter 7 covers some of these disorders.

WHERE INTESTINAL GAS COMES FROM

Intestinal gas (also called *flatus*) is a completely normal part of digestion. Even though some gas may come from air entering the stomach during swallowing, especially after consuming fizzy drinks, most gas comes from the activities of bacteria in the colon. Most of the gases produced there are hydrogen and carbon dioxide. Your gut produces far more gases than you know — around 80 percent of the total gases are absorbed back into the gut mucosa. Only about 20 percent of the gases remain to be released at an opportune time. The release of gas is more likely when the muscles in the rectum are active, such as shortly before a bowel movement.

The smell of flatus is caused by the mixture of gases produced, which in turn depends on the foods you consume as well as the microbes you have in your digestive tract. Some high-fiber foods containing sulfur may cause foul-smelling gas. Other factors affecting the smell include food intolerances (because in lactose or gluten intolerance the inability to break down dietary substances can lead to gas), medications, or infections. Chapter 6 discusses intestinal gas in greater detail.

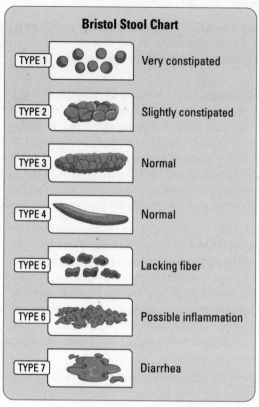

FIGURE 2-3: The Bristol Stool Scale, showing different categories of stool forms.

Delving into gut chemistry

Chemical processes play a big role in digestion. Enzymes and other digestive juices transform the food components creating smaller pieces or joining them to different substances.

Furthermore, some of the cells lining your stomach and small intestine create hormones to help control digestion. These hormones trigger your body to make digestive juices and send signals to your brain that you're hungry or full. Your pancreas also makes hormones that are important to digestion.

A chemical reaction critical to digestion is called *hydrolysis* — the process in which water molecules are merged with larger molecules such as proteins, fats, or carbohydrates, making these large molecules easier for your cells to absorb. Hydrolysis happens slowly, but your body can produce enzymes that speed up the process.

AN IMPORTANT SATIETY HORMONE: GLP-1

Several hormones contribute to digestion and metabolic health, but *glucagon-like peptide 1 (GLP-1)* has received more attention than most. L cells in the human gut (in the colon and terminal ileum, mostly) produce GLP-1 after a meal, and it's known for stimulating the release of insulin and inducing a feeling of satiety, making you feel full and refraining from consuming more food. GLP-1 is rapidly degraded in the body, but drug scientists managed to overcome this challenge so that GLP-1 could be harnessed for new medicines such as semaglutide (Ozempic), which improve metabolic health and induce weight loss.

Knowing about immune system interactions

Many immune cells reside in the gut, especially in a section of the small intestine called the *gut-associated lymphoid tissue (GALT)*. These immune cells participate in various activities related to digestion. They primarily interact with the microorganisms of the gut (see Chapter 3 for more information). Further, some fatty acids and vitamins are absorbed through the lymph system, which is a network of vessels carrying white blood cells and *lymph* (a colorless fluid) throughout your body to fight infection.

Meanwhile, the layer of intestinal epithelial cells have a radar that can sense whether the bacteria nearby have the potential to cause trouble. Specifically, they sense molecular patterns from microbes (called *pattern recognition receptors*). When they detect a possible pathogen, they stimulate the immune system into inflammation mode to try to combat the threat.

DETOXING YOUR GUT: YES OR NO

The idea of cleansing or detoxifying (detoxing) your gut goes way back to 19th-century ideas of autointoxication — a belief that intestinal waste products poisoning the body are major contributors to disease. Indeed, something is universally appealing about the narrative that you can somehow cleanse your insides and start fresh. But in fact, there's no scientific benefit behind this concept. You can spend a lot of money on fancy detox programs or put yourself through strict digestive cleansing regimens and end up with a gut that's no better off. Your gut detoxes itself naturally, so there's no need for any special detox efforts. However, increasing your fiber consumption and drinking sufficient water can bulk up your stool and help your digestion proceed more cleanly. For simple, science-backed ways to improve your gut health, refer to Chapters 10 and 11.

Chapter **3**

Getting to Know Your Gut's Ecosystem of Microbes

You may have thought your body was made up of only human cells. But in truth, your human form is incomplete without its 38 trillion *microorganisms* (living things too small to be seen without a microscope), which invisibly make up about one pound of your weight. Overall your microbial cells slightly out-number your human cells. It's a codependent relationship: The microbes need a safe place to call home, and you need them to help your body to thrive.

You have distinct groups of microbes living in or on different parts of your body, including your skin, your nose and lungs, and your genital tract. But where do the vast majority of these microbes hang out in your body? Your digestive tract (also known as your gut). All along the length of your gut, from your mouth to your anus are living, thriving collections of microorganisms.

In this chapter, I introduce you to these gut microorganisms and how they came to call your body home. I explain the crucial tasks these organisms perform to keep your body running smoothly and some general principles for shaping them up to support your health.

Meeting Your Gut Microbiome

If you could look through a window into your digestive tract, you'd see a dynamic and complex community of microbes. The dark, crowded world of the colon, for example, is teeming with all manner of *bacteria, archaea, fungi,* and *viruses* (which I describe in this section) in fantastical shapes that range from tiny squid to pearl necklaces to balloons on strings. All these microbes are packed together in one colorful mass, with each one vying for its own space and nutrients to thrive and multiply.

You'd see tiny viruses hang off the bacteria like leeches. Each new influx of food would send some of the microbes into a feeding frenzy, whereas other microbes would hang around the edges and feast on the by-products. Yet others would run out of their preferred food and abruptly shut down their systems. You'd witness a captivating continual cycle of life and death and regrowth.

Here I explain the types of microorganisms in your gut microbiome and the techniques scientists use to find out information about them.

Getting acquainted with your gut's inhabitants

The community of microorganisms in one particular place, such as the colon, is referred to as a *microbiota* or at times as a *microbiome.* (Among scientists, the word *microbiome* refers more specifically to the genes of the microorganisms in a community, but this definition isn't used outside the scientific realm.) Most scientists now avoid using the outdated word *microflora,* because flora denotes all plant life, making an incorrect parallel between microorganisms and plants. Note that the words *microbes* and *microorganisms* are generally used interchangeably.

REMEMBER

What exactly are the microorganisms in this gut community? The four main categories are as follows:

>> **Bacteria:** Single-celled microorganisms that reproduce independently

>> **Fungi/yeasts:** Microorganisms consisting of either single or multiple cells, which reproduce independently using spores

>> **Archaea:** Ancient (early-evolving) microorganisms that look similar to bacteria but often have a differently structured cell wall, helping them thrive in extreme environments such as volcanoes or the deep ocean

>> **Viruses:** The tiniest microbes, which are only active and able to reproduce when they latch onto the cells of other living things, such as bacteria

Getting acquainted with the microbes

Scientists today have two main ways of finding out about the microbes living in your gut or any other environment.

Culturing

Culturing is a technique for growing microbes under controlled laboratory conditions, generally in a petri dish with a growth-supporting material called a *culture medium*. Different microbes have different requirements for growth, so scientists tailor the conditions to the microbe they want to reproduce. Many microbes are so finicky that they've never been grown in a lab to this day.

BACTERIA'S BAD REP

Bacteria and other microbes have had a pretty bad reputation over the years. This regrettable status came about because the first microbes to be made famous by scientists were *pathogens*, the ones that cause sickness. A scientist named Robert Koch published a paper in 1876 providing proof that anthrax was caused by the bacterium *Bacillus anthracis*, providing the first proof for the germ theory of disease. In subsequent years, more than a dozen other bacterial pathogens were pinpointed as causing disease.

This discovery was a big breakthrough because knowing how people got sick helped save a lot of lives over the next decades. But focusing so intensely on the bacteria that caused disease had a downside — it solidified the reputation of bacteria and other microbes as bad and harmful. This rep persisted for almost a century and a half and produced a lot of *germophobes* (people who are afraid of germs and obsessed with cleanliness).

Yet now, with the emergence of microbial science, the paradigm is starting to shift. With scientists able to interrogate the entirety of microbial communities, it's clear that the sickness-causing microbes are a tiny fraction of all microbes. The majority are clearly benign or even beneficial to humans, so they deserve to be celebrated and met with curiosity rather than feared.

Gene sequencing

Microbes have genes, just like humans do. *Sequencing* these genes means determining the order of the nucleic acids, which carry the genetic information that gets interpreted in cells to carry out life-sustaining functions.

Microbial gene sequencing allows scientists to find out the identity of all microbes in a sample without having to culture them. This ability to take a complete microbial snapshot based on genetic information is the basis of microbiome science over the past two decades and has made new complex worlds visible.

The two main types of sequencing are

» **16S rRNA gene sequencing:** A method that analyzes one small ID tag in each cell

» **Whole-genome sequencing:** A method that breaks up all the DNA into pieces, analyzes it, and fits it back together into a complete picture by looking for regions of overlap between pieces

Both methods generate a large amount of data — and *bioinformatics* is the field of science concerned with turning large, complex sets of biological data into useful information such as microbe names.

Even though awareness of microbiomes and beneficial microbes existed since at least the early 1900s, only in the early 2000s did the technology advance so microbial genes could be sequenced on the large scale and with the economic efficiency that made microbiome science possible.

Identifying what's in your gut

The first thing scientists can find out about a microbiome is what's there, or the identity of the microbes. This information is known as the microbial *composition*, and it can be gained from either 16S rRNA gene sequencing or whole-genome sequencing. Whereas 16S gives a big-picture overview and general categories of microbes, whole-genome sequencing can give a more detailed picture of the microbial identities.

REMEMBER

Microbes are classified into groups and named based on their similarity to other microbes. Today's method for classification of all living things, including microbes, derives from a system proposed in 1758 by the Swedish botanist Carolus Linnaeus. From general to specific, scientists identify microbes according to the following groups:

- » Domain
- » Phylum
- » Class
- » Order
- » Family
- » Genus
- » Species
- » Strain

REMEMBER

Starting with the most specific, bacteria of the same strain are exact clones of one another. Moving up the classification ladder, bacteria that are the same species (but different strains) may share genes and act similarly under certain conditions. At higher and higher levels of classification, the microorganisms in each group become less similar to each other. Figure 3-1 provides an example of the levels at which a microorganism (in this case a bacterium) can be classified and named.

Level of classification	Name
Domain	Bacteria
Phylum	Pseudomonadota
Class	Gammaproteobacteria
Order	Enterobacterales
Family	Enterobacteriaceae
Genus	*Escherichia*
Species	*Escherichia coli*
Strain	*Escherichia coli* O157:H7

© John Wiley & Sons, Inc.

FIGURE 3-1:
Example of how a bacterium is classified at different levels.

Why does this discussion focus on bacteria, when archaea, fungi, and viruses also abound in the gut? The answer is that bacteria have been the most frequently studied microorganisms in the microbiome by far. They also make up the largest biomass in a gut microbiome, so they've been the priority for scientists around the world. But as the science progresses, expect to hear more about the other types of microbes, too.

REMEMBER

Any specific microorganism is properly referred to by its genus, species, and strain. This triple-barreled name becomes important when talking about probiotic microorganisms and finding out what health benefits they provide.

This list introduces you to a few specific groups of microorganisms you may come across on a regular basis when talking about gut microbiomes:

>> **Lactobacilli:** This diverse group of bacteria is shaped like little rods, similar to the classic sprinkles you'd see on a cupcake. You may even think of Earth as one big cupcake with lactobacilli scattered all over because members of this bacterial group are found in countless settings, from soil and rotting leaves, to fermented milk and other foods, to the human gut and skin. All lactobacilli were previously classified under the genus *Lactobacillus*, but in 2020 scientists subdivided this group according to new discoveries about their genetic relationships. Now lactobacilli is a loose, unofficial term for a group of 25 different genera of bacteria that (cleverly) still all have names beginning with "L." Many common types of lactobacilli are found in yogurt and probiotic supplements.

>> **Bifidobacteria:** In 1899 a French scientist named Henri Tissier got curious about the bacteria in babies' dirty diapers and discovered the first species in this group of bacteria, most of which are Y-shaped. Since then, many other bifidobacteria have been identified as important members of gut microbiomes — not only in babies, but also in healthy adults and in a variety of other mammals as well as birds. In humans, bifidobacteria have the very important job of assisting the body with fiber digestion. All bifidobacteria are currently members of one official genus, *Bifidobacterium*, and certain strains are found in foods and probiotic supplements.

>> *Escherichia:* I won't blame you if the words *Escherichia coli*, or *E. coli*, bring up feelings of fear or revulsion. Bacteria of this species are regularly pinpointed as the cause of terrible outbreaks of illness, lurking in Romaine lettuce or undercooked ground beef. But it's not quite fair to paint all *E. coli* with the same brush. Even though all *E. coli* share some features in common, the hundreds of strains are highly diverse and the effects on the human body can be drastically different from strain to strain. So although the strain *E. coli* O157:H7 can definitely cause a nasty gut infection, for example, the strain *E. coli* Nissle 1917 has the opposite effect: It's a probiotic that can prevent or treat diarrhea.

Each of these bacterial groups are the focus of multiple scientific conferences and books, but this list doesn't even begin to describe the vast number of diverse microorganisms that exist, nor even the ones that specifically affect human health. On the other hand, if you remember these three groups you'll be well on your way to discovering the wonders of the microbial world. I introduce you to some other important groups of bacteria in other sections of this book.

PREVENTING GUT MICROBIAL TAKEOVER

Microbes naturally multiply given the right environment. If your body is mostly microbes, what stops them from completely taking over? The answer is that each microbe requires specific conditions to grow and multiply, such as certain levels of oxygen or acidity. Because these factors vary along the length of the digestive tract and other parts of the body, they limit the types of microbes that can grow in each part. In addition, microbial competition for limited food supplies, as well as immune system monitoring, ensures that things stay under control in this complex community.

At first glance, the names of microorganisms can be long and intimidating. But wait, who hasn't met a 5-year-old who can rattle off the complicated multi-syllable names of 18 dinosaurs? Learning the names of life forms isn't impossible if you connect them to what you know and get excited about what they can do. I hope this book helps you increase your appreciation and excitement for microorganisms — that way, maybe a few of the names will stick and you'll be able to talk about them with confidence.

Exploring the microbes in your digestive tract

Here's a quick tour of the microbial communities in the major parts of the digestive tract:

>> **Mouth:** Many of the oral microbes originate from the outside world (through activities such as eating, breathing, and chewing your nails) but they don't last long because of the antimicrobial defenses in the saliva. Overall the community changes constantly as microbes come and go, but specific microbes grow consistently in different mouth geographies. Some microbes team up and grow on your teeth in spiny hedgehog configurations that you need to destroy regularly by brushing your teeth.

>> **Esophagus:** The microbes in the *esophagus* (the tube connecting your mouth to your stomach) are mainly the same as those found in the mouth, and they also change constantly with the passage of food and saliva en route to the stomach.

>> **Stomach:** Because the stomach is highly acidic, many microbes from the mouth and esophagus call it quits here. The stomach microbiome is much more sparse than elsewhere in the digestive tract. But on the other hand, acid-tolerant microbes exist and thrive in the stomach for a longer amount of time. This microbial community, too, is constantly changing.

>> **Small intestine:** Microbes are quite populous in the small intestine, but because most of your digestion occurs here, your body has ways of keeping them in check to make sure they don't overstep their bounds and digest things they shouldn't. Although it seems the microbes at this site are highly dynamic over time, the location of the small intestine makes sampling difficult so scientists know relatively little about this microbial community overall.

>> **Large intestine (particularly the colon):** The large intestine, the main part of which is the colon, is a gathering place for the biggest variety and number of digestive tract microbes. The population is relatively stable over time here, unlike the other digestive tract sites. If you analyze the microbiome of your large intestine, you'll find anywhere from 180 to 1,000 different species represented, but in a group of 100 people, chances are that not a single species is universally present in every person.

Determining what microorganisms can do

Just as a human child can have a genetic predisposition for athletic or musical skill, microorganisms are equipped with certain abilities depending on the genes they have — in other words, their *function*. For example, some microorganisms have genes that enable them to make molecules called *short-chain fatty acids (SCFAs)*, which feed the gut lining and are important for realizing the benefits you get from consuming fiber. Whole-genome sequencing (which I describe in the section "Getting acquainted with your gut's inhabitants" earlier in this chapter) can give information about microbial functions.

BEYOND "GOOD" AND "BAD" MICROBES

Although it's true that some microbes called pathogens have specific talents for causing sickness or harm to humans, I try to avoid the trap of talking about "good" and "bad" microbes. Even though you'll see this dichotomy very frequently in materials about gut health, it just doesn't measure up to the scientific reality.

If you imagine all the life forms in an ecosystem such as a rainforest, none of these life forms are inherently good or bad. The same applies to microbial ecosystems; a great many of the microbes in your gut are harmless most of the time but turn harmful when certain conditions are met. Instead of saying microbes are either good or bad, like superheroes or villains, you can say microbes have relationships with each other. For each type of microbe and for the other life forms it interacts with, the outcome of these relationships can be either beneficial, neutral, or harmful to each player. Investigating the outcomes of human-microbe relationships is one of the primary tasks of scientists in the microbiome field.

Although the function of an individual microbe within a vast community may not matter much, the collective functions of an entire community are important. The totality of microbial functions is your labor pool: Do you have the right microbes to do all the jobs required for your body to thrive? Carrying further the example of SCFAs, several different bacteria can produce these important molecules — so as long as you have some SCFA-producing microbes in your gut such as *Faecalibacterium prausnitzii* or *Roseburia intestinalis* when you consume fiber, you're likely to have a supply of this molecule to support your health.

Even though no two people have the same gut microbial composition, microbial functions may be more universal. In essence, scientists believe a basic set of functions must be provided by your gut microbes to best support your health, regardless of which exact microbes provide these functions. At the same time, however, there may be specialist species required in the gut to carry out functions that no other species can provide.

Finding Out What Your Gut Microbiome Does for You

A germ-free human has never existed so scientists don't know what life would be like without a person's microbes. But countless creatures that evolved before humans have outsourced essential life functions to their accompanying microbes over time, so probably humans are no exception. All available evidence suggests you couldn't get by without your microbes pitching in on some key activities that keep you healthy and well.

REMEMBER

Gut microbes are local residents of the digestive tract, so as you may expect, they contribute significantly to keeping your gut healthy. However, these gut microbes manage (you may even say micromanage) some very important processes elsewhere in the body that are necessary for maintaining day-to-day health. Chapter 5 provides more detail on how the microbes' hard work influences the functioning of various organs in the body, including the brain. But for now, here are the essential tasks your gut microbes tirelessly carry out so you can maintain your health every day.

Fortifying your gut barrier

A strong gut barrier not only helps keep the chemical environment of the gut stable, but it also helps you by thwarting any sickness-causing microbes nearby that may be looking for an opportunity to cause trouble.

If you took a cross-section of your small or large intestine, the gut barrier — which divides the space inside the intestines from your blood circulation and the rest of your body — would look like a four-layer cake. The two main layers (refer to Chapter 2) are the mucus layer and the epithelial cells. These layers have microbes on top and immune cells underneath. From top to bottom (with bottom being adjacent to blood circulation), the layers are as follows.

A thick dusting of gut microbes

A community of microorganisms lives on top of the gut barrier, nestled in the part of the mucus layer that faces the inside of the intestine. The microbes are suited for living in this mucus and make use of it in different ways, as a habitat or sometimes a food source.

A spongy layer of mucus

The mucus layer, with its constant turnover of fresh mucus, is essential for the integrity of the gut barrier. It provides physical distance between the sensitive epithelial cells and the complex mix of digestive enzymes, bacteria, and even toxic substances inside the intestine.

Scientists have learned from *germ-free mice* (mice born and raised in a sterile capsule, with no microbes in their guts or elsewhere) that the gut microbes living in the mucus layer, such as bifidobacteria, are essential for its proper formation. These microbes regulate the constant turnover of the mucus, making sure it's produced and secreted into the intestine and degraded at appropriate rates to maintain its optimal function in protecting the body. Certain bacteria sitting atop the mucus layer use the mucus as their food, earning the name *mucolytic bacteria*. For instance, *Akkermansia muciniphila* is one group of mucus-loving bacteria that chow down and multiply on the mucus layer, likely providing metabolic benefits in the process. (See the section "Pulling the strings of your metabolism" later in this chapter for more information on metabolism.)

When pathogens try to fight their way through by degrading the mucus layer to reach the epithelial cells and infect the body, the bacteria on the mucus layer may sense this and employ different strategies, such as:

>> Giving the signal to ramp up mucus production so the pathogen is kept farther away from the epithelial cells

>> Occupying the binding sites (which are like empty seats) available on the mucus proteins, leaving nowhere for the pathogens to latch onto

A thin sheet of epithelial cells

Epithelial cells underneath the mucus layer form a thin sheet that's only one cell thick, making up the internal gut lining. The epithelial cells are connected to each other by protein structures called *tight junctions*, which can increase or decrease their permeability depending on what needs to be kept inside or let out. This function allows the gut barrier accomplish its tricky job of letting nutrients pass through into the body while keeping out pathogens and other harmful materials.

A layer of mixed immune cells

Right below the epithelial cell layer is a diverse mix of immune cells. These cells communicate with each other and with the epithelial cells to guard the gut barrier and activate against any threats.

Keeping your immune system on a leash

Your immune system is, at its core, a way for your body to figure out what its own boundaries are. If you think of yourself as a walking, talking ecosystem made up of human cells and trillions of microbes, the immune system's job is to keep that ecosystem thriving and intact. Its jobs include carrying out regular repairs, tossing out what's no longer needed, incorporating new substances into that ecosystem if they'll help it thrive, and rejecting or destroying substances that disrupt the ecosystem. Essentially it's a force field surrounding you as you move through the world, constantly making the call about whether to accept or reject the things it encounters. In doing this work, it defends you from sickness-causing microbes and cell changes that could cause harm.

REMEMBER

The gut is one of the largest immune organs in your body because it houses the immune system structure called the *gut-associated lymphoid tissue*, which contains around 70 percent of your body's immune cells. Microbes are in close proximity to the immune cells of the gut barrier, and they help regulate the immune system in complex ways — ensuring under normal circumstances that immune activity doesn't become overactive or underactive.

TECHNICAL STUFF

Here are some important immune cells found at the gut barrier and how the gut microbes help control them:

>> **Macrophages:** These cells can capture and destroy any unwanted material that gets past the epithelial barrier, and they also clean up dead cells and help repair damaged tissue. Gut microbes influence the function and development of these cells, and their failure to do so can lead to chronic inflammation, cancer growth, or *fibrosis* (thickening and stiffening of body tissues).

» **T cells:** These important cells orchestrate *adaptive immunity*, the search- and-destroy mission that happens when your immune system has previously identified something as a threat. Specific gut microorganisms have the ability to command T cells to develop into several different specialized types such as helper T cells and regulatory T cells, and also to regulate their responses against threats.

» **Dendritic cells (DCs):** These clever cells have a system for discriminating between harmless and harmful microbes and generally help keep the peace (for instance, by promoting tolerance) in the intestine. Their signals help defend against harmful microbes and protect against injury to the intestinal wall. Pathogenic bacteria in the gut can activate DCs to induce inflammation in an attempt to protect the body, while resident gut microbes can activate DCs to create a signal for more T regulatory cells, which limit inflammation.

SCIENTIST
SAYS

Immune cells have ways of identifying harmful bacteria as immediate threats, and they also rely on nonharmful bacteria to fine-tune immune activity. This regulation of immunity is accomplished in a variety of ways. Ed Ishiguro, Professor Emeritus of Biochemistry and Microbiology at University of Victoria, Canada, explains that when gut microbes eat, they produce by-products that trigger the protective functions of the various classes of the immune cells, which ends up stabilizing the immune system. He says the microbes communicate to the immune cells directly, too, because the immune cells have sensory receptors that detect different features of microbes. Moreover, certain chemicals that come directly from the microbial cell structures (for example, a chemical fragment from the cell walls of bacteria called muramyl dipeptide) regulate the activities of immune cells.

When the resident bacteria fail to regulate the immune system properly, gut barrier damage and rampant inflammation can ensue. Chapter 5 lists some of the conditions associated with out-of-control inflammation.

Making vitamins

To function properly and avoid a deficiency, your body requires a range of vitamins on a regular basis. Gut microbes can be mini factories for producing essential vitamins: vitamin K as well as some B vitamins (biotin, cobalamin, folate, nicotinic acid, panthotenic acid, pyridoxine, riboflavin, and thiamine). The majority of your vitamin B is supplied through your diet and absorbed from the small intestine, but a small portion is synthesized by the microbes in the colon and absorbed directly from that region of the digestive tract.

Transforming your food

Another constant occupation of your gut microbes is to consume components of your diet, creating waste products called *metabolites* that can directly benefit your health. *Substrate* is the technical term for a food component that gut microbes come in contact with and consume (or metabolize). Some of the resulting metabolites become food for yet other microbes, in a food chain interaction known as *cross-feeding*, or if they don't get consumed, they can go on to directly affect your physiology by finding their receptors and fitting in like a key in a lock.

Gut microbial metabolites can have receptors in the body either locally (in the gut), or they can get shipped around the body to affect health in different places. Thousands of different metabolites are careening around your body at this very moment, and although the ones produced by your gut microbes account for only a small percentage overall, they have some important functions for maintaining your health.

The gut microbial composition you currently have can influence the metabolites you produce in response to your food — so two people can eat the exact same thing and produce very different sets of metabolites. Scientists think this could partially account for why the same diet can seem to affect people's health differently. In other words, your gut microbiota's ability to transform dietary compounds can influence the benefits you get out of your diet.

However, individuals do consistently produce some types of metabolites in response to foods. Here are two key examples of your gut microbes transforming parts of your diet into health-promoting metabolites:

>> **Turning fiber into SCFAs:** Specific forms of indigestible dietary fiber (also known as *fermentable fiber*) reach the colon, where microbes break them down to produce SCFAs — with three of the most important types being acetate, propionate, and butyrate. These powerhouse metabolites not only provide energy to the cells of the colon and reinforce the all-important gut barrier, but they also have receptors in many different parts of the body.

>> **Turning tryptophan into serotonin:** Tryptophan is an *amino acid* (a broken-down component of protein) found in foods such as milk, turkey, chicken, and oats. Gut microbes turn this compound into serotonin, which functions locally to influence *motility* (movement of materials through the digestive tract; see Chapter 2 for more about motility) and a number of other gut functions. Gut-produced serotonin is identical to brain-produced serotonin, and although the two types operate in different spheres, the gut serotonin may be able to influence certain brain functions, too.

Modifying your medicines

Xenobiotic metabolism is the breakdown of external substances, including drugs, by the body. Your body prepares to excrete any medicines you take, often by transforming them into different compounds. Your gut microbial community has the job of transforming many of the medicines you consume — and sometimes these transformations either help or hinder the effect of the drug on your body.

Scientists have discovered examples where microorganisms either activate or inactivate medicines. For example, some cancer immunotherapy drugs fail to work in germ-free mice because they need assistance from gut microbes. In humans, these immunotherapies are found to be more effective at eliminating cancer cells when certain bacterial species are present in a person's gut.

SCIENTIST SAYS

Sahar El Aidy, Professor of Host-Microbe Interaction at University of Groningen in the Netherlands discovered a way in which gut microbes inactivate a medicine. She found that levodopa, a very common and effective medicine for Parkinson's disease, is broken down by gut microbes to become less effective. Although this line of research on medicines is fairly new, the research from her lab and others shows that the gut microbiome significantly impacts medication effectiveness and safety by doing any of the following:

» Influencing how drugs get metabolized or absorbed

» Generating toxins in some cases

» Changing the body's immune responses when the drug is taken

The power of gut microbes to transform medicines is becoming a big deal in the field of pharmacology, with more studies underway.

Pulling the strings of your metabolism

Every living being acquires nutrients and other substances from its surrounding environment and uses them for energy to move and to grow — whether it's a bird in the park digging in the grass for a beetle, or you're opening a take-out box for some pad Thai. Ingesting a tasty morsel is part of your *metabolism*: a set of interconnected processes whereby the body breaks down food components and builds up energy and body tissues — the basic activities that keep it functioning.

Gut microbes help control many aspects of metabolism, contributing to how you digest and extract energy from your food, absorb nutrients, and excrete by-products. Scientists first observed a connection to body weight in mouse studies in the early 2010s: Given the exact same diet, mice who harbored the gut microbiota of a lean person gained less weight than mice who harbored the microbiota of a person with obesity. Later, human research showed that changing a person's gut microbiota could alter *insulin resistance* (a state in which your cells stop responding to signals they should take up glucose from the blood). Studies in the Netherlands showed a fecal microbiota transplant from a lean, metabolically normal person helped someone with disordered metabolism to slightly improve their responsiveness to insulin (although they didn't lose weight). Although no miracle cures have been discovered, the research does indicate gut microbiota is part of maintaining healthy metabolism.

As for how the gut microbes exert this control over metabolism, the SCFAs appear to play an important role. When SCFAs are produced by gut microbes after they feast on certain types of fiber, these molecules provide a source of calories that the body either absorbs or excretes. The complicated balance between SCFA production, absorption, and excretion may account for different effects on metabolism and body weight.

Another example of how gut microbes exert control over metabolism is through regulating important gastrointestinal hormones. Some of the tryptophan from your diet, for example, is turned into a compound called indole, which calls the shots on secretion of glucagon-like peptide 1 (GLP-1) — a hormone that floods the intestine to regulate blood sugar and insulin after a meal (in part, by getting the pancreas to produce insulin). SCFAs are another metabolite that trigger the intestinal cells to produce more GLP-1.

A secure gut barrier, which I discuss in the section "Fortifying your gut barrier" earlier in this chapter, is also a major factor in regulating your metabolism. When the microbes fail to help maintain a strong gut barrier, intestinal permeability increases. This leakiness allows forbidden substances past the epithelial cell layer and leads to *low-grade inflammation,* overactivation of your immune system throughout your body, which wreaks havoc on your overall metabolism and ability to stay lean. As Chapter 5 discusses, this phenomenon may contribute to disordered metabolism, spurring weight gain and elevated blood sugar levels.

Guiding your development

No exaggeration — your microbes have gotten you to where you are today. From the very first days of your life, they guided the development of some key parts of your physiology: primarily your immune system and your central nervous system.

Research suggests that the immune system fails to develop properly in the absence of a gut microbiota (such as in germ-free mice) and that an early-life window of opportunity exists, during which the gut microbes must teach the immune system the difference between harmless and harmful substances. The gut microbiota appears to send out chemical signals to help guide the development of the immune system. If this immune education doesn't occur within the appropriate window of time, impairments in immune function occur in young animals and may last into adulthood. Chapter 18 explains how this may play out in humans.

Central nervous system development is an intricate process that happens rapidly in humans' early life. Scientists have found clues that many basic developmental processes in the brain are modulated directly or indirectly by gut microbes. These processes include formation of the *blood-brain barrier* (which separates the brain from blood circulation), *myelination* (the formation of an insulating layer around nerves to help signals travel faster), and the growth of neurons.

Understanding How You Get Your Unique Gut Microbiome

At this moment, the types and amounts of microbes in your gut microbiome are unique to you, similar to a fingerprint. Many different forces converged to give you the unique microbiome you have today. You get your gut microbiome starter pack during birth, and these starter microbes change rapidly in the first few months of your life along with the rest of your body. The pace of change slows around age three but continues little by little until adulthood, when it becomes relatively stable. However, different aspects of your lifestyle and experiences continue to shape it to this day.

Here's the story of how you got your gut microbiome, from the very beginning.

ADDING UP THE FACTORS SHAPING YOUR GUT MICROBIOME

If scientists knew your detailed health status and tracked your every move — what you ate, what medications you took, where you travelled, how soundly you slept, and even your bowel movements — they'd only be able to predict about 10 to 15 percent of your gut microbiome composition compared to other people. However, when one group of scientists added this kind of information to people's 26-year health history, they were able to account for 33 percent of the microbiome variation between people. This supports the idea that your unique collection of gut microbes is the cumulative result of many health and lifestyle factors, extending over a long stretch of time.

Microbes influencing you before birth?

For many years the sealed pouch of the womb in which a fetus develops was thought to be a microbe-free zone. But sequencing studies started to emerge in the 2010s showing microbial DNA inside the womb, leading some scientists to conclude the fetus already had a starter microbiome in utero. More recently, scientists in the field identified two problems with these studies:

>> The list of microbes supposedly detected in the womb looks suspiciously like a list of common laboratory contaminants.

>> If the fetus had a microbiome in utero, it would need to know how to distinguish between pathogens and harmless microbes, but its immune system doesn't have the capacity to do that yet.

The up-to-date thinking is that the fetus doesn't have a true microbiome. However, a mother's microbes still influence the fetus in utero, in ways that scientists are beginning to figure out. Find more information on Chapter 17.

Bathing in microbes at birth

Say you're about to be born, floating in a watery pouch inside your mother. Her water suddenly breaking is a big turning point for you microbially: The container that kept you separated from the microbial world has been punctured. Your mother no longer filters your interactions with microorganisms and your little body must face them yourself. Consider the following:

>> If you were born vaginally, you received a generous coating of microbes on your way through the birth canal. The microbes were mostly lactobacilli (refer to the section "Identifying what's in your gut" earlier in this chapter). As you moved farther and farther down the birth canal, more microbes staked their claim on your body, nestling in your nose and mouth and forming a layer on your skin. Other microbes that you inhaled established in your little lungs. A whole lot were swallowed, and the ones that thrived without oxygen (primarily bifidobacteria) took up residence in your digestive system. Voila, your entire body was seeded with microorganisms before you took your first breath.

>> If you were born by C-section, as one in five of babies are worldwide, you had a slightly different experience. The womb was punctured by the surgeon's knife, and your body was initially occupied mostly by the microbes on your mother's skin and on the hospital surfaces. You ended up with fewer bifidobacteria than a baby delivered vaginally.

Nevertheless in both cases, the microbes on your body (including in your gut) changed rapidly after birth, leading to a very different configuration after several weeks or months. Few of your earliest microbes stayed with you through to adulthood. I discuss in Chapter 17 the establishment of the gut microbiota and some possible health consequences.

Identifying early-life influences

Although your range of behaviors as a newborn was basically limited to eating, crying, sleeping, and filling diapers, you were already a complex biological system whose microbiome was rapidly changing. As for your gut microbiome specifically, it came to be dominated by bifidobacteria.

Diet — what a newborn eats

Overall your diet, whether breastmilk or formula, was the most influential factor on your gut in your first months of life, as I discuss here:

>> **For breastfed infants:** The gut microbes were specially shaped by indigestible sugars in breastmilk called *human milk oligosaccharides (HMOs)*. These HMOs are the perfect food for specific bifidobacteria in a baby's gut that have the right genes for breaking them down. Recent research notes that when the HMOs are metabolized, the by-products help the development of the baby's immune system.

>> **For formula-fed infants:** Although these infants receive good nutrition, they don't typically ingest HMOs, resulting in slightly different gut microbes overall.

The switch to solid foods, leading to a more diverse diet, triggers the next big change in the child's gut microbiota and starts the gradual shift towards an adult-like composition. Chapter 18 goes into more detail on how you can take care of the gut microbes during the first year of life.

Environment — what a newborn encounters

The environment around you had a minor influence on your gut microbes in your first year of life as well. Factors such as sharing your space with family members and pets, and your outdoor exposures contributed to how your gut microbiota shaped up in your first year.

Tracking microbes as you age

As you grow from childhood into adolescence and from adulthood into older adulthood, your gut microbes naturally change with each life stage. Throughout childhood the ecosystem is dynamic, becoming more and more diverse. It reaches a relatively stable state in adulthood. Later in life, once-rare microbes increase in number, making the gut microbiome more eclectic. Proinflammatory microbes also increase in older age and correlate with the extent of frailty. Chapter 19 covers specific ways to take care of your gut microbiome in older age.

Considering the genetic connection

Your human genes also account for a portion of your gut microbiome composition. That is, some microbes are *heritable* (passed from one generation to the next) — so people with certain genes (for example, ones that confer a lean physique) tend to have some of the same gut microbes throughout their adult lives.

When scientists have studied large groups of people and tried to find patterns between their human genes and their gut bacteria, they've found that specific gut microbes tend to occur with genes that determine your digestion of lactose in dairy products and others with genes that encode blood type.

TECHNICAL
STUFF

The fascinating part about these observed gene-microbe co-occurrences is that they seem to extend back through evolutionary time. Apparently over a span of 15 million years, some bacterial lineages diversified at the same time as the humans and primates that harbored them. Scientists still see evidence of this co-evolution today, with specific strains of *Helicobacter pylori*, for example, occurring in genetically similar human populations worldwide. This evidence suggests gut microbes and humans have undergone parallel evolution and that certain lineages of bacteria have been paired with the same human genes from generation to generation over time.

Aiming For Diversity and Resilience of Your Gut Microbiome

The next question about your gut microbes may be: "How do I know if I have a healthy microbiome?"

I wish I could give you an easy answer to this question, but the truth is that scientists are still stumped. After billions of dollars spent on microbiome research and millions of healthy people sampled, they still haven't been able to uncover any specific compositional or functional features that clearly signal a healthy microbiome — because the gut microbiomes of healthy people are just too varied. Currently, if scientists looked at ten different microbiome samples, already knowing that five were from perfectly healthy people and five were from people diagnosed with a chronic disease, they would be hard pressed to accurately predict which samples were from which people.

But surely there's some indicator that one microbiome is healthier than another? This is where the concept of a *health-associated microbiome* comes in. Some general gut-microbe patterns tend to be observed or inferred in healthy people, so they're said to be associated with health. Those two patterns are diversity and resilience, which I discuss here.

Recognizing diversity in the gut ecosystem

Diversity refers to how many different types of organisms exist in a place. Mathematically, diversity is like this: Pluck a microbe from a community at random, without knowing what all the other microbes are. Based on what you picked, what's the probability you'll be able to predict the name of the next microbe you pick out of the community? In a less diverse community (with lots of the same microbes), the probability of making a correct prediction is higher, and in a more diverse community, the probability is lower.

REMEMBER

Diversity as a sign of a healthy and thriving ecosystem makes intuitive sense. In a forest with diverse tree species, an invasive beetle that attacks only one species won't bring down the whole forest ecosystem. The same principle applies to gut microbiomes. In a diverse gut microbiome, chances are that some microbes may have the skills to overcome threats or disruptions that emerge. (Chapter 4 discusses some of these possible threats.)

Lo and behold in real life gut microbiomes, scientists find over and over again that diversity is associated with better health. In most (although not all) cases, people who have a disease have less diverse microbiomes than those who are healthy.

You may be wondering "Just how diverse should my gut microbiome be?" And even though this question is valid, scientists haven't yet found a diversity cut-off that marks the difference between healthy and unhealthy. Sure, you can do a consumer gut microbiome test that gives you an official-looking diversity score, but in truth that rating is no guarantee of health. Rather, diversity is a general aim: If you live in a way that fosters gut microbiome diversity, you're more likely to maintain your health. Chapters 10 and 11 cover how to foster increased gut microbiome diversity.

Knowing what makes a resilient gut community

Resilience is the tendency of an ecosystem to maintain its original state and recover from any disruptions. A gut microbiome that bounces back to a normal or baseline state after a disruption is considered resilient.

Inevitably in your adult life, you'll encounter certain gut microbiome disturbances (refer to Chapter 4). Given that adults have a relatively stable gut microbiome over time, resilience of the gut microbiome in healthy people is considered desirable because it indicates a stable ecosystem that will continue to provide the services your body needs.

TECHNICAL STUFF

Studies that back up the idea that gut microbiome resilience is necessary for health are few because resilience is challenging to study scientifically. The timing of the measurements can make a big difference to the results, and at least three gut microbiome measurements per person are needed, spaced out over time:

>> One at baseline

>> One immediately after the disturbance

>> One later on to check how closely it returns to baseline

But some studies show gut microbiota stability and resilience are reduced in certain diseases such as Crohn's disease and ulcerative colitis, so substantial gut microbiome fluctuations over time may not be a good sign for your health. With more studies in the future looking at gut microbiomes over time, researchers will find out how resilience truly supports health.

Researchers do know some people's gut microbiomes are more resilient than others. But instead of aiming for a certain percentage of restoration — for example, the gut microbiome returning to 95 percent of its original state after a disturbance — think of resilience more as a general aim. You can apply some strategies to increase your gut microbiome resilience, which I cover in Chapters 10 and 11.

WHAT HIGH-PERFORMANCE ATHLETES SHOULD KNOW ABOUT GUT HEALTH

High-performance athletes are those who are motivated to compete and do their personal best. These athletes need to be especially cautious about their gut health, taking steps to manage it alongside their athletic performance. Intense exercise has the potential to damage the gut, leading to diminished thickness of the mucus layer in the gut as well as gut permeability and increased inflammation. At the same time, elite athletes are shown to have signs of gut health such as higher gut microbial diversity and increased production of anti-inflammatory molecules such as SCFAs. Athletes show increases in the biological pathways and metabolites associated with greater muscle turnover and overall health compared to people who aren't athletes.

As with other individuals, diet and exercise work in tandem to influence gut health in high-performance athletes. One research study showed that gut microbial instability was observed in elite endurance athletes when they consumed a short-term high-protein diet, which hindered their performance. Overall the research seems to show that irregular, exhausting, or long-lasting training may have negative effects on the gut microbes and may contribute to the impaired immunity that's seen in elite athletes.

Studies have attempted to identify bacteria in the guts of elite athletes that may be performance-enhancing; for example, the bacteria *M. smithii* are found in greater abundance in professional cyclists compared to amateurs. Also, in an Ironman competition the highest concentrations of some well-known health-associated bacteria such as *A. muciniphila* were observed in athletes with the fastest finishing times. However, these observations are too general to be of interest and much more research needs to be done to confirm the effectiveness of these microbial candidates if turned into probiotics.

In the meantime, some experts point out that several existing probiotics are shown to decrease intestinal permeability, which may occur in athletes following intense, prolonged exercise. But by managing diet and sticking to a regular training routine, high-performance athletes may be able to avoid the shock effects of intense exercise on the gut.

IN THIS CHAPTER

» Understanding the way that lifestyle changes can affect gut health

» Untangling how the medication you take affects gut health

» Examining how your diet shapes your gut environment

» Finding out how exercise and stress impact gut health

» Looking at why sleep is important to your gut

» Considering how infections can cause gut issues

Chapter **4**

Discovering What Influences Gut Health

The Colombian pop singer Shakira famously pointed out that "Hips Don't Lie." Well your gut doesn't lie, either. Your gut microbiome bears the traces of what you eat, whether you exercise every day, whether you have pets, and more. Shakira herself may even be a proponent of listening to the truth of what your gut is telling you: In a 2014 yogurt commercial, she enacted the role of cells in the gut waking up and dancing energetically when they're fed yogurt. The message of the scene was, "Feeling good starts from within."

Whether your digestion is A-okay or whether you're experiencing major digestive symptoms, your gut health is complex and influenced by multiple, overlapping factors. You've probably noticed firsthand that some of the main influences on your gut health can be medications and what you eat. But beyond the obvious, all the individual contributing factors to gut health can be difficult for scientists to untangle. For example, a student who moves to campus may experience changes in bowel habits and maybe even weight gain related to a change in gut health. But were these changes ultimately triggered by the student's new living quarters, the cafeteria food, staying up late to study, or the stress of coursework deadlines? Or perhaps a little bit of everything? All these factors individually can induce a shift in the gut microbiome, with possible consequences for gut health. Although everyone's gut health and gut microbes are unique, meaning the exact same factors may affect one student differently from another, scientists are starting to identify some of the distinct factors that can reliably shift gut health.

This chapter covers what's known to alter gut health in adulthood, either for better or for worse. You can come away with a new appreciation for how your everyday choices and habits have measurable effects on your gut and how many of them you can control.

Some of the gut-altering factors in this chapter actually cause digestive symptoms, but others invisibly alter your gut microbiome. And even if gut microbiome changes may not have consequences in the short term, the tight connection between your gut microbiome and overall health (see Chapters 3 and 5 for more information) means that you may indeed see the health impact of gut microbiome alterations over the long term. These factors, all together, are likely to have a cumulative effect. Similar to car engine maintenance, if you ignore your gut microbiome for too long, your gut health is bound to break down at some point.

Before this chapter delves into what shifts your gut microbiome, allow me to clarify how much of your gut microbial community is actually changeable. Truth be told, the vast majority of your gut microbiome is stubborn to change and doesn't correlate with anything about your lifestyle that scientists can measure. According to the best estimates, you probably have the power to change around 10 percent of your gut microbiome's makeup (in other words, composition) by altering different aspects of your lifestyle. Even if that seems a small percentage of your overall gut community, those changed microbes can in theory have important and noticeable impacts on your health. Part 3 gives you more direction on how to push your gut microbial composition in a direction that benefits your health.

In materials about gut health, you may have seen the word *dysbiosis*, which refers to a gut microbiome that's different from a healthy or normal state. For example, a study may compare the gut microbiomes of people with type 2 diabetes to those of healthy people without a diagnosed disease and discover a difference in the people with diabetes, which they call dysbiosis. But scientists still have no idea how to define a healthy microbiome — and defining an unhealthy one is similarly difficult because there's no standard to compare it against. Because dysbiosis can take so many different forms, it's only a general description for research purposes and not something that can be diagnosed for an individual.

Eyeing How Medications Alter Your Gut

As I discuss in Chapter 3, your gut can help determine your response to medicines. Actually the effects go both ways because, in turn, the medications you ingest can lead to noticeable differences in your gut health.

Firstly, if you take a medication to address some digestive symptoms, such as a laxative for constipation or eluxadoline for irritable bowel syndrome (IBS), you can normally expect it to affect your gut health — and likely for the better. (If the medication is supposed to work for people similar to you but doesn't, you're known as a *nonresponder*.)

The following sections focus on the main types of medications that may be taken for a reason other than gut health, which can nevertheless provoke either gut symptoms or significant changes in your gut microbiome as side effects. This list isn't comprehensive because this is an emerging field with lots of ongoing work, but it includes the main drugs affecting gut health that scientists have found to date.

WARNING

The fact that these medicines change your gut microbiome doesn't mean you should always avoid them. If a qualified medical professional prescribes you any of these medications, you should absolutely take them to address whatever health problem has been targeted. If you're worried about gut-microbiome-related side effects, check out some of the strategies in Chapter 10 and Chapter 11 for mitigating the gut microbiome changes and run them by the medical professional to see whether they're appropriate for you.

THE HISTORY AND OVERUSE OF ANTIBIOTICS

Once upon a time, humans lived without antibiotics. Up until the early 1900s, picking up an infectious illness very often resulted in death. Furthermore, any surgical procedure was incredibly risky and often led to life-threatening infections. Even a small cut on your hand from opening the wire gate of the chicken coop had a chance of being fatal.

By the late 1800s, scientists were wise to the fact that microorganisms caused serious diseases. The concept of antibiotics was of interest scientifically but didn't really go anywhere until 1928, when the Scottish physician Dr. Alexander Fleming returned from a holiday to his lab in London. He noticed a Petri dish of *Staphylococcus* bacteria that had gone moldy in his absence and saw that the mold seemed to prevent the bacteria

(continued)

(continued)

around it from growing. He figured out the mold was producing a chemical that could kill bacteria and named the chemical penicillin. You can imagine Fleming's excitement at this discovery. But the enthusiasm waned when he and his colleagues were unable to purify penicillin from the mold. After much painstaking work and many more years, they finally came up with a process for purifying it. Yet the process remained painfully inefficient, requiring huge quantities of mold broth to produce a tiny bit of penicillin.

But then came a melon to the rescue. When scientists put out the call for strains of mold that would produce penicillin more efficiently, a lab assistant named Mary Hunt brought in a rotting cantaloupe melon she had found at a market. The melon's mold turned out to produce six times more penicillin than the original strain the scientists had been working with. World War 2 provided the impetus to scale up production of penicillin in the United States, and soon it was being used around the world. Today antibiotics are a mainstay of medicine and many of us would not be alive today without them.

This story drives home the fact that, over a relatively short span of time and due to several chance occurrences, antibiotics revolutionized how medical professionals treat infectious diseases and radically diminish the threat they pose in people's lives. However, the pendulum has swung the other way with antibiotic use. Antibiotics are too frequently used when they're unnecessary, or the wrong type of antibiotic is used. Estimates show a large proportion of today's antibiotic prescriptions — 30 percent or more — are unnecessary.

Antibiotics

Antibiotics are a group of medications specifically used to kill bacteria. They can reduce damage from infections and can often be lifesaving, but they're too often used unnecessarily, leading to detrimental effects on gut health. Antibiotics can cause the following gut-related issues:

» **Diarrhea:** The most frequent downside is the occurrence of diarrhea when people take antibiotics, which happens between 5 percent and 35 percent of the time. This antibiotic-associated diarrhea (AAD) varies depending on the type of antibiotic and the overall health of the person taking them. Part of the reason that AAD occurs may be the disturbance that antibiotics cause in the gut microbial community.

>> **Bacterial infections:** Individuals who take antibiotics are more susceptible to infections by a bacterium called *Clostridioides difficile* (also called *C. difficile* or *C. diff*), which tends to take advantage of disruptions to the gut microbial community to cause sickness. *C. difficile* infection can lead to severe diarrhea and pain, and in some cases, it starts a nightmarish cycle of debilitating digestive problems that occur weeks or months apart.

>> **Colon cancer:** Across the population, taking antibiotics frequently is associated with the development of colon cancer years later. The association is especially strong for younger people: In a large study from the United Kingdom, for individuals younger than 50 antibiotic use was associated with a 49 percent higher risk of developing colon cancer. The exact reasons for this association are unknown, but they may relate to antibiotics' ability to disturb the intestinal microbes and their immune-regulating functions.

>> **Other digestive-related symptoms:** Some other commonly documented side effects from antibiotics are

- Nausea

- Vomiting

- Bloating

- Stomach pain or cramping

- Loss of appetite

What's happening to your gut microbiome when you consume antibiotics? Given that many antibiotics kill a range of bacteria, the targeted sickness-causing microbe may be defeated but lots of your other gut microbes take a hit, too. Studies show a reduced diversity of species in the gut after ingesting most types of antibiotics, which may not come as a surprise. Bifidobacteria and lactobacilli often dramatically decrease. Normally these effects are temporary; within about 30 days the community bounces back to its original state. However, sometimes the gut microbes take much longer to bounce back — up to 6 months — and other times the original state is never again reached.

The disrupted gut microbes could play a role in some of the gastrointestinal symptoms that crop up after antibiotics. They're likely the reason people are more susceptible to bacterial infections after antibiotic treatment. For potential pathogens lurking in the gut, the antibiotics are enough to disturb the microbes and metabolites normally keeping the pathogens in check, allowing them to grow to problematic levels.

ANOTHER ANTIBIOTIC THREAT: RESISTANCE

Leaving your gut microbial community undisturbed is one good reason to avoid unnecessary antibiotics, but another very important reason to reduce antibiotic use overall is the danger of antimicrobial resistance (AMR) — when microorganisms (bacteria, but also viruses, fungi, and parasites) change over time so they no longer respond to medicines designed to eliminate them.

AMR happens when disease-causing microorganisms develop new defense strategies (when they're faced with antibiotics and under pressure to adapt) that enable them to resist being killed by the antibiotic. This phenomenon is happening all around the world and could potentially bring humans back to an era when antibiotics can't be used for serious diseases — not because they're unavailable, but because they're ineffective. The World Health Organization (WHO) has declared AMR one of the top ten global public health threats. To prevent the worst-case scenario, reducing unnecessary antibiotic use is crucial.

Here's how to do your part to reduce unnecessary antibiotic use:

- Don't seek an antibiotic prescription for conditions such as a respiratory infection because the common cold is caused by a viral infection and antibiotics are only effective for treating a bacterial infection.

- When an antibiotic prescription is being considered for either prevention or treatment of a condition you have, ask your doctor if any alternative treatments are possible. In some cases, careful monitoring of symptoms may be sufficient.

- When you must take antibiotics, follow the prescribed direction as specified.

Chemotherapy and radiation therapy

For many individuals who have been diagnosed with cancer, chemotherapy and radiation therapy prove effective treatments that reduce or eliminate the cancer cells that are proliferating in their bodies. Here's how each affects gut health:

>> **Chemotherapy:** This treatment, which uses powerful chemicals to kill the cancer cells, commonly can cause nausea, vomiting, and diarrhea, but another common occurrence is *intestinal mucositis,* which is inflammation or ulcers affecting the mucus layer inside the digestive tract.

The effects of chemotherapy on the gut microbiome depend on the specific type of chemicals used, but overall, it appears to reduce the quantity of bacteria as well as certain health-associated bacteria. This gut bacterial damage is associated with intestinal mucositis as well as chemo-induced weight gain in those with breast cancer.

>> **Radiation therapy:** Also referred to as radiotherapy, this treatment uses X-rays or other forms of intense energy (radiation) in a local area to damage the DNA of cancer cells. Intestinal mucositis is a particularly common side effect of radiation therapy, affecting 80 percent or more of individuals receiving it in the pelvic area. Others may experience diarrhea.

This therapy also affects the gut microbes, reducing overall numbers and diversity as well as health-associated species. Radiation causes inflamed tissues, increasing intestinal permeability and allowing some gut microbial metabolites to cross the gut barrier and exacerbate the inflammation.

WARNING

Chemotherapy and radiation therapy are often lifesaving, with gut-related side effects being of minor importance overall. The decision to go ahead with these treatments should be based on their likely effects on the cancer cells, as discussed with your doctor.

Metformin

Metformin is a commonly prescribed blood-sugar-lowering medication for type 2 diabetes. Side effects in the gut sometimes include abdominal discomfort, nausea, vomiting, or diarrhea.

Metformin changes the composition of the gut microbiome, and in this case the changes appear to be beneficial for health. Proportions of bacteria in groups such as lactobacilli and *Akkermansia* are increased. Digging in further, scientists have found metformin ends up suppressing the bacteria that break apart a certain bile acid that has beneficial effects, allowing that bile acid to increase. In fact, metformin may exert its hypoglycemic effects in part by shifting the gut microbiota in ways that help maintain a strong gut barrier and promote the production of short-chain fatty acids (SCFAs).

Nonsteroidal anti-inflammatory drugs

Pain can be a real pain, which is why many people have a trusty bottle of over-the-counter (nonprescription) pain-relieving medicines tucked away in a drawer or medicine cabinet. Nonsteroidal anti-inflammatory drugs (NSAIDs) are a common group of medicines taken for reducing pain and inflammation. Examples of NSAIDs are ibuprofen, naproxen, and aspirin.

One side effect of NSAIDs is indigestion, with common symptoms being stomach pain or bloating. Taken over a long term at high doses NSAIDs may damage the gut, leading to peptic ulcers.

What's more interesting is how NSAIDs affect your gut microorganisms. A study in 2020 tested how people's microbiomes from fecal samples changed in response to different medications in test tubes. Scientists were surprised to find that different types of NSAIDs, which offer similar pain-relief potential, had significantly different effects on the gut microbiomes. For example, ibuprofen was seen to wipe out bacteria in a fashion similar to antibiotics, reducing the overall quantity of microbes and decreasing *Akkermansia* as well as other common gut residents. A different NSAID, indomethacin, enriched some bacteria known to cause infections.

Overall, NSAIDs can undoubtedly be useful for pain relief; consult your doctor about alternatives if you find you're using them frequently.

Proton pump inhibitors

Proton pump inhibitors (PPIs) are medicines that reduce stomach acid production by blocking an enzyme that's necessary for acid secretion into the stomach. They're often prescribed to alleviate acid reflux or treat peptic ulcers as well as other conditions, and they're one of the world's most prescribed drugs.

Some possible gastrointestinal side effects of PPIs include nausea or vomiting, abdominal pain, flatulence, constipation, and diarrhea. Both children and adults who use PPIs may be at risk for severe infections — primarily gastrointestinal infections. Used over the long term, PPIs appear to bring an increased risk of gastric cancer, but scientists need more data to confirm this association.

These gut-related side effects may be linked to how PPIs dramatically alter the gut microbial community. In the fecal microbiome, they can change up to 20 percent of the bacteria present and reduce diversity. Interestingly, PPIs shift the fecal microbiome toward bacteria that are normally found in the oral cavity. Scientists believe this shift occurs because PPIs make the stomach less acidic, allowing more bacteria from the oral cavity to survive all the way through the digestive tract.

PPIs apparently change the microbiota of the small intestine as well, allowing a higher quantity of bacteria to survive. And in the stomach, which is the site that PPIs target, bacteria increase in diversity and previously rare bacteria increase dramatically.

A QUICK GUIDE TO MESSING UP YOUR GUT HEALTH

Just in case you were wondering, here's a quick guide to what it takes to really mess up your gut health: Pop antibiotics like candy. Avoid fiber at all costs (put down that apple!) and fill up on sugary and high-fat foods such as soda, french fries, and donuts. Don't bother with yogurt, sauerkraut, or other fermented foods. Make sure you maintain a completely erratic sleep schedule and do nothing to manage the stress in your life. You're likely to end up with perfectly terrible gut health.

Be honest though, how closely does your lifestyle resemble this description? Maybe it's actually time to do some navel-gazing to see what you can do to improve your gut health. I've been there and I can tell you: Better gut health is definitely within your reach. Part 3 shares some useful advice you can use to implement good health choices for your gut and your entire body.

WARNING

Despite these gut-related effects, PPIs are an important and useful medication. If you already take PPIs, never decide to stop taking them without first speaking with your doctor because doing so may lead to serious bleeding in the stomach or the first part of the small intestine.

Linking Eating Habits to Gut Health

Here's a no-brainer for anyone who has ever experienced heartburn after a meal of fish and chips or bloating after a large ice cream cone: What you eat can cause gut symptoms.

But beyond these personal experiences, this phenomenon stacks up scientifically too. What you eat is the second leading factor accounting for your gut microbiome differences compared to other people. As I discuss in the following sections, the specific foods you eat or the overall balance in your diet can have a measurable influence on your gut microbiome and gut health.

Your daily bread — The foods you eat

Specific foods you eat can affect your gut health in the short term — the classic case of a food that disagrees with you and causes some kind of gastrointestinal symptom. Or as my grandma used to say, certain foods tended to "repeat" on her. Everyone has their own personal list of foods in this category. In many cases, you can't tell if gut microbes are driving the symptoms you get after eating a certain food.

Specific foods you consume day to day that don't cause any digestive symptoms can also affect the microbes you harbor in your gut. Across an entire population, different people who prefer (and consume) milk chocolate over dark chocolate may share several types of microbes whereas the dark chocolate lovers may share a few other types of microbes.

Understanding how macronutrients can impact your gut

Broadly, foods with different proportions of the three macronutrients (carbohydrates, proteins, and fats, which I outline in Chapter 10) affect your gut microbes in different ways as follows:

>> **Carbohydrates:** The body's main energy source can be either simple or complex:

- **Simple:** These carbohydrates are made up of shorter chains of molecules that the body can break down and absorb easily. Sugar is a simple carbohydrate and is mainly a problem for gut health when it makes up too much of your diet proportionally or isn't balanced with enough fiber (as I explain in the section "Patterns prevail — The balance in your diet" in this chapter).

- **Complex:** These carbohydrates consist of longer, more complex sugar molecules that take longer to digest. Dietary fibers are complex carbohydrates. Many types of dietary fibers are digested by the microbes living in your colon, producing beneficial SCFAs as a fortuitous by-product.

>> **Proteins:** They're substances made up of chains of amino acids, which build and repair body tissues. They're mostly broken down in the small intestine, but some of them reach your colon and are transformed by microbes. The exact microbes that increase with high-protein foods depend on the type of food, but if you feed your colonic microbes too much protein, they end up producing potentially toxic by-products, such as ammonia and p-Cresol, which are linked to higher inflammation and intestinal diseases.

>> **Fats:** Oily or greasy, these energy-rich substances don't dissolve in water. They're crucial to many aspects of physiological function. The effect of fats on your gut microbes depends on the type of fat, with saturated fatty acids (found in palm oil, for example) leading to higher levels of possible sickness-causing bacteria, and monounsaturated fatty acids (found in olive oil) increasing health-associated bacteria.

Identifying the common culprits

Individual foods and beverages that appear to have a negative impact on gut health include the following:

>> **Emulsifiers:** Some of these dietary components, used to improve the texture and shelf life of some ultraprocessed foods, appear to promote intestinal inflammation by weakening the gut barrier and allowing bacteria to get through.

>> **Artificial sweeteners:** Although artificial (noncaloric) sweeteners such as saccharin, sucralose, and aspartame ostensibly benefit metabolism and control weight, their effects on the gut microbes and blood sugar appear to be personalized. Saccharin especially seems to have the paradoxical effect of worsening blood sugar in tandem with gut microbiota changes.

>> **Alcohol:** More than seven drinks of any kind per week are associated with health risks such as liver disease and cancer. Meanwhile, alcohol decreases key microbes that reduce inflammation and maintain the gut barrier. However, wine may have some benefits for the gut and overall health if consumed in moderate amounts as part of a Mediterranean diet (detailed further in Chapter 10).

Chapter 10 also covers the effect of different foods on gut health, as well as probiotics, prebiotics, synbiotics, and postbiotics.

Patterns prevail — The balance in your diet

Dietary pattern refers to the big picture of what you eat: the types and amounts of foods you consume on a regular basis over a longer term. Cake once a year on your birthday doesn't establish your dietary pattern, but cake twice a week is a part of your dietary pattern, establishing that you consume sugary foods on a regular basis. The research is fairly well established showing your dietary pattern may protect your health, or it may put you at risk for digestive diseases and other chronic illnesses.

WARNING

Your dietary pattern puts long-term pressure on your gut microbial ecosystem. Many different dietary patterns lead to good health, but without a doubt, one pattern is the worst for your gut microbes and your overall health. This pattern is known as the *Western diet* or *standard American diet* — characterized by a lack of fiber and a high intake of both sugary and fatty foods. When you consume this diet, your gut microbes can't do their job of maintaining a strong gut barrier (refer to Chapter 3), making the gut overly permeable. As a result, some microbes encounter sensors of the immune system (known as dendritic cells), which give the red-alert signal to ramp up inflammation. This process disrupts your metabolic health and weight and can even affect brain function.

On the positive side, a dietary pattern high in fiber seems to support your health and your gut microbial community. The gold-standard example is the *Mediterranean diet pattern* — rich in plant foods with some fish, poultry, and dairy, and very little red meat and only occasional sweets. (Check out the latest edition of *Mediterranean Diet For Dummies* for more in-depth information.) Otherwise, simply including 30 or more different plant foods in your diet every week is associated with high gut microbiome diversity, which is associated with better health across many parameters.

SCIENTIST SAYS

How quickly can your gut change in response to a dietary shift? Lawrence David, Associate Professor of Molecular Genetics & Microbiology at Duke University in Durham, North Carolina, published some of the first work showing a dramatic change in dietary pattern could affect the gut microbiome. "A big diet change can affect the gut microbiome in one to two days," he said. "Such changes could be eating a lot more (or a lot less) fiber, as well as switching to a primarily meat-based diet." So, if you find yourself locked into a Western diet pattern, you're only a couple of days away from being able to change your gut microbes to better support your health.

Connecting Exercise and Fitness to Gut Health

The amount you move has effects on your gut and your overall health, too. Physical activity reduces your chance of being diagnosed with a range of chronic diseases and effectively extends your life. As the following sections discuss, both physical activity and your overall fitness level can change your gut microbial community in a way that is likely to benefit health.

Working out

Exercise is physical activity you undertake on purpose to maintain or improve your health or fitness. Regular exercise brings about positive changes in your immune response and reduced inflammation over a long term.

REMEMBER

Across many human and animal studies, exercise leads to increased diversity in the gut microbiome, with modest shifts in its composition and more SCFA-producing organisms. In another episode of "your gut doesn't lie," these positive changes go away after you stop regularly exercising — even if you keep your gym membership active.

The exception to exercise being supportive of gut health may occur with marathon runners or other elite athletes who push their bodies hard and experience symptoms such as diarrhea, nausea, vomiting, or heartburn. These symptoms generally go away after a short time and with good fluid intake.

Achieving fitness

Fitness is the result of exercise — a measurable level of health or of skill achievement. One measure of fitness, for example, is how far you can run before you become exhausted. Another measure of fitness often used by scientists is VO_2 max, the maximum rate of oxygen your body consumes during exercise. Individuals with a high fitness level tend to have higher microbial diversity and SCFAs in the colon.

Nevertheless, a high fitness level isn't required to get the benefits of exercise. One study compared people who did longer bouts of moderate exercise compared to short bursts of intense exercise. The short, intense exercise led to noticeably better fitness, but both types of exercise modified the gut microbiota and dampened inflammation in the body over time.

Seeing How Your Brain Influences Your Gut

As Chapter 5 discusses, two-way communication exists between your brain and your gut. What happens in your gut affects your brain, but does the opposite happen — the state of your brain influencing your gut health?

The answer is yes. As I explain in these sections, both stress and overall mood can have top-down effects and either trigger symptoms or change the microbial makeup of your gut.

Coping with worry — a stressed gut

Although stress is a normal part of the human experience, too much worry or mental tension can affect your entire body. When you experience stress, the hormones cortisol, epinephrine (adrenaline), and norepinephrine flood your body. Digestively speaking, your gut transit time and gastrointestinal secretions may increase or decrease, and your gut may become more sensitive to pain. You may even experience diarrhea from the digestive changes that occur.

Stress in small doses can be a good thing, pushing you to perform your best. But longer-term stress can have a negative impact on your health, contributing to the development or worsening of digestive diseases such as IBS, inflammatory bowel disease, and gastroesophageal reflux disease. Chronic stress during pregnancy is especially detrimental (check out Chapter 17).

Stress also alters the gut microbiota composition, reducing the levels of health-associated bacteria. Complex studies have also found gut microbes have a role in bringing about some of the consequences of stress on the body, including increased inflammation and impaired cognitive performance. Further, if you turn to ice cream or alcohol overconsumption to help cope with stress, your gut microbiota will change as a result.

Monitoring mood

Given the existence of the gut-brain axis, you may wonder whether depression or anxiety can change your gut microbiota and trigger digestive disease. Evidence shows that people with depression do have higher rates of IBS, acid reflux, peptic ulcer disease, as well as stomach and colon cancer. And those with a diagnosed anxiety disorder are more prone to digestive symptoms and inflammation as well as ulcers. The gut microbes are also altered in anxiety and depression, but scientists don't yet know if they cause the associated gastrointestinal symptoms. Chapter 5 discusses in greater detail the connection between gut and mood disorders.

Tying Sleep Habits to Gut Health

Not just your human body needs a good night's sleep — your gut microbes do, too. Microbes in the gut fluctuate according to the day-night cycle and your eating times. Most adults and their microbes need seven to nine hours of sleep per night, and either shorter or interrupted sleep can have negative effects on the gut. The following sections discuss how sleep duration, sleep quality, and jet lag can leave their marks on your gut.

Sleeping enough

Sleep duration is one measure of your sleep that matters for the gut. Longer duration of sleep in a night is associated with more gut microbiota diversity whereas sleep deprivation tends to change bacterial groups associated with metabolic problems and weight gain. A study in older adults found a shorter duration of sleep led to proinflammatory bacteria.

Sleeping well

Quality of sleep — meaning how restful it is, regardless of how long you sleep — is another factor that can affect gut health. *Insomnia*, or difficulty falling asleep or staying asleep, is a marker of poor sleep quality. Studies have found that poor sleep quality goes hand in hand with digestive symptoms: primarily abdominal pain, but also acid reflux, distention, and belching.

Overall, people with diagnosed gastrointestinal disorders tend to have more insomnia, although it's not completely clear if poor quality sleep causes more symptoms or the other way around. But one study showed the connection, for example, where people with IBS who had poor sleep showed more severe symptoms the next day.

Sleep quality also affects your gut microbial community: Diversity increases with more restful sleep.

Dealing with jet lag

Jet lag is a short-term sleep problem, often leading to extreme tiredness, that can affect you after travelling quickly across several time zones. A similar condition called *social jet lag* (changing the midpoint of your sleep by 90 minutes or more) happens when you're at home but disrupt your routine by going to sleep and waking up at different times, such as on the weekend. When sleep is disrupted by jet lag, typically your eating routine is also shifted.

Both types of jet lag negatively affect your gut by disturbing the day-night rhythms of your gut microbiota and decreasing diversity while also messing with your blood sugar levels. A 2023 study found that social jet lag influenced gut microbes, specifically increasing the bacteria associated with health problems.

Exploring How Infections Alter Your Gut

Your body has some sophisticated defenses against sickness-causing bacteria, but sometimes they do in fact manage to overcome your defenses and make you sick. An infection can be sudden, as when you have food poisoning, or the microorganisms can affect you slowly over the long term. Either way, infections can have lasting impacts on your gut microbiome and gut health. Here I explain how both short-term and longer-term gut infections can impact gastrointestinal health.

Experiencing sudden sickness due to infectious diarrhea

A sudden (or *acute*) gastrointestinal infection can really shake things up in your gut. Food-borne pathogens such as *Salmonella* species, *Campylobacter* species, *Listeria monocytogenes*, and specific strains of *E. coli* can cause short-term diarrhea and other gastrointestinal symptoms.

During such acute infections, the diarrhea-causing microbes remain at low levels in your gut despite causing the troubling symptoms. But your gut sees the impact overall — the composition changes drastically and its diversity decreases.

After the acute infection resolves itself, gut health can go one of two ways:

>> In some cases, scientists have found, infection seems to leave your gut microbiota in a better position overall. That is, your resident microbes after an infection may remodel themselves to protect you even better from a subsequent infection. In one study, scientists worked out that a gut infection triggered the body to produce more taurine (a sulfur-containing amino acid), which nourished the bacteria in the gut that enhanced defenses against the next infection.

>> On the other hand, after acute infection some people may suffer from longer-term gastrointestinal symptoms — for example, in the case of post-infectious IBS. Likely in these cases, the gut microbiota is permanently altered by the infection. A marked shift in the gut microbiota persists, which can disrupt the gut barrier, make the gut more sensitive to pain, and bring about other gut changes that leave you with sustained IBS symptoms.

Wreaking havoc — stealthy microbes

Microbes infecting your gut over a longer term also have the power to cause issues in gut health at various times. These two gut residents normally behave themselves — until they don't:

>> *Helicobacter pylori*: A stomach-dwelling bacterium called *H. pylori* infects 50 to 80 percent of people globally, depending on the region, and tends to be mostly asymptomatic. Immune cells in the stomach called ILC2s, which depend on signals from the gut microbiota, help contain the effects of *H. pylori*. With these bacteria present, the gut microbiota becomes less diverse and changes in gastric acidity alter its composition. Over a longer term, *H. pylori* infection causes gut inflammation as well as ulcers and stomach cancer.

>> *Clostridioides difficile*: These bacteria in the colon, mentioned in the section "Antibiotics," tend to take over when the gut has been annihilated by antibiotics. They're present at a low abundance in the guts of healthy individuals and are normally suppressed by the microbial community. When infection occurs, however, they tend to flourish in the gut microbiota, accompanying other changes in composition as well as lower microbiome diversity.

Influencing Gut Health — Other Factors at Play

Some other relatively minor influences on gut health also exist: geography and your outdoor and indoor environments. I delve deeper into these factors here.

Looking at geography: Where in the world?

Your geographical location in the world can affect your gut health. On a very broad level, certain digestive diseases and illnesses are more common in different areas of the world. For example, the rates of diarrheal illness in Africa and South America can be as high as 80 percent whereas in Europe and North America this figure may be around 30 percent.

Paralleling these digestive disease discrepancies is the discovery that people's gut microbiota varies by geographical location as well. That is, individuals in different areas of the world have different features of their microbiota composition, especially in relation to diseases. And when immigrants come to the United States, for example, their gut microbiota soon loses diversity and looks more like that of U.S. longtime residents. (Some of these changes can be chalked up to dietary shifts, but other changes are likely due to the geographical shift.)

During travel, gut microbiota diversity remains stable, but the composition fluctuates. Yet how about when someone from a higher-income country travels to a country where infrastructure around hygiene isn't as established, and is among the 40 to 60 percent of people who experience a dreaded bout of traveller's diarrhea? In that case, the person experiences a major gut microbiota shift right away. Their gut may also gain a high number of antimicrobial resistance genes that can remain high for weeks afterward.

Going wild: How nature impacts gut health

Contact with nature has been proposed as a factor that affects the gut, although this area of study is relatively new. Scientists have wondered how to account for the fact that people growing up in a farm environment are protected from certain immune-related diseases. Possibly through animal contact and time outdoors their gut microbiomes are exposed to more environmental microbes during an important time of life, teaching their immune systems to deal appropriately with them. One study looking at children in a ten-week nature play program found their fecal microbes were altered after the program, and in addition they showed a reduction in stress and anger. See Chapter 18 for more discussion.

Some researchers have proposed that increased exposure to soil microbes, as our human ancestors would have had, is important for gut health. Others have hypothesized that pollution and toxins in the environment today might negatively impact gut health and overall health. Research on this topic is ongoing.

Investigating house and home

The people and animals with whom you share your indoor space can have traces in your gut, too. People who live under the same roof have more similar gut microbiomes, with longer cohabitation leading to greater similarity. Roommates share gut microbes more frequently than do people who live separately. Parents and children (including siblings) living together also share microbes. Living with a spouse is associated with greater diversity of gut microbes than living alone, and cohabitating spouses — especially those reporting a close relationship — share many more gut microbes than do siblings who live in the same home. Chapter 18 touches on microbes shared with family members in early life.

Your furry friends can also impact your gut microbes: Having a dog or cat changes the composition of your gut microbiome, although it may not alter the diversity overall. The impact of pets on gut health is seen the most in early life — once again, refer to Chapter 18.

Chapter **5**

Connecting the Dots from Gut Health to Overall Health

What happens in the gut definitely doesn't stay in the gut. That is, the complex activities happening inside your digestive tract have effects throughout the rest of the body — even at sites distant from the digestive tract.

As I discuss in Chapter 1, among the reasons gut health is hot right now is that scientists are discovering more and more connections to aspects of health outside the gut. By managing the core body activities of immune and metabolic function, gut microbes end up having effects on many other diseases and conditions.

This chapter gets you up to speed on the major communication channels between the gut and other organs or organ systems. I delve into specific conditions, giving you an idea of how closely they are (or aren't) connected to what goes on in the gut. I also cover how all this information heralds a new era when you can be empowered to prevent health problems before they even show up — a brighter future made possible by your gut microbes.

Seeing How the Gut Connects with Other Organ Systems

Think of a single tiny blood cell, making its way through your entire body in about 45 seconds. In that time, it encounters thousands of metabolites and other types of messages sent from the gut. All of your body's major organs have permanent channels of communication with the gut so they can both send and receive these messages.

Here are the main channels of communication that exist between the gut and other organs:

>> **Immune system:** Gut microbes influence the activities of immune cells in the gut, which can have a cascade of effects throughout the body.

>> **Metabolites:** Molecules called *metabolites,* produced by gut microbes after they consume different substances, cross the gut barrier and are sent all around the body via the bloodstream.

>> **Hormones:** Hormones produced in the gut (for example, glucagon-like peptide 1, involved in metabolism) can signal to other areas of the body.

These channels account for the gut's back-and-forth chatter with the organs I describe in the following sections. The word *axis* refers to a two-way (or even multidirectional) pathway by which one part of the body sends biochemical signals to another part of the body. The axes (plural for axis) in this section are the most frequently studied for the role that gut microbes play.

Gut-skin axis

Skin is your body's largest organ — the one that holds all your parts together. Not only does it protect you, but it also regulates your body's water and temperature levels. Your skin has its own microbiota, which differs according to the conditions (for example, heat and moisture) at different skin sites such as your forehead, elbow, or the sole of your foot.

Overlap exists between skin and gut conditions. Psoriasis, a condition characterized by rough, scaly patches of skin, occurs in 7 to 11 percent of people with inflammatory bowel disease (IBD) compared to 1 to 2 percent of the general population. Furthermore, some interventions targeting the skin end up having effects in the gut; an example is skin-focused narrow-band UVB light changing gut microbiome diversity.

REMEMBER

The skin (along with the gut and lungs) is considered an *epithelial barrier organ*, which means it has tightly packed cells that cover and protect a specific area from the outside world. Across the animal kingdom, examples are found of signals from microorganisms that influence the status of epithelial tissues. It's true in humans too — both gut and skin microorganisms have effects on skin health. The gut and skin send signals back and forth via the immune system and endocrine system, with microbes being key switchboard operators.

Gut-lung axis

The lungs take care of the crucial function of breathing: that is, exchanging carbon dioxide in the blood for oxygen. Your lungs have their own diverse microbial community, which has a much lower number of microorganisms than the gut. Microbes often reach the lungs from higher up in the respiratory tract, but they're quickly cleared away through coordinated motion of the *cilia* (hairlike structures) as well as through coughing and immune system activities.

The gut-lung axis is a relatively new area of study, but already scientists have documented that bacteria can move from the gut up to the lungs via reflux and then be inhaled into the respiratory tract. Molecules produced in the gut such as short-chain fatty acids (SCFAs) can also hitch a ride through the bloodstream and end up in the lungs to meddle with immune activities there. Immune cells themselves also move through the *lymphatic duct* (a tube that carries fluid) back and forth between the gut and lungs, affecting immune responses in both organs.

Gut-brain axis

Your brain is an enormously complex supercomputer that manages at least three main jobs at once:

>> Supervising your thoughts and emotions

>> Controlling your conscious movements

>> Regulating your automatic activities such as breathing and digestion

Although the gut and the brain are fairly close together in the body, many people think of the brain as operating separately from the rest of the body — after all, it's sealed off from the rest of the organs and blood circulation by the blood-brain barrier. However, the brain is in active communication with the digestive tract at all times.

REMEMBER

Apart from the central nervous system (CNS), which includes the brain, the gut has its own nervous system called the *enteric nervous system (ENS)* with between 200 and 600 million neurons. The ENS oversees the gamut of gut functions, including the following:

>> Blood flow

>> Gut barrier function

>> Secretion of fluids

>> Transit of food through the intestine

The ENS and the CNS are connected through a main superhighway, the vagus nerve, with 90 percent of vagus nerve fibers conveying messages upward to allow the brain to keep tabs on all aspects of gut function: hunger, metabolic activities, inflammation, and more.

Doctors have long known about the higher rates of psychiatric conditions such as depression and anxiety in those with diagnosed gastrointestinal disorders, as well as the higher rates of gastrointestinal symptoms in people with diagnosed psychiatric disorders. This supports the existence of a gut-brain axis, but only recently are scientists figuring out the role that microbes play.

TECHNICAL STUFF

Recent research has shown that the microbe-gut-brain connection goes way back into humans' evolutionary history. At some point in the evolution of complex life on earth, microbes found their way inside the digestive tube of an ancient (early-evolving) marine creature called the hydra, which still thrives today. This simple animal shows the origins of the ENS — and just how closely the microbes are related to its functioning. From the hydra onward through evolution, a communication system between microbes and the ENS was maintained.

REMEMBER

Today researchers know that the microbes interfacing with the gut-brain axis influence many aspects of brain function in humans. (I discuss more about specific brain-related conditions in the section "Linking the Gut to Specific Diseases and Conditions" later in this chapter.) Examples of how microbes influence brain functions are as follows:

>> **Affecting neurons directly:** Certain microbes appear to influence neurons, making them either more active or less active. In mice, for example, a strain of *Bifidobacterium* directly activated ENS neurons to send signals to the brain via the vagus nerve and increase anxiety-like behaviors.

>> **Modulating immune cells:** Some microbes affect the brain by way of the immune system. For example, stressed mice were given a probiotic strain of *L. johnsonii*, which lowered their previously high levels of immune cells called gamma delta T cells, thereby normalizing their behaviors.

>> **Producing hormones and neurotransmitters:** Strains of bifidobacteria produce gamma-aminobutyric acid (GABA), which helps modulate signals to the brain that affect mood, cognition, sleep, and other functions.

Gut-liver axis

Your liver makes and secretes bile to digest fats, so it's considered an organ of digestion even though food doesn't pass through it directly. In general, the liver works to filter your blood and convert substances so your body can function effectively.

MY MICROBES MADE ME EAT IT?

In 2014, several scientists published an article in the scientific journal *Bioessays* proposing that gut microbes may have ways of controlling cravings and eating behavior through the gut-brain axis, with the purpose of increasing their own survival and growth. As cute as it is to imagine trillions of hungry little microbes in your gut scheming to make you march down to the bakery and pick up a cupcake, nearly a decade later very little evidence in humans has emerged to back up this theory.

On the other hand, gut microbes may be part of the bigger picture of how cravings emerge; for example, one study published in *The American Journal of Clinical Nutrition* found that when people consumed a diet high in prebiotic foods (which alter the gut microbiota), they had a reduced desire to eat sweet, salty, and fatty foods. Certain probiotic strains may also have the effect of reducing food cravings. But rather than being an effect of the microbes directly, the craving reduction is likely achieved through complicated mechanisms that involve satiety hormones and psychological influences, alongside microbes' global influence on metabolism.

Symptoms of liver disease may include fatigue, loss of appetite, nausea and/or vomiting, abdominal pain and swelling, sleep reversal (daytime drowsiness and nighttime insomnia), easy bruising, and a pale stool color.

REMEMBER

Gut microbiota contributes to the back-and-forth communication between the gut and the liver, mainly by producing chemical messengers (metabolites) that enter the bloodstream and become detoxified in the liver. The liver produces molecules called primary bile acids, which help digest fats, that the gut microbes convert into secondary bile acids. Some of these secondary bile acids are reabsorbed in the colon and circulated back to the liver. As another example of reciprocal influence between the liver and gut microbes, when the gut barrier is damaged, bacterial components called pathogen-associated molecular patterns (PAMP) can reach the liver and may cause injury to liver cells.

Gut-kidney axis

Even your kidneys, those hard-working organs that remove waste and extra fluids from your body and maintain the balance of water, salts, and minerals, have their own special communication channels with the gut. Kidney disease is associated with multiple gastrointestinal symptoms.

One channel of gut microbiota influence on the kidneys is through the production of metabolites — notably, uremic toxins that can contribute to kidney dysfunction. Gut microbes also influence immune system activation: When bacterial components or metabolites get into circulation through a permeable gut barrier, the process activates immune cells that infiltrate the kidneys and produce chronic inflammation that interferes with normal kidney function.

Researching the Gut and What May Cause Diseases

For most diseases and health conditions, researchers have uncovered something about the genes and lifestyle factors that increase your risk of developing them. But over the past 20 years, microbiome research has opened a whole new possibility: Your gut microbiome might also put up red flags that signal your risk of developing certain diseases. And because (as I discuss in Chapter 4) many of your lifestyle choices leave their imprint on your gut microbes, this internal ecosystem could in some cases be the biological link between your everyday actions and your disease risk.

Chapter 3 covers some general ways that the gut microbes affect body functions and health. This section gets into a very hot area of research: whether the activities in the gut can cause specific diseases and conditions. New gut-focused diagnostics and treatments are more likely for some diseases than for others. Slowly scientists are untangling whether microbes cause some aspects of each disease or whether microbes simply react to other processes that are driving a disease.

Having followed the microbiome biotech space for a decade, I want to caution that the process of taking gut microbiome knowledge and turning it into actionable medical treatments is incredibly slow. Some researchers have come up with great concepts for gut-focused treatments and started to develop them as drugs, only to find out they don't work in humans. The microbiome won't solve everything, but over time it may point in the direction of new options for diagnosing and treating some diseases.

Examining the missing microbes hypothesis

If you look at a graph of disease patterns in the global population over the past several decades as in Figure 5-1, you may notice an interesting trend. As the burden of infectious disease has decreased because of antibiotics, vaccinations, and other medical innovations, chronic health problems (otherwise known as noncommunicable diseases) running the gamut from diabetes and heart disease to IBD, have skyrocketed. On a global level, medical innovations have successfully reduced death due to infection, but despite living longer, humans today live with more illness. What factors could be contributing to this increase in chronic disease?

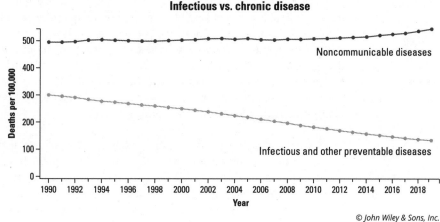

Infectious vs. chronic disease

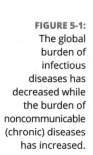

FIGURE 5-1:
The global burden of infectious diseases has decreased while the burden of noncommunicable (chronic) diseases has increased.

© John Wiley & Sons, Inc.

In his 2014 book *Missing Microbes: How the Overuse of Antibiotics Is Fueling Our Modern Plagues* (Henry Holt and Company), Dr. Martin Blaser proposed a theory about why the incidence of chronic diseases is increasing rapidly, especially in the industrialized world. He hypothesized that the increasing use of antibiotics and practices such as C-section birth in industrialized nations, despite their benefits, exert "collateral damage" on the gut microbes. Blaser pointed to emerging evidence that antibiotics, by depleting the gut microbiota (especially in early life), could have negative effects on both the immune system and metabolism and that this depletion could lead to the emergence of chronic diseases and obesity. In other words, he believed "missing microbes" in people's guts were responsible for increasing chronic disease. The observation that people in industrialized societies have lower-diversity gut microbiomes than those with other lifestyles (such as hunter-gatherers) supports this conjecture.

Blaser's idea is related to previous ideas such as the "hygiene hypothesis" proposed by David Strachan in 1989: that infection in early childhood and sharing microorganisms with siblings may be protective against allergic diseases. Although Strachan didn't specifically identify the gut microbiome connection, he proposed that "higher standards of personal cleanliness" and other aspects of more hygienic lifestyles were rendering people susceptible to chronic disease. Later came the similar "old friends hypothesis" advanced by Graham Rook and colleagues in 2006, hypothesizing that exposure to microorganisms that co-evolved with humans serve to protect us against immune-related disorders. Carrying the ideas through to today, the point is that inappropriate engagement of the immune system is the basis of chronic disease — and this may start in the gut.

Although antibiotics and other factors can deplete microbes from people's guts, diet also contributes to microbial exposures. The immune system must react in one way or another to everything it encounters in the gut. In previous eras, humans presumably consumed a much higher quantity of microorganisms in food; both because fermentation (producing foods with live microbes) was a ubiquitous way to preserve and increase the safety of foods and because sterile, industrialized food didn't exist. Leading scientists are exploring the possibility that the gut immune system is accustomed to seeing far more food-associated microorganisms than it sees today, causing it to overreact in the absence of these microorganisms and leading to chronic disease.

The lower consumption of microbes in modern Western diets doesn't mean people should try to eat unwashed or contaminated food to replenish some of the missing microbes. In industrialized food systems, food safety is paramount because practices that generate a higher volume of food product (such as crowded livestock pens) have led to pathogens frequently contaminating food. Nor should people let go of hygienic practices and purposely expose themselves to more pathogens. Chapters 10 and 11 cover ways to increase exposure safely and healthily to microorganisms.

Looking to the gut for the cause of diseases

To truly uncover the relationship between the gut and a complex disease, scientists must connect evidence from different types of studies, each with their own strengths and limitations. Only by putting together these puzzle pieces of evidence over many years will they discover the role of the gut.

Here are some types of studies that count as proof that the gut microbiome is involved in causing a condition (or a symptom of that condition):

>> Showing that germ-free animals don't develop the condition

>> Discovering that animals with the condition can be treated effectively if they receive a fecal transplant or some other gut microbiome-altering intervention

>> Showing in a laboratory setup mimicking the digestive tract, called a *gut model system,* that gut microbes affect some biological marker relevant to the condition in humans

>> Demonstrating in humans that some deliberate method of gut microbiome modulation (for example, prebiotics) improves the condition

Linking the Gut to Specific Diseases and Conditions

Time to get into the nitty gritty — the specific diseases and conditions linked to the gut and its microbes. No doubt as you read through this list, you may notice a theme: People with these diagnosed conditions show differences in their gut microbiota composition or function compared to healthy individuals. Most of the time, they also have a lower-diversity gut microbiome.

The exact bacteria that are disrupted in a disease, however, tend to differ from study to study. Why would this be? Some of it can be chalked up to the different techniques for sequencing the gut microorganisms. Or it may be that many different gut microbiome patterns can have the same negative influence on health. But more importantly, people have complex lives and regardless of how a human study tries to account for all the relevant factors that can affect results, otherwise known as *confounders*, every study has a limited ability to get at the truth (whatever that may be).

The following contains an alphabetical list of diseases and conditions that have been linked to some aspect of gut health — and gut microbes, in particular. I focus on the general trends rather than the exact microorganisms that are increased or decreased in these conditions because the microorganisms tend to vary from study to study, and moreover, their names can be red herrings given that their effects are dependent on how they operate within the complex microbial ecosystem. This list isn't exhaustive, but it does cover the major conditions that have been researched for their connection to the gut.

Allergies

An *allergy* is a tissue-damaging immune response to a substance that's harmless to most people. The most common type of allergy occurs when the allergen triggers production of IgE *antibodies* (proteins that fight harmful substances), which are specific to the allergen. These antibodies attach to receptors on *mast cells* (tissue-dwelling immune cells), which then release proinflammatory chemicals like a red alert, causing allergic symptoms such as itching, swelling, and difficulty breathing. Sometimes gastrointestinal symptoms also occur — typically nausea, vomiting, abdominal pain, or diarrhea.

Gut microbiome differences are seen in people with allergies compared to people without allergies, and these differences emerge even before allergy onset. Further, increased microbial exposures in early life through siblings and pets is associated with a lower risk of allergy. (Chapter 18 discusses this topic.)

This area of research is quite established, with both prevention and treatment strategies being explored. Live microbial drugs are being tested, both to increase the success of oral immunotherapy (ingestion of small amounts of an allergen to increase the body's tolerance of it), and for broadly modulating the immune system to prevent allergic diseases in children who are at risk.

Alzheimer's disease

Alzheimer's disease (AD) is a brain disorder characterized by memory deficits and gradual loss of cognitive function over time, eventually leading to the inability to respond appropriately to the surrounding environment. Researchers don't fully understand the causes of this disease, but they've documented abnormal proteins in the brain of some AD patients.

In mice, the gut microbes are a necessary ingredient for the abnormal buildup of Alzheimer's-like proteins in the brain. And in humans with AD, the gut harbors reduced levels of SCFAs compared to healthy people, as well as increased proinflammatory bacteria from the groups *Escherichia* and *Shigella*. Researchers think the gut microbes affect the brain by increasing inflammatory markers in the blood, which signal to the brain.

A moderate amount of research exists on this topic, but microbiome-focused therapies don't appear to be among the most promising in the entire list of drugs currently being tested for AD.

Amyotrophic lateral sclerosis

In 2014, the Ice Bucket Challenge went viral on social media where people filmed themselves dumping buckets of ice water over their heads to raise awareness for amyotrophic lateral sclerosis (ALS). The trend raised $115 million in donations for the ALS Association, allowing it to fund 130 research projects and support the development of 40 potential treatments.

ALS is a disorder involving progressive degeneration of nerve cells in the spinal cord and brain, causing a loss of voluntary muscle movement over time. Gastro-intestinal symptoms that accompany the progression of the disease include con-stipation, abdominal pain, a feeling of fullness, and nausea.

Some ALS research is focusing on the role of the gut microbiota. Studies are con-flicted on whether people with ALS have a different gut microbiome compared to healthy people (not attributable to gastrointestinal symptoms) around the time of disease onset, suggesting that gut microbes may not trigger the onset of disease. However, some gut microbial patterns are associated with an increased risk of death in ALS, meaning the microbes could be responding to the progression of the disease.

Only a handful of studies have been done in this area, but at least one company is testing a gut-targeted therapeutic for ALS involving two live bacteria found in the human gut. Researchers are also exploring ALS drugs based on metabolites produced by *Akkermansia muciniphila*.

Anorexia nervosa

Anorexia nervosa (AN) is a psychiatric disorder in which a person experiences a strong and persistent fear of gaining weight. Digestive symptoms are common for people with AN, and (particularly in women) the condition may be linked with IBD and other autoimmune diseases.

Certainly it's logical that the changes in food intake and dietary pattern in AN would influence the gut microbiota composition, and this pattern is in fact seen in the available research studies. Patients show great variability from person to person in their gut bacteria, and they tend to have decreased levels of serotonin, GABA, dopamine, and SCFAs in their stool samples compared to healthy people.

Some research indicates the pre-illness gut microbiota potentially influences the risk of developing AN.

Although few studies have been conducted on this topic, probiotic treatments may hold potential.

Anxiety

Feeling anxious from time to time is a normal part of life and is an appropriate reaction to some circumstances. But these feelings become a clinical anxiety disorder when feelings of worry are excessive or persistent and may become worse over time. Uncontrollable worry may cause distress and affect the activities in a person's daily life. Gastrointestinal disorders and anxiety are closely related; each may accentuate the other.

Studies show those with anxiety disorder have different bacteria in their guts compared with healthy people, and these tend to be proinflammatory bacteria that correspond with overall inflammation in the body. SCFA-producing bacteria are decreased.

This topic is an active area of study in the broader area of the microbiota–gut–brain axis, with potential new therapies in the future.

Arthritis

Arthritis is a collection of different conditions, all of which usually involve inflammation and swelling of the joints. Types of inflammatory arthritis include

» **Ankylosing spondylitis (AS):** A condition causing inflammation in the joints and ligaments of the spine as well as some other joints throughout the body. Over time some of the spinal vertebrae may fuse, reducing flexibility in the spine. Between 5 and 10 percent of people with AS also have IBD and a much larger percentage have observable inflammation in the gut. People with AS have a different gut microbiota composition than healthy people, with more inflammation-associated bacterial groups.

» **Psoriatic arthritis (PA):** This type of arthritis affects some people with psoriasis (a condition causing rashes on the skin that are red with dry, whitish scales). The arthritis involves painful, swollen joints and stiffness that can affect any part of the body. Psoriatic arthritis increases the risk of IBD, especially Crohn's disease. In this condition gut microbiome diversity appears to be reduced.

>> **Rheumatoid arthritis (RA):** This is a body-wide autoimmune condition that ends up damaging joints over time. Gastrointestinal symptoms such as nausea, abdominal pain, bloating, swallowing difficulties, and stool leakage are more common in people with RA than in people without RA.

Decreased microbial diversity is a hallmark of the gut microbiota in RA, along with altered composition characterized by reduced anti-inflammatory groups and increased *Prevotella* and *Collinsella*. The gut microbiota pattern may even correspond with the severity of RA.

A recent study found specific gut microbiota changes in composition and function — including increased bacterial groups from the mouth — that are seen across different types of arthritis. However, these changes are likely a response to system-wide inflammation rather than the cause of it.

Overall, arthritis and gut microbiota is an active area of research, with live bacteria being explored as new drug treatments.

Asthma

Asthma is a disease in which the airways become narrow and inflamed at certain times, causing shortness of breath, coughing, wheezing, and other symptoms. Gastrointestinal symptoms occur at higher rates in those with asthma, and many individuals with asthma also have gastroesophageal reflux disease.

An intriguing study in 2015 found that early warning signs of developing asthma at the age of one year could be seen when a child was only 3 months old, by the absence of four groups of bacteria in their fecal samples. This finding, along with the fact that antibiotic use in early life increases asthma risk, back up the missing microbes idea that early-life bacterial exposures influence asthma development (refer to the section "Examining the missing microbes hypothesis" earlier in this chapter for more information). In general, those with asthma have a lower-diversity gut microbiome and increased bacteria from the group Pseudomonadota (formerly known as Proteobacteria). Children with normal levels of SCFAs in their stool at one year are less likely to develop asthma than those who have lower levels.

Research in this area is robust and promising for preventing the inflammation-related processes that underlie several allergic diseases, including asthma.

Atopic dermatitis

Atopic dermatitis, also known as *eczema*, is a long-lasting disease that causes skin dryness, irritation, and itching. The condition most often emerges in childhood but can occur at any age. Children with eczema commonly manifest gastrointestinal symptoms, especially diarrhea, vomiting, and regurgitation.

Beyond interest in the skin microbiome as a target for eczema treatment, researchers have targeted the gut to dampen the skin inflammation at the root of the disorder. An altered gut microbiome affects immune system activity that can affect the skin. And studies have found that the gut microbiome in early life correlates with eczema's age of onset, severity, remission, and flares.

Few studies on this topic are published annually, and most of the research with eczema relates to prevention; for mothers of children who are susceptible to eczema, taking certain probiotics during pregnancy may provide a protective effect.

Autism spectrum disorder

Autism spectrum disorder (ASD) is a neurodevelopmental condition, often diagnosed in childhood, that's characterized by three observable characteristics:

» Abnormal social interaction

» Disordered communication

» Repetitive behaviors

ASD often co-occurs with gastrointestinal symptoms. These symptoms aren't considered a core feature of the disorder, nor is there any biological measurement for diagnosing ASD. Nevertheless, the search is on for biomedical interventions that may make a difference for these individuals.

Children with ASD show an altered gut microbiota, but the nature of the alterations lack consistency. In addition, levels of some metabolites that originate in the gut are associated with behaviors typical of ASD. However, a large study found the restrictive diets typical of children with ASD, rather than ASD itself, accounted for their gut microbiome alterations. According to the research so far, any claims that targeting the gut microbiota (through interventions such as fecal microbiota transplantation) can improve autism behaviors should be viewed with extreme caution.

As far as ASD prevention, another line of research focuses on how maternal diet affects the gut microbiota and offspring social behavior. Scientists found in mice that shifts in the mother's microbiota caused abnormal social behavior in the mouse pups, but a single strain of bacteria corrected these social behaviors.

ASDs and gut microbiota is an active area of study, and a gut-targeting therapeutic to alleviate autism-associated irritability is under development.

Cancer

Cancer occurs when abnormal cells grow uncontrollably in a part of the body and spread to other parts of the body.

The connections between different cancer types and the gut microbiota would need an entire book to explain, but across different cancers — lung, skin, colorectal, pancreatic, and others — scientists observe an altered gut microbiota. Moreover, the gut microbiome in several cancers (including the presence of specific species) predicts how individuals will respond to immunotherapy drugs.

The cancer connection is one of the hottest areas related to the gut microbiome at present, with more than a thousand scientific studies published on the topic annually. New treatments or ways to enhance the success of immunotherapies may be around the corner.

Cardiovascular disease

Cardiovascular disease is a general term that describes a disease of the heart or blood vessels. Atherosclerosis occurs when fatty deposits build up inside an artery, leading to hardening and narrowing, and if a blood clot forms, it can block the flow of blood and cause a heart attack or stroke. Cardiovascular disease is the leading cause of death globally.

The gut microbiota structure and function are altered in cardiometabolic diseases, with lower diversity being a main finding, and the changes occurring before the onset of disease. Metabolites of the gut microbiota seem to play a big role. In particular, a molecule called trimethylamine N-oxide (TMAO), which is produced by gut microbes from dietary substrates and circulates in the blood, appears to promote atherosclerosis and predict the risk of a heart attack.

A large number of published studies address the cardiovascular disease-gut microbiota connection, and new therapies such as metabolites or live microbes are being tested.

Celiac disease

Celiac disease is a disorder in which *gluten* (a protein found in wheat and some grains) causes an immune reaction that damages the small intestine. The damage may prevent the body's absorption of nutrients. A range of gastrointestinal symptoms are typical in this disease, including bloating, diarrhea, constipation, gas, stools with poor consistency, nausea, vomiting, and abdominal pain.

People with celiac disease show lower microbial richness in the small intestine. Before diagnosis, children who would go on to develop the disease showed a distinct gut microbiota composition, accompanied by specific blood metabolites and cytokines. Also, certain bacteria isolated from the small intestines of those with celiac disease show abnormalities in how they metabolize gluten, causing increased immune reactions.

Not many research groups are focusing on celiac disease and gut microbiota, but immune-targeting therapies and probiotics may be promising.

Chronic kidney disease

Chronic kidney disease (CKD) is characterized by damaged kidneys that can't filter blood appropriately. People with CKD frequently experience gastrointestinal symptoms, including feelings of fullness, nausea, and upper abdominal pain. An inflamed stomach and reflux are also common.

Decreased microbial diversity in CKD is a consistent scientific finding. Furthermore, the gut microbiota produce metabolites that are circulated around the body and eventually cleared by the kidneys. When dietary proteins are metabolized by an altered gut bacterial community, high levels of uremic toxins can be produced, which accumulate and cause inflammation and kidney damage. An altered gut microbiota (for example, decreased *Akkermansia muciniphila*) in kidney disease may independently promote body-wide inflammation as well.

This area of research is active, with several gut-inspired therapeutics under development.

Clostridioides difficile infection

Clostridioides difficile infection (also known as *C. difficile* or *C. diff* infection) is a debilitating gastrointestinal condition that often occurs when individuals receive antibiotics, involving symptoms such as watery diarrhea, severe abdominal cramping and pain, and nausea. After treatment of the condition with specific antibiotics the infection may clear up and recur multiple times.

Recurrent *C. difficile* has been the flagship success story of gut microbiome research. Individuals with recurrent *C. difficile* have a severely depleted gut microbial community, and a fecal microbiota transplant from a healthy person is a highly effective treatment. Because fecal transplants have unknown safety outside of established donor programs, several companies have developed ways to test and process donors' fecal samples in a standardized way to produce two approved drug treatments.

A high number of studies focus on gut microbiota and new-onset *C. difficile* infection or recurrent *C. difficile* infection, and an eventual movement away from donor-based drug products and toward cocktails of probiotics is likely.

Depression

Major depressive disorder, or depression, is a mood disorder characterized by long-lasting feelings of sadness and loss of interest. These feelings can interfere significantly with the activities of daily life. Depression can influence digestive health, with constipation being a frequent symptom.

The gut microbiota in individuals with depression shows a higher abundance of proinflammatory bacteria and fewer SCFA–producing bacteria.

A high number of studies are published annually on the topic of depression and gut microbiota, and already some probiotics show modest effects for improving depression symptoms.

Diabetes, type 1

Type 1 diabetes is an autoimmune disease in which cells in the pancreas that normally create the hormone insulin are destroyed, so the body produces little to no insulin. This hormone normally allows sugar (glucose) to enter cells and produce energy.

Lower bacterial diversity is seen in the colon of people with type 1 diabetes compared to people without the disease. In fact, some gut microbiota alterations (primarily in function, not composition) as well as increased gut barrier permeability seem to precede the onset of type 1 diabetes.

This area of research has steady interest and a fair number of studies per year but whether microbiome-targeted therapies will be successful remains to be determined.

Diabetes, type 2

Type 2 diabetes is a disorder affecting how your body manages glucose for energy. In this disease the body's cells don't respond properly to insulin, leading to a high level of blood glucose. Rates of most gastrointestinal symptoms in people with type 2 diabetes are about the same as in the general population — except that high blood sugar is known to lead to *gastroparesis* (the delayed emptying of the stomach).

SCFA-producing bacteria are consistently depleted in individuals with type 2 diabetes, and overall the gut microbiota has an altered composition and lower diversity. As Chapter 3 mentions, SCFAs prompt intestinal cells to secrete GLP-1, which affects pancreatic function and insulin release.

Many studies focus on type 2 diabetes and gut microbiota. One medical probiotic for type 2 diabetes exists in the United States with microbiome-focused drug products likely in the future.

Fatty liver disease

Fatty liver disease (sometimes called *hepatosteatosis*) is a buildup of fat in the liver, which can cause liver dysfunction and serious complications. This condition tends to be more common in people who are overweight or obese and/or those who consume high amounts of sugary and fatty foods. Non-alcoholic fatty liver disease (NAFLD), which is now called metabolic dysfunction-associated steatotic liver disease (MASLD), can occur in people who drink little to no alcohol; alcoholic fatty liver disease can occur in those who drink heavily.

Lower gut microbiota diversity, as well as higher levels of possibly harmful metabolites such as TMAO, are seen in fatty liver disease. SCFAs contribute to the regulation of inflammation and insulin resistance and are considered protective against MASLD. Moreover, an altered gut microbiota in MASLD may trigger increased gut barrier permeability, causing an inflammatory state that may damage the liver.

This area of research is active and growing and new therapeutics are in development.

Graft-versus-host disease

Graft-versus-host disease (GvHD) is a serious and frequently occurring complication of allogeneic hematopoietic cell transplantation (allo-HCT), which is a life-saving treatment for blood cancer in which a healthy donor's stem cell or bone marrow (known as a *graft*) is transferred to a patient. In GvHD, the graft's immune cells attack the patient's own body.

GvHD can affect tissues in the gastrointestinal tract, resulting in a range of symptoms, including nausea, appetite loss and weight loss, a feeling of fullness, gas, bloating, diarrhea, and abdominal pain.

Gut bacteria are associated with the risk of GvHD and its complications; for example, in one study the lower the fecal bacterial diversity after HCT, the lower the person's chance of survival. Other work has shown individuals undergoing HCT might have overactive or underactive inflammatory responses to their resident microbes. Some metabolites from gut bacteria such as indoles may be protective against GvHD.

This condition is the focus of a low number of published studies per year, but at least one company is developing a microbiome-based therapeutic to address GvHD: a live microbial treatment derived from a donor's fecal sample with high diversity plus a specific group of bacterial species that produce anti-inflammatory SCFAs.

HIV infection

Human immunodeficiency virus (HIV) infection can, over time, lead to acquired immune deficiency syndrome (AIDS) if untreated. A range of gastrointestinal symptoms can accompany HIV infection, including nausea, vomiting, swallowing difficulty, diarrhea, and problems with nutrient absorption.

Germ-free animal studies show that the lack of a microbiota seems to increase both HIV acquisition and levels of HIV in the body, which intensifies HIV infection. After HIV infection is established, patients have an altered gut microbiota (compared to people with no HIV infection), which contributes to sustaining chronic inflammation even in people who receive standard antiretroviral therapy. When severe immunodeficiency occurs in HIV infection, the gut's community of viruses expands while the diversity of the (already-less-diverse) gut bacteria decrease even further.

The scientific literature in this area is fairly robust. One company is developing a live bacterial therapy to prevent HIV infection in women, using a probiotic bacterium to neutralize/inhibit HIV in the vagina, the possible site of infection.

Inflammatory bowel disease

IBD is a group of conditions involving chronic inflammation of the gastrointestinal tract. The two main inflammatory bowel diseases are

>> **Crohn's disease (CD):** In CD, the inflammation shows up in different locations as distinct patches of damaged tissue and extends through multiple layers of the digestive tract walls. This inflammation can occur anywhere from the mouth to the anus.

>> **Ulcerative colitis (UC):** UC is characterized by inflammation localized in the colon with continuous (nondefined) areas of damage that are only in the innermost layer of the colon wall.

REMEMBER

The inflammation in IBD causes cycles of gastrointestinal symptoms as well as weight loss and fatigue. CD and UC each have a different relationship with the gut microbiome, but what ties them together is lower gut microbial diversity and a composition that changes erratically over time. Although gut microbiome targeting interventions such as probiotics and fecal microbiota transplantation show some promise for UC, they don't seem to work well in CD.

IBD remains one of the most popular areas of gut microbiome research, and a number of companies are developing new therapeutics based on microbiome modulation, making it likely that new treatments are just around the corner.

Irritable bowel syndrome

Irritable bowel syndrome (IBS) is a functional disorder because there's no observable biological cause of the symptoms. However, IBS is characterized by persistent gastrointestinal symptoms that include excessive gas, abdominal pain, cramps, as well as either diarrhea or constipation.

Research shows differences in gut microbiota composition in a subset of patients with IBS compared with healthy controls. In general, individuals with IBS have a gut microbiota with lower diversity and stability. Furthermore, the gut fungal community is also altered in IBS and may contribute to hypersensitivity of gut tissues.

Published studies on IBS and gut microbiota are fairly numerous, and several scientifically supported treatments that target the microbiome exist. These include probiotics, prebiotics (for example, inulin), non-absorbable antibiotics, and dietary interventions. Over time, these interventions may become more targeted and effective. At least one company is developing a drug treatment for severe IBS, which so far seems safe and effective.

Multiple sclerosis

Multiple sclerosis (MS) is a condition of the brain and spinal cord in which the immune system attacks *myelin* — the insulating layer of fat and protein covering the nerves — causing communication problems between the brain and the rest of the body.

Individuals diagnosed with MS have a higher rate of gastrointestinal symptoms than the general population, with common symptoms being bloating, reflux, and nausea. As for bowel problems, individuals with MS may deal with either constipation, or on the other extreme, diarrhea and loss of bowel control.

The gut microbiota differs in people with MS compared with people who don't have MS — reduced diversity being the primary difference. The exact nature of the compositional changes varies in different studies, but many report a lack of SCFA-producing bacteria.

A landmark study published in 2022 confirmed in a large population of U.S. military recruits tracked over 20 years that infection with Epstein-Barr virus (EBV) sharply increased the risk of later being diagnosed with MS. It's still unclear whether the gut microbiota, as modified by EBV, could influence the emergence of MS.

A fair number of studies have been completed in this area, and one therapeutic of interest is based on a damper for the immune system that's dysfunctional in people with autoimmune diseases. The therapy involves genetically engineered bacteria that produce a molecule called lactate, which tames immune activity.

Necrotizing enterocolitis

Necrotizing enterocolitis (NEC) is a serious condition affecting preterm infants with underdeveloped intestines, involving portions of the bowel tissue becoming inflamed or dying.

Scientists have identified a shift in both gut bacteria and gut viruses that occurs before onset of NEC. Probiotics are also effective in reducing risk, although the gut microbiota contributions to this efficacy aren't certain.

Steady interest in the gut microbiota and NEC has existed since around 2015, although relatively few studies are published per year on the topic.

Obesity

In the reality TV show competition *The Biggest Loser,* weight loss is a game filled with workouts, weigh-ins, and watermelon-kiwi salsa. But in real life, weight loss can be highly challenging. Obesity (defined as a body mass index higher than 30) is increased fat accumulation, which poses a risk to health.

As for how the gut is involved in obesity, the gut microbiota does seem to be altered but not in a consistent manner. As I discuss in Chapter 3, the gut microbiota is intertwined with metabolic health and can sometimes trigger damage to the gut barrier, which leads to body-wide inflammation and weight gain. So far scientists haven't found effective ways of reversing weight gain through gut microbiome modulation. Studies have shown fecal microbiota transplantation isn't effective for prompting weight loss.

The connection between obesity and the gut microbiota is a very active area of research with more than a thousand published studies annually in recent years. However, few interventions focused on the gut microbiome have succeeded in helping people lose weight. The idea that the gut microbiome can solve the obesity crisis is unlikely, but it does seem plausible that doctors will eventually add a few new tools to the toolbox for weight loss through the gut. Across the obesity research done to date — related to the gut microbiome or not — the best medicine is prevention.

Parkinson's disease

At the age of 29, the actor Michael J. Fox was diagnosed with Parkinson's disease (PD) — a progressive disease involving damage to brain cells that make *dopamine* (a chemical that helps coordinate body movements). Fox subsequently became one of the most prominent patient advocates for this disease and launched a PD research foundation in 2000.

Individuals with PD experience both motor symptoms (such as tremors and slowed movement) and nonmotor symptoms (such as cramps and constipation). The gastrointestinal symptom of constipation, incidentally, may precede the development of PD by many years.

The gut microbiota of individuals with PD is altered, with a reduced capacity to create SCFAs. *Akkermansia muciniphila* bacteria, which are normally associated with healthy states, are increased in PD.

PD and the gut microbiome is an active area of research, and several companies are developing potential new PD therapies, including live microbial drugs.

Severe acute malnutrition

Severe acute malnutrition (SAM), a type of undernutrition resulting in sudden weight loss or fluid retention, affects 45 million children under the age of 5 globally. SAM causes children to have a very low weight for height, and over time it can cause stunted growth.

Researchers investigated whether the gut microbiota had something to do with SAM-related irregular growth in a group of children from Bangladesh. They found that children with SAM had an "immature" gut microbiome for their age, which corresponded with their growth. They also discovered the gut microbiome maturity could be partially fixed when the children were given two types of widely used diet interventions. As a next step, the same researchers experimented with combinations of local foods that had the ability to normalize the gut microbiota trajectory of children with SAM and growth stunting. When these foods were administered, the gut microbiota for those children with SAM looked more like that of healthy children and their growth pattern became more normal.

This area of research is fairly active, given its potential importance in the lives of vulnerable children globally.

Systemic lupus erythematosus

Systemic lupus erythematosus (SLE), or lupus for short, is a complex autoimmune disease in which the body attacks some of its own healthy tissues, triggering inflammation and organ damage.

Because gastrointestinal symptoms aren't a hallmark of lupus, researchers didn't previously focus on the gut when studying lupus. However, they've now found that gut microbiome diversity is decreased in lupus and the gut barrier integrity is compromised. Some of the features of altered gut microbiome composition are consistent across individuals with lupus in several countries (for instance, Spain and China). One emerging theory is that gut microbiota may contribute to the disease by prompting the immune system to stop tolerating (or start reacting to) autoreactive T cells or B cells in the gut.

Even though few studies have been completed on lupus and gut microbiota to date, the number has increased in recent years and the topic remains worthy of further investigation.

Preventing Disease through the Gut

If you could look into a crystal ball and see the future of your personal health, what would you see?

Medicine does have a crystal ball of sorts, but it's very cloudy and only allows you to see the basic outlines of what might happen health-wise. This crystal ball is called *risk factors* — that is, facts about you and your lifestyle that increase your likelihood of ending up with a specific disease. For example, say you live in a big city within an industrialized country, have a parent with IBD, currently smoke, and don't consume much dietary fiber — in this case, you could say there's a possible future where your crystal ball shows you're diagnosed with IBD. But then again, you may have factors that protect you personally, so you may actually not develop IBD.

SCIENTIST SAYS

The promise of the gut microbiome and gut health over the long term is to make this crystal ball — well, crystal clear. Even though the gut microbiome doesn't cause every disease, it may be responsive enough to the nuances of your lifestyle and environment that predispose you to diseases that it could foretell your future health better than existing methods. After researchers learn to decipher what your gut microbiome is revealing about your future health, they may be able to pinpoint your personal risk for disease to an unprecedented extent. At the very least the gut microbiome could be used to track progression toward or away from disease, and in some cases, it may even be leveraged to delay or prevent the disease altogether. Scientist Rob Knight likens this predictive ability to a "microbial GPS" guiding you to health.

This concept brings new energy to the idea of prevention — empowering you to veer away from a disease, even if you may be at risk of being diagnosed with it.

REMEMBER

As anyone whose car has broken down in the middle of a highway can attest, most of the time you're better off preventing problems than dealing with them after they happen. The gut microbiome is a possible opportunity for everyone to rally around prevention in healthcare, letting your microbes guide you to healthier lifestyle choices. So far, the way they guide you is general, but as the research advances over time, the guidance is likely to become more personalized to your unique health situation. The following sections explain why the gut, especially during certain times of life, is a good target if you want to prevent disease.

Aiming to prevent disease by maintaining gut health

Gut health is a reasonable target to aim for if you want to live a longer and healthier life. Not that a healthy gut will protect you from every possible disease, especially if you have strong risk factors for developing a certain disease, but gut health can serve as newfound motivation to implement lifestyle choices that positively support your overall health.

TIP

For an individual to grasp the connection between eating fries regularly and a future diagnosis of fatty liver disease may have been difficult in past decades given scientists' reliance on population-wide data; but today researchers have shown that your gut microbes directly respond to your choices and influence many diseases. It's a new way to think about your health: Stay healthy from the inside out and you'll be more likely to sidestep chronic disease and live a healthier life.

Important times of life for paying attention to gut health

The research on asthma that I discuss in the "Asthma" section earlier in this chapter hints at the idea that specific times of life are important for your gut health, in that they set the course for some aspect of health later in your life. These so-called *critical windows* are times when the state of your gut may have an amplified effect on your health.

Early life — particularly the first 90 days — is one of these critical windows for immune development. The entire first year of life is important, in fact, because of the rapid body and brain development that occurs during this time, partially in response to signals from gut microbes. Older age is another critical window for gut health that affects quality of life as you age. Read more about these specific times of life in Part 5.

2

Restoring Your Gut Health

Chapter **6**

Demystifying Digestive Symptoms

According to the stories of Greek mythology, Kronos, King of the Titans, suffered from severe digestive pain. This all-powerful ruler of the cosmos thought he had everything figured out; because of a prophecy that his own son would one day overthrow him as ruler, he simply gulped down each of his children whole as soon as they were born. The first five went down the hatch without incident, but the sixth seemed to cause him terrible stomach pain. Little did he know the sixth was actually a stone wrapped in swaddling clothes; his wife Rhea had hidden the baby away to be raised in secret on the island of Crete. When the child Zeus grew up, he eventually did fulfill the prophecy and usurp his father, while also mercifully putting an end to Kronos's digestive pain by causing him to regurgitate the stone and all of Zeus's swallowed siblings. With digestion — unlike with overthrowing a powerful ruler, I suppose — all's well that ends well.

If digestive symptoms can happen to the ruler of the cosmos, they can happen to anyone. And they do — because starting with a newborn's early days digesting milk and progressing to solid foods and onward through childhood, adulthood, and older age, tummy troubles are a part of the human condition.

The word *symptom* means an outward sign of a change or condition inside the body. This concept highlights that a symptom must be observable in some way and that the underlying cause may not be immediately apparent. The explanations of symptoms in this chapter make clear that these outward signs can have many potential causes and that identifying these causes often requires further investigation by a healthcare practitioner. (Certain symptoms may in fact be part of a digestive disease, as Chapter 7 outlines.)

This chapter goes over the prevalence of digestive symptoms, and then provides definitions and descriptions of specific gut symptoms in plain language so you can clearly communicate what you're experiencing. I flag when you should see your healthcare practitioner for each symptom, and finally, I highlight some nonscientific labels that some people try to put on gut-related symptoms despite a lack of evidence.

Throughout this chapter, remember that normal functioning of the digestive tract looks very different from person to person. For example, when it comes to the frequency of bowel movements, anywhere from three times per day to three times per week can be considered normal. A well-formed stool can be on the harder side for some and loose for others. And even for the same person, digestion can vary over time because of diet, daily activities, and even the hormonal changes of the menstrual cycle. Ultimately the body's skillful adaptations to what you encounter and ingest every day are what create the fluctuations in your digestive functioning from day to day.

Understanding Who Gets Digestive Symptoms

Digestive symptoms are more common than you may realize — because they often go hidden and unmentioned. In any given week, more than 60 percent of Americans may have at least one gastrointestinal symptom. Typically symptoms fall into one of two categories: occasional symptoms or those that are part of a digestive disease.

Occasional symptoms

When people without a digestive disease experience gut symptoms, they're known as occasional symptoms. Everyone deals with them at one point or another.

If occasional symptoms sounds like a phrase you'd hear in a yogurt commercial, that's because it is. And deliberately so. Because yogurt is a food rather than a drug, regulators typically don't allow companies to claim that yogurt can cure, mitigate, treat, or prevent a specific disease. So yogurt companies must use vague language that stays in the domain of healthy people — for example, a probiotic added to the yogurt may be said to support healthy digestion or improve occasional gas or bloating, but it may not be said to cure irritable bowel syndrome (IBS). So when an intervention is for occasional symptoms, it applies across the general population.

Symptoms as part of digestive disease

Researchers estimate that 20 percent or more of Americans experience their gut symptoms as part of a digestive disease diagnosis. The risk for having a digestive disease varies worldwide according to age, sex, and geographical region.

Diagnoses of certain digestive diseases are increasing — partly because of more awareness, but also because they're becoming more widespread in the population. Among the top conditions leading this increase are gastroesophageal reflux disease, stomach irritation, and celiac disease. Chapter 7 explains how healthcare practitioners diagnose digestive disease.

Clarifying Specific Digestive Symptoms

The everyday language for talking about digestive symptoms includes vague phrases such as "tummy trouble" and "stomachache" that aren't precise descriptions of symptoms. This section gets into the ABCs of different gut symptoms, spelling out exactly what they are and their typical frequency in the population. The list may help you become more aware of what constitutes a symptom and may also help you describe them clearly should it become necessary to consult a healthcare practitioner.

REMEMBER

Before delving into the symptoms, it's worth knowing some basic criteria for when to seek a medical opinion on your digestive health:

>> A sudden or dramatic change occurs in bowel habits or the appearance of your stool

>> Rapid weight loss happens

>> Digestive symptoms start affecting your quality of life and make you miss out on activities you enjoy

Your healthcare practitioner can recommend appropriate treatment for your gut symptoms, tailored to your individual situation. This book doesn't offer medical advice, but some general categories of treatments are found in Chapter 7.

Abdominal pain or discomfort

Abdominal pain/discomfort is any uncomfortable sensation occurring near your belly region, in the space between your ribs and your pelvis. It includes sharp pain as well as aching or cramps.

REMEMBER

Many important organs are located in this area of your body, so multiple causes can exist for abdominal pain or discomfort. Some are digestion-related and some aren't. To pinpoint the cause of the problem, a healthcare practitioner needs to know some details about the sensations you're experiencing, including:

>> When the pain started

>> Whether or not you experienced the same pain in the past, and if so what the outcome was

>> Whether certain activities (for example, eating or bowel movements) alleviate the pain or make it worse

>> Its location and whether it moves to other parts of the abdomen or back

>> Severity

>> How it progresses over time

TIP

Only you can describe this symptom, so using clear language to talk about your abdominal sensations is essential for a proper diagnosis. Here are some ways you may describe your symptom:

>> *Localized* (in one area of the abdomen) or *generalized* (all over)

>> Dull (aching), sharp, or burning pain

>> Severe pain (preventing you from doing everyday activities) or mild pain

>> Continual over time, or intermittent

>> *Colicky* pain (felt in a single area, starting and stopping abruptly)

Abdominal pain or discomfort is completely normal from time to time and often resolves on its own. Frequently caused by other digestive symptoms such as gas or loose stool, it's a highly common digestive symptom, second only to heartburn. On the other hand, abdominal pain that's more persistent or severe often prompts an emergency room visit. In fact, abdominal pain is the top reason for visiting the emergency room in the United States, accounting for around 7 percent of all such visits.

REMEMBER

If you encounter one of these serious signs, you should see a healthcare practitioner about your abdominal pain:

>> The pain is so severe you have difficulty moving, eating, or drinking.

>> The pain comes on suddenly or gets worse over several hours.

REMEMBER

Get immediate medical attention if the pain is accompanied by a high fever, blood in your stool, or shortness of breath. Also, see a healthcare practitioner immediately if you experience abdominal pain while pregnant, after digestive tract surgery, or after abdominal trauma (for example, being hit while playing a sport).

Bloating and distension

Bloating is a word that's often used incorrectly to refer to an expanded belly. In fact, *bloating* is when the belly feels uncomfortably full and tight, whereas *distension* is the correct word for a visible expansion (and sometimes hardness) in the abdominal area. Bloating is what you feel, and distension is what you see. One of these symptoms can occur without the other, but often they occur together, which may account for why bloating is used as the catch-all term.

Bloating and distension are normal to experience on a fairly regular basis. Whereas sometimes these symptoms may be triggered by gas, constipation, or water retention, other times they happen after simply eating a meal. An Instagram challenge in 2017 tried to normalize bloating and distension and demonstrate how bodies changed shape throughout the day: Glamorous Instagrammers posted two side-by-side belly pictures from the same day, one showing a flatter belly and another showing the expansion that had occurred throughout the day.

Bloating and distension sometimes cause other difficulties such as incontinence if the belly expansion puts excessive pressure on the pelvic floor. Often, however, these symptoms resolve on their own in a short period of time.

REMEMBER

Here are signs to see a healthcare practitioner about bloating and distension:

>> The symptoms persist over time and don't seem tied to your eating cycle.

>> They're accompanied by severe abdominal pain, fever, or vomiting.

Constipation

When my kids were toddlers, I overheard them playing one day in a pretend battle against some kind of monster. One of them issued a battle cry, which I think was supposed to be "Let's conquer the monster!" but instead came out as "Let's constipate the monster!" An unusual battle tactic, for sure. But then again, anyone who's experienced constipation, which is virtually everyone at some point in time, knows what a monster punishment it can be.

Constipation is a condition that involves effortful or infrequent bowel movements. Someone who is constipated may have a bowel movement less than three times per week, typically straining to pass small amounts of hard stool.

REMEMBER

Anyone can experience constipation periodically, especially when they travel or change their habits temporarily. Chronic constipation, however, is a problem for about 15 percent of individuals in the population, with a higher proportion of females to males, and more adults over the age of 65.

Besides making bowel movements frustrating and time-consuming, constipation may cause significant pain and discomfort that affects people's quality of life. Repeated straining can lead to further problems such as *hemorrhoids* (swollen, painful veins in the anal/rectal area) or rectal bleeding. If that's the case, seeking medical help is advisable.

REMEMBER

Intermittent constipation is often resolved with a conscious effort to increase water intake, exercise, and dietary fiber. But you should see a healthcare practitioner about constipation when:

>> It occurs with severe abdominal pain.

>> It comes on suddenly and doesn't go away.

Diarrhea

Diarrhea is loose or watery stools that occur three or more times per day (or more frequently than is normal for you). Stools on the looser side don't necessarily count as diarrhea unless they're also passed often throughout the day; and at the same time, frequent passing of formed stools isn't diarrhea. Both the stool form and its frequency are relevant.

Many causes of diarrhea exist — with infections being the most serious cause. According to WHO/UNICEF, approximately four billion cases of diarrheal disease occur every year around the world, mainly caused by poor infrastructure around sanitation. In industrialized countries with good sanitation, acute episodes of diarrhea may be the result of food poisoning or other types of infections. Other times it's triggered by a dietary change such as an extra-spicy meal. In such cases, diarrhea typically lasts one to two days and resolves on its own. Overall, people in industrialized countries tend to have, on average, one or two episodes of diarrhea per year (although children under five may have more), while those in non-industrialized countries may have 5 to 12 episodes of diarrhea per year.

Diarrhea lasting 48 hours or less isn't usually cause for concern. But you should see a healthcare practitioner when:

>> Diarrhea persists for more than seven days.

>> Diarrhea is accompanied by fever, pain, or nausea after taking antibiotics.

Get medical attention right away if you find you become dehydrated (have dark urine or dry mouth or are light-headed) because of frequent diarrhea.

Gas and burping

The gases inside the digestive tract have to go somewhere, and they can come out as gas (otherwise known as *flatulence*, or farting) or burping.

First, flatulence. Your digestive tract is a gas-producing factory, with the gut microbes in your colon being mainly responsible for the amount and type of gases that are produced. As the microbes carry out their metabolic activities and ferment the components of the diet that humans can't digest, they produce gases (hydrogen and carbon dioxide, and occasionally methane) as waste products. The amount they produce depends on the exact microbes living there but also on the type of dietary substrates because some components of the diet lead to more gas production than others.

When these gases are produced in the colon, about 80 percent of them are seamlessly absorbed through the colon's inner lining where they enter into circulation and end up being excreted via exhaled breath. Other gases are recycled by different bacteria in the colon that use them. But the gases left over need to be expelled somehow, so they come out as flatulence.

Noble are the scientists who study flatulence: A scientific paper from 1998 begins with "the social significance of flatus derives mainly from its odor," and then goes on to explain how sulphur-containing gases are the main (but not the only) malodorous component. Overall, scientists have shown that the mix of gases produced in the intestines determines the smell. Unfortunately, some of the same bacteria that contribute to intestinal health by feeding on dietary fibers are implicated in producing foul-smelling gases. Pinto bean eaters, beware.

Burping, which scientists call *eructation,* occurs when you swallow excess air, sometimes via carbonated beverages. You may swallow more air when you eat or drink quickly, talk while eating, chew gum, suck on candies, or smoke. Burping can also be caused by too many bacteria in the small intestine, stomach inflammation, or *H. pylori* infection.

Like it or not, gas and burping are normal daily occurrences for anyone with a digestive tract. Healthy people may discharge gas from the bottom end between 8 and 20 times per day (letting go of about one quart of gas in total) and from the top end up to 30 times per day. These occurrences may be inconvenient or embarrassing, but they're not cause for concern. Sometimes dietary adjustments can decrease the frequency of these symptoms.

REMEMBER

See your healthcare practitioner about flatulence or burping if:

>> You suddenly experience these symptoms much more than normal, without a major dietary change.

>> You experience excessive gas with abdominal pain.

>> You experience excessive burping or gas along with diarrhea, constipation, or vomiting.

>> The frequency is impacting your quality of life.

Individuals who drastically increase their fiber consumption may experience more gas in the short term, but the frequency of gas should return to normal after the microbes in the colon adapt to the new substrates within a couple of weeks.

Gastrointestinal bleeding

Gastrointestinal (GI) bleeding is any bleeding that starts in your digestive tract. Acute bleeding comes on suddenly, whereas chronic bleeding may be mild and ongoing or may be intermittent. GI bleeding can be a symptom of digestive diseases such as ulcers, gastroesophageal reflux disease, colonic inflammation, or cancer, so it should never be ignored. However, most people recover from GI bleeding with timely treatment.

How GI bleeding looks depends on the site and severity of the bleeding. Your stool may be dark/black in color, or it may be a normal color with red streaks of blood. Occult (hidden) bleeding in the GI tract is microscopic so it can't be observed in your stool, but it can be detected through laboratory tests that a healthcare professional orders.

Before you panic about seeing blood in your stool, make sure you think about whether you've eaten beets in the past few days because they can be responsible for the bright red hue.

Bleeding in the digestive tract is a relatively rare symptom experienced by less than 0.5 percent of the population. GI bleeding, unless it's clearly due to hemorrhoids, should prompt you to make an appointment with your doctor.

Seek immediate medical care if:

>> You see blood mixed within your stool instead of only on the outside (which is likely due to hemorrhoids) or you have black, tarry stools.

>> You're suddenly vomiting blood or discharging it into the toilet.

Heartburn

Heartburn is a painful or burning sensation in the mid-chest, which tends to occur after meals or while lying down. Most of the time heartburn is the result of *reflux* — digestive acid leaking from the stomach upward into the esophagus — but some other conditions can cause a heartburn-like sensation. Heartburn caused by reflux may be mild or severe and may be accompanied by a sour taste in your mouth, burping, nausea, or sometimes regurgitation of food. If reflux occurs repeatedly, it can cause irritation and damage to the esophagus, sinuses, mouth, or vocal folds.

Heartburn is the most commonly reported GI symptom, with 30 percent of American adults experiencing it in any given week. When triggered after a rich, acidic, or spicy meal, it usually goes away within two to five hours. Chronic heartburn, on the other hand, may be the result of gastroesophageal reflux disease (GERD) — a condition affecting around 20 percent of the population. Aging, weight gain, or certain medications can increase the chances of developing GERD.

See a healthcare practitioner about your heartburn if you experience it repeatedly (more than twice a week) for an extended period of time, or when:

>> The symptom doesn't go away with common over-the-counter medications.

>> You experience heartburn with unexplained weight loss.

>> The symptom is accompanied by frequent coughing, choking, or hoarseness.

>> You have severe chest pain or pressure and/or difficulty breathing.

Incontinence

Incontinence is a loss of control over the bladder or bowel. Mild fecal incontinence can lead to minor leakage and soiled underwear, and more severe incontinence can mean having a bowel movement before you can reach a toilet. Fecal incontinence can result from muscle or nerve damage in the rectum, large hemorrhoids, or some chronic diseases. It can sometimes accompany other GI symptoms such as diarrhea or constipation. Besides being embarrassing, this symptom can interfere with people's quality of life.

A population-wide survey in 2009 found more than 8 percent of American adults experience fecal incontinence, and the risk is higher in older people and in people who tend to have loose or watery stools. Even though minor fecal incontinence can be a normal part of aging, seek medical advice if fecal incontinence is frequent (happening twice a month or more) or severe.

Nausea

Nausea is a feeling that you may vomit, which may be felt in your stomach or the back of your throat. It may be accompanied by sweating, weakness, and/or increased saliva. Vomiting may or may not occur.

REMEMBER

Nausea is quite common, particularly during pregnancy or as a side effect of certain medications (such as Ozempic).

See a healthcare professional if you experience any of the following:

>> Nausea that lasts for more than three days or comes back repeatedly.

>> Nausea that prevents you from carrying out your normal daily activities.

>> Nausea usually goes away on its own.

Regurgitation

Regurgitation is when undigested or partially digested foods come back up the esophagus and into the mouth. It's similar to vomiting but typically less forceful.

Regurgitation occurs in around 80 percent of people with GERD and can also be the result of a condition called rumination syndrome. You should talk with your healthcare practitioner if you experience frequent regurgitation.

Small intestinal bacterial overgrowth

Small intestinal bacterial overgrowth (SIBO, pronounced "see-bow") is the presence of too many bacteria in the small intestine — more than 100,000 organisms/mL. Testing for SIBO relies on the fact that bacteria produce gases as they carry out their metabolism. These gases are measured in the exhaled breath, via noninvasive glucose or lactulose breath testing.

Even though SIBO can be measured, its significance is debated by researchers and medical professionals. Some view it merely as a consequence of *poor motility* — that is, the movements that normally sweep bacteria down the digestive tract toward the colon are impaired, allowing bacteria in the small intestine to multiply. Others believe SIBO is the underlying cause of nutritional deficiencies, chronic diarrhea, bloating and distension, and other gastrointestinal complaints. The latest research suggests that both scenarios can occur — slow motility as the root cause of SIBO and SIBO as a phenomenon in itself that causes GI symptoms.

The prevalence of SIBO in healthy populations is unknown. However, it may occur in as many as 80 percent of people with IBS. The likelihood of experiencing SIBO increases with age and taking certain medications. See your healthcare practitioner for advice on testing and possible treatment for SIBO.

Swallowing difficulties

Swallowing is a complex process involving tightly coordinated muscle movements with high stakes if things go wrong: choking or complications if food enters the airway. Difficulty swallowing, known medically as *dysphagia*, is the sensation that foods or liquids are hard to swallow. People with dysphagia may have problems swallowing specific consistencies of food or liquid, or they may not be able to swallow at all. Signs of dysphagia include pain while swallowing, coughing or choking while ingesting food and drink, or regurgitation through the mouth or nose.

Dysphagia can be caused by problems with the structures of the digestive tract or altered neural control of the swallowing muscles. In a large U.S. study of more than 32,000 participants, one in six adults (around 17 percent of the population) reported having difficulty swallowing sometimes. The risk of dysphagia increases with age.

See your healthcare practitioner if dysphagia occurs on a regular basis. The following are reasons to call for immediate medical help:

>> Incompletely swallowed food makes it hard to breathe.

>> You're unable to swallow because food is stuck in your throat.

>> You can't swallow anything.

Vomiting

Vomiting, known medically as *emesis*, is forceful ejection of the stomach contents through the mouth. It differs from regurgitation, which is the slower ejection of food from the throat or esophagus. Whereas vomiting can happen at any time, regurgitation usually happens right after eating.

Vomiting is never pleasant — either for the person experiencing it or for others in the vicinity. It may occur because of infection, GI tract irritation, or as a side effect of some medications. If the symptom lasts only a day or two, it's typically not a cause for concern. However, continual vomiting can lead to dehydration so care should be taken to replenish fluids and electrolytes.

REMEMBER

Vomiting that lasts longer or recurs in cycles or vomiting accompanied by unexpected weight loss is cause to seek medical attention. Find help right away if:

>> You vomit blood.

>> Your vomit is dark in color and resembles coffee grounds.

Identifying Charlatan Conditions

It's a classic schtick in the wellness industry: Invent a new entity, test people for it, and then purport to treat them using various special pills and potions. The mainstream medical world doesn't generally recognize these conditions for good reason; little to no evidence suggests that they exist, let alone that they can or need to be treated. In the gut health world, several so-called conditions fall into this category. This section gives you a heads-up on three red herrings for your gut health.

Candida overgrowth

A wide range of symptoms, from digestive issues to brain fog and joint pain, are often blamed on overgrowth of *Candida*, a genus of fungi, in the gut. This so-called *Candida* infestation is diagnosed in a rudimentary way by spitting in a glass of water, or is identified through stool, blood, or urine tests in the natural healthcare industry. Addressing the infection often means adopting a complicated and restrictive low-sugar dietary regimen (often with an array of supplements you need to purchase, too).

In truth, *Candida* is a normal resident of a healthy GI tract and scientists don't yet know what amount could constitute an overgrowth. A true infection with *Candida* is called candidiasis. If the infection happens in your mouth or throat, it's called oral thrush; it's esophagitis if it affects the esophagus, and if the infection enters your bloodstream, it's called candidemia. Invasive candidiasis is a serious condition that happens when *Candida* infects your blood and/or different parts of your body in which *Candida* shouldn't be present, such as your bones, central nervous system, heart, liver, kidneys, or eyes. These need to be treated medically.

Candida has been detected in individuals with severe diarrhea or other symptoms, but the symptoms don't seem to go away with a medically administered antifungal treatment protocol. More research needs to be done to link amounts of *Candida* in the GI tract (when no infection occurs) with various digestive symptoms.

No one is denying that diverse symptoms such as digestive issues and brain fog can occur together. But there's little evidence that *Candida* is the culprit. So instead of embarking on a 3-month *Candida* cleanse, go ahead and cut down on sugar and bring your list of symptoms to your healthcare practitioner. You can also try some of the gut-friendly diet and lifestyle changes in Chapters 10 and 11.

Dysbiosis

Dysbiosis is said to be an imbalance in the gut microbiota between good and bad microorganisms. Gut microbiome testing companies, for a few hundred dollars, are happy to analyze the microbes living in your gut and diagnose you with dysbiosis. They'll give you a detailed list of foods to seek out or avoid, and many of them provide a line of probiotics or prebiotics that will supposedly solve the problem.

As I explain in Chapter 3, the idea of balancing good and bad microorganisms is simplistic and doesn't match with what scientists know: that there can be no good or bad life forms and the activities of microorganisms always depend on context. Furthermore, none of the brilliant scientists working in the microbiome field for more than two decades have managed to define a healthy microbiome, so the definition of an unhealthy or dysbiotic microbiome is similarly elusive. Some microbiome testing companies tell you how your sample compares to the average sample of a healthy person, but even this gives no guidance on what diet or probiotics would make your gut microbiome healthier or stronger. The concept of dysbiosis is sometimes useful in studies to refer to a large group of people with a disease who have different gut microbiomes compared to a group of healthy people. But dysbiosis means little on an individual level.

Because dysbiosis isn't a diagnosis, you're better off saving the money you would have spent on a gut microbiome test and buying yourself a wealth of cabbage and chickpeas instead. The evidence-based ways to change your diet and lifestyle for better gut health — essentially pushing your gut microbiome in a direction that's more supportive of your health — are in Chapters 10 and 11. See your healthcare practitioner about any specific GI symptoms.

Leaky gut syndrome

Leaky gut syndrome supposedly occurs when your gut barrier is overly permeable, letting toxins leak through into your bloodstream. The leakiness is said to lead to a grab-bag of symptoms, including food sensitivities, poor mood, and skin conditions. Alternative health practitioners sometimes diagnose this condition based on a symptom questionnaire and/or an intestinal permeability test, and then recommend an anti-inflammatory dietary and supplement regime to address it.

The kernel of truth in leaky gut is that your gut barrier can truly vary in its permeability. As Chapter 3 outlines, your gut barrier has the tricky job of letting required nutrients and water pass through while keeping harmful bacteria and other substances out of your bloodstream. To do these jobs, the gut barrier cells tighten and loosen accordingly. Various medical and research tests can measure intestinal permeability, and researchers have found that certain chronic diseases are associated with increased permeability of the gut barrier.

But where leaky gut syndrome falls apart is when it's claimed to be the root cause of various symptoms. No evidence exists that leaky gut occurs independently (apart from the chronic diseases it's associated with) or that altering a leaky gut will make symptoms go away. Rather, if you think you have leaky gut, it really means you need to see your healthcare practitioner about the possible cause of the symptoms you're experiencing. Don't let this unproven obscure entity get in the way of seeking medical attention for your GI problems.

IN THIS CHAPTER

» Comprehending how digestive
  diseases are diagnosed

» Demystifying some of the specific
  digestive disorders that exist

» Knowing what to do with a digestive
  diagnosis

» Recognizing the main categories of
  treatments

Chapter **7**

Understanding Digestive Diagnoses

The next time you're in a public place, look around you. For every ten people you see, chances are that one or two of them has a diagnosed digestive disease. Even though conditions affecting digestion are common, they're often invisible when you see someone walking by you on the street. Neither are they a favorite topic of conversation among friends and family.

This chapter is all about what happens when you go down the path of getting a digestive disease diagnosis (plural: diagnoses). Through the chapter, I focus on the experiences of you, the patient. I discuss what a diagnosis is, who can make a diagnosis, and the information necessary for making a diagnosis, including the types of tests that may be involved. Then I get into the specifics of some major digestive disorders and offer some guidance on embracing your diagnosis and how to move forward with the best knowledge possible. Finally, I cover the broad categories of treatments available for digestive disorders.

REMEMBER

This chapter is chock-full of information, but please don't take any of it as medical advice. Above all, you should seek care and guidance from a qualified, licensed medical professional.

Diagnosing Digestive Disorders

Modern medicine is the most advanced, scientifically based, statistically guided system of care available to humans today. This type of medicine is based on treating symptoms using well-tested medical interventions and procedures that are designed to work across populations. *Diagnosis*, or characterization of illness, is a crucial part of this medical model. After the diagnosis, treatment appropriate to the specific illness can be initiated. If no diagnosis is appropriate, an individual is considered a generally healthy person with specific symptoms (as Chapter 6 discusses).

The following sections delve deeper into what happens when you visit your healthcare practitioner's office — who makes the diagnosis and then how they make that diagnosis by looking at your medical history and your symptoms, and by examining you and conducting tests.

Identifying who makes the diagnosis

A qualified medical professional — most commonly a primary care doctor or a gastroenterologist — diagnoses digestive disorders. These professionals are qualified to order the appropriate tests and have the training to put all the information together into a diagnosis, and the ability to prescribe medications for the diagnosed conditions.

REMEMBER

Digestive disorders are medically diagnosed conditions that affect your gastrointestinal (GI) tract, anywhere from your mouth to your anus. To make a diagnosis, a medical professional collects information about an individual — first to determine whether they fall into the normal range on certain parameters, and if not, which of several broad diagnostic categories they fall into. Digestive diagnoses aren't made based on the doctor's opinion, but rather according to concepts and criteria widely accepted in the medical literature. Most digestive diseases fit into a known category that doctors frequently assign people to. (However, because of the great individual variability in how symptoms and clinical signs show up, in reality many individuals don't fit neatly within a specific diagnostic category.)

A diagnosis depends on observed or reported information from any of the following sources (which I discuss in the following sections):

>> Your medical history

>> Your reported symptoms

>> A physical exam

>> Laboratory and diagnostic imaging tests

>> Upper endoscopy and/or colonoscopy

Sometimes these sources of information are used to confirm you have a condition, and other times they're used to rule out a condition.

REMEMBER

Gastrointestinal diseases fall into two basic categories:

>> **Structural:** The digestive tract looks abnormal when examined and may not work properly.

>> **Functional:** The digestive tract looks normal, with no observable physical reason for the symptoms. These disorders are often responsive to treatments, underlining that they have a biological cause.

Digging into your medical history

A *medical history* is a set of information about the past health of you and your biological family members. To complete this aspect of medical care, the doctor may ask you a series of questions about operations, hospitalizations, and the diagnosed conditions of your biological family members. Because you share genes with those in your family of birth, this information can help your doctor understand any genetic contributions to digestive disease that you may have.

REMEMBER

A comprehensive medical history requires knowledge of the major medical conditions that are affecting or have affected the following family members, including the approximate age at which the conditions were diagnosed (with the first three categories of family members being the most relevant):

>> Parents

>> Siblings, including half-sisters and half-brothers

>> Children

>> Grandparents

>> Aunts and uncles

>> Nieces and nephews

You may have to call up some family members to find out this information. Don't worry, you don't have to make it awkward by getting into all the details. Even knowing the basic facts about a diagnosis can give you valuable information that's relevant to your own health.

Detailing symptoms

Symptoms are features that indicate a disease — in other words, the telltale signs in and on your body that something isn't functioning the way it should. Symptoms related to the digestive system, as well as those outside the digestive system, may be useful for diagnosing a digestive disease.

TIP

Before you go into the doctor's office, make a short note about your symptoms as follows:

>> The symptom(s) you experienced, whether gut-related or not gut-related

>> The time and place you first experienced the symptom

>> The most recent time and place you experienced the symptom and what happened just before it occurred

>> How you typically handle the symptom or how long it takes to resolve

Also be prepared to talk about any changes you've experienced in your symptoms, such as what the change is, when you noticed it, and whether it was a sudden or gradual change. The doctor may request more details about the symptoms, too. For example, belly pain is a common symptom for many different digestive disorders or sometimes may not be related to a digestive disease at all. Your doctor may ask you to describe the precise location of the pain and its characteristics.

Undergoing a physical examination

Your doctor may want to conduct a physical examination to determine how certain parts of your digestive system are working. It may involve checking or touching certain parts of your body to look for abnormalities. If any parts of the examination are uncomfortable for you, the best strategy is to communicate calmly and openly with the doctor about how your discomfort can be minimized.

Taking tests

Certain biological parameters are impossible for you to personally observe, and even if you could observe them, you wouldn't know if they're within the normal range. For this reason, medical tests are often necessary for making a digestive disease diagnosis. Numerous medical tests for assessing digestive diseases exist, and your doctor may want information from certain ones.

Here are some of the tests that provide information relevant to a digestive diagnosis.

Abdominal ultrasound

This painless test uses a small device pressed against the outside of your abdomen, which sends sound waves that are used to image the structures inside. The test is especially good for identifying gallstones in the gallbladder and looking for dilation in the bile ducts.

Colonoscopy

A colonoscopy is a type of *endoscopy* (a procedure for looking inside the body) that focuses on the lower GI tract. Often done with sedation, this test uses a scope (tube) with a camera inserted through the anus and up into the colon to visualize what's inside. Instruments inserted through the tube can remove polyps or take samples of tissue. Prior to the test, the bowel must be cleaned out using a bowel preparation technique.

Computerized tomography (CT) scan

A CT scan uses a computer to combine a series of X-ray images and is useful for finding structural abnormalities within the abdomen.

Endoscopic retrograde cholangiopancreatography (ERCP)

Done under sedation, this test involves a scope with a camera inserted through the mouth and down into the small intestine, with contrast dye inserted via a smaller tube into the bile ducts or pancreatic duct. The test helps diagnose and treat gallstones.

Esophageal pH monitoring

For this test, you keep a small tube inserted through your nose and into your esophagus for 24 hours to measure acid and fluid in the lower esophagus. The test helps evaluate gastroesophageal reflux disease (GERD) or the origin of certain chest symptoms.

Fecal calprotectin test

This is a noninvasive test that requires giving a stool sample and sending it to the lab for analysis of *calprotectin*, a protein that marks intestinal inflammation. It helps diagnose or monitor inflammatory bowel disease (IBD).

Gastric emptying study

This type of test uses high-energy radiation passed through body tissues to generate an image. For the test, you ingest a solid labeled with a marker (called *technetium-99m sulfur colloid*) that can be seen on an X-ray. The test assesses how quickly the food moves out of your stomach — after four hours, normally only 1 to 10 percent of the food is left — and helps investigate unexplained nausea, persistent reflux, and other conditions.

Intestinal permeability test

For this test, you drink a solution with two sugars:

>> **Mannitol:** A small sugar that normally passes through the gut barrier and is detectable in the urine

>> **Lactulose:** A larger sugar that has trouble passing through the intact gut barrier

The ratio of lactulose to mannitol in the urine shows whether permeability is increased. This test gives information about intestinal permeability that is relevant in conditions such as diarrhea, celiac disease, or IBD.

Lactulose breath test

For a lactulose breath test, you ingest a poorly absorbed sugar that's fermented by gut bacteria. When there are too many bacteria in your small intestine, the bacteria feed on the sugar to produce greater levels of methane and hydrogen gases, which are expelled in the lungs and measured. This test measures the overgrowth of bacteria in the small intestine, which can indicate poor *motility* (how substances move through the GI tract — refer to Chapter 2 for more about motility).

Magnetic resonance cholangiopancreatography (MRCP)

This noninvasive test uses magnetic resonance imaging (MRI) with a contrast dye to produce high-resolution images of the bile ducts, gallbladder, liver, and pancreas to identify abnormalities.

Tissue transglutaminase (tTG) immunoglobulin A (IgA) antibody test

This blood test helps diagnose celiac disease in people who are currently eating gluten. People with celiac disease often make antibodies that attack an enzyme called tTG, which helps repair damage in the body. This test shows the levels of anti-tTG antibodies circulating in the blood. Doctors consider the results of this test alongside other criteria such as diarrhea and malabsorption to make a celiac disease diagnosis.

Upper endoscopy

This test involves a scope with a camera that goes through your mouth all the way to your *duodenum* (the first part of the small intestine, right after the stomach) with anesthetics used to minimize discomfort. The test is used to evaluate GERD or to investigate conditions such as swallowing difficulties, ulcer disease, stomach cancer, or celiac disease.

X-ray tests

Various X-ray tests use high-energy radiation to visualize the structure or function of your digestive tract:

>> **Static abdominal X-ray:** Used to spot any obvious abnormality such as a bowel obstruction.

>> **Defecogram:** Gives information on constipation. *Barium* (a chalky white substance) is inserted into the rectum and sigmoid colon (and possibly the vagina) and is pushed out while the X-rays are taken.

>> **Barium swallow:** Requires you to ingest barium during the X-ray to examine the function of the esophagus.

>> **Video swallow:** An expanded version of a barium swallow, requiring you to ingest different liquids and solids to evaluate the functioning of the throat and upper esophagus.

Putting the information together

All the relevant information your healthcare professional gathers must be pulled together and compared against the categories of digestive disorders. Even though the list of tests and information in this section isn't exhaustive, it gives you an idea of what the health professional must do to confirm whether you fit within a known diagnostic category. Thus, when all the pieces fit together, you may receive a diagnosis.

Looking At the Major Digestive Disorders

Dozens of digestive disorders exist, and a complete list would take up this entire book. However, this section covers some of the major digestive disorders that are most frequently diagnosed.

Celiac disease

Celiac disease (CD) is an autoimmune disease in which ingestion of *gluten* (a protein in wheat, rye, barley, and other grains), damages the lining of the small intestine. Currently the only treatment for CD is strict lifelong avoidance of gluten in the diet. Many individuals are diagnosed as children.

TECHNICAL STUFF

The disease was first observed centuries ago, but doctors didn't have the knowledge about what dietary item was causing the diarrhea, chronic indigestion, and malnutrition in affected children. In 1934 the American doctor Sidney Haas zeroed in on carbohydrates as the culprit and treated ten children with what he called a banana diet. Several years later, a Dutch pediatrician named William Dicke noticed during World War II that the health of affected children improved when they lacked access to wheat — so the responsible dietary item was finally identified.

Clostridioides difficile infection

Infection by bacteria called *Clostridioides difficile*, or *C. difficile* (sometimes shortened to *C. diff*), usually occurs after taking antibiotics. *C. difficile* frequently live in guts of healthy individuals but are normally kept in check by a diverse gut microbial community. It's only when the gut microbial community is damaged by antibiotics or other conditions that *C. difficile* go on a pathogenic rampage and cause diarrhea and inflammation of the colon. The infection is normally treated with specific antibiotics, but it may crop up again and again, requiring multiple rounds of antibiotics and further decimation of the gut microbial community.

Colorectal cancer

Colorectal cancer, or colon cancer, occurs when cells in the inner lining of the colon or rectum grow out of control. The cancer often starts as polyps (growths), and removing these polyps can prevent development of the cancer. Medical organizations recommend screening for colon cancer via colonoscopy approximately every five years, starting at the age of either 45 or 50.

Crohn's disease

Crohn's disease is a type of IBD. The disease entails inflammation anywhere in the GI tract, from mouth to anus, but often occurring in a specific location: the lower part of the small intestine and upper part of the large intestine. The inflammation affects all layers of the gastrointestinal tract wall and commonly causes weight loss and diarrhea. The pattern of inflammation tends to be patchy, involving various noncontiguous segments of the intestine.

TECHNICAL STUFF

Crohn's disease was identified less than a century ago. A doctor named Burrill Crohn from Mount Sinai Hospital in New York first published a paper in 1932 describing 14 patients with a particular pattern of small intestinal findings during surgery. The disease was called terminal ileitis and later became known as Crohn's disease. Interestingly, some doctors initially suspected Crohn's disease was caused by a bacterial infection because bacteria called *Mycobacterium avium* subspecies *paratuberculosis* (MAP) were present in some patient samples; the same bacteria were known to affect the ileum in cows, causing a condition called Johne's disease. But the theory fell apart when further investigation revealed MAP were present in many individuals in the population who didn't develop Crohn's disease.

Diverticular disease

Diverticular disease in the colon is when small marble-sized pouches (called diverticula) form anywhere along the colonic lining. In diverticulitis, these pouches become blocked or inflamed. The condition may be caused by increased pressure in the intestine. A high-fiber diet helps diverticulitis, but during flare-ups (periods of intense symptoms, including sharp abdominal pain) switching to clear liquids and low-fiber foods promotes healing.

Functional dyspepsia

Functional dyspepsia is diagnosed when symptoms of stomach upset occur for at least three months with no observable physical cause. Common symptoms include stomach pain or burning, feeling full after ingesting a small amount of food, or feeling over-full after a meal.

Gallbladder disease

The gallbladder is a sac that sits under the liver, toward the right side of your trunk, and its function is to store and concentrate bile from the liver. Gallbladder disease can refer to inflammation, infection, stones, or blockage of the gallbladder. In gallbladder disease, pain may occur in the upper abdomen radiating to the back, especially after meals. Gallstones are a frequent cause of gallbladder disease, with women being twice to three times as likely to develop them as men.

Gastroesophageal reflux disease

Gastroesophageal reflux disease (GERD), referred to as acid reflux for short, occurs when the ring of muscle at the bottom of the esophagus called the lower esophageal sphincter doesn't work properly and allows the stomach contents to leak up into the esophagus. The stomach's mixture of food and digestive juices such as hydrochloric acid can damage the lining of the esophagus, triggering symptoms such as heartburn (a burning sensation behind the breastbone), regurgitation, and sometimes throat and voice irritation.

Gastroparesis

Gastroparesis is an uncommon functional disorder that involves a slower than normal emptying of the stomach into the small intestine, without an observable blockage in the stomach or intestines. Improperly functioning stomach nerves and muscles account for this disorder (which is also known as stomach paralysis) and can cause a range of digestive symptoms such as bloating, abdominal pain, nausea, vomiting, and a general loss of appetite.

Irritable bowel syndrome

Irritable bowel syndrome (IBS) is a common functional digestive disorder in which an individual experiences persistent digestive symptoms. IBS is diagnosed when the symptoms occur at least three days per month; even though the diagnosis is centered around abdominal pain and either constipation or diarrhea, an individual may experience belly distension, flatulence, nausea, and even mood alterations. IBS is a diagnosis of exclusion, so other problems need to be ruled out before confirming its presence.

IBS sometimes occurs after a viral or bacterial infection — and in this case it's called post-infectious IBS. The working hypothesis on how post-infectious IBS occurs is that the gut bacteria become damaged by the infection and trigger symptoms long after the intense infection has cleared up.

Lactose intolerance

Lactose intolerance is an inability to digest the sugar (lactose) in milk products, which is attributable to your small intestine not making enough of a digestive enzyme called lactase. This scarcity of lactase leads to symptoms such as bloating, diarrhea, or gas. Certain probiotics can reduce the symptoms.

Peptic ulcers

Peptic ulcers are sores on the lining of your stomach, small intestine, or esophagus that are caused by digestive juices. The most common cause of ulcers is stomach infection by the bacteria *Helicobacter pylori*. Some ulcers are associated with abdominal pain, but others have few or no symptoms.

Ulcerative colitis

Ulcerative colitis (UC) is a major type of IBD involving inflammation that's mostly confined to the innermost lining (mucosa) of the colon. The inflammation is usually continuous rather than patchy and starts in the rectum but may spread to other parts of the colon.

Another condition called pouchitis occurs when inflammation happens in the lining of a pouch created during a surgery to treat ulcerative colitis.

Embracing Your Diagnosis

If you end up receiving a digestive diagnosis, you may wonder what's next. After diagnosis you may have a mix of emotions — perhaps experiencing relief at having a label for what you're going through, but also grieving the loss of your disease-free self and perhaps feeling overwhelmed with information and choices available to you.

Many digestive diagnoses are conditions you'll have to live with for the rest of your life, but they don't have to define your life. Some days you may forget all about your diagnosis. By accepting your diagnosis and dealing with the fact that you'll have good and bad days, you can get the most out of life. A diagnosis may even motivate you to aim for healthier living than ever before. Your best opportunity for thriving with a digestive disease is to accept and understand your diagnosis, and to look for scientifically-backed ways to manage it.

Coming to terms with your condition

Accepting your condition and what it means for your life can be a gradual process. However, going through this process is important because it allows you to meet each new situation in a strong and composed manner and advocate for what you need. Your self-advocacy efforts may even raise awareness and make the world a little better for individuals who are diagnosed in the future.

REMEMBER

Here's what experts say you can do to come to terms with a digestive disease diagnosis:

>> Focus on the here and now, rather than dwelling on what you could or couldn't have done in the past to avoid your diagnosis.

>> Find a doctor who listens, problem-solves, and doesn't shy away from talking about the tough issues.

>> Connect with a supportive community. These communities come in many forms — in-person support groups, virtual meetings, or online groups or chats. Not only will you feel less alone in your diagnosis, you also may meet some digestive health dynamos and pick up useful tips for dealing with your condition. Chapter 8 has more information on finding community.

Arming yourself with scientific knowledge

As soon as you have a diagnosis, you may become aware of a whole industry out there, full of products and services that promise to be the magic bullet for curing you of your condition. The marketing materials often use sciency-sounding language to convince you to make a purchase, even though scientific evidence is actually lacking.

REMEMBER

Too many of these so-called miracle cures are based on little or no scientific evidence. Knowing what interventions are scientifically supported is crucial as you discover more about your condition. Regulatory bodies try to do their part — for example, products in the realm of dietary supplements aren't allowed to have claims that they address any particular disease. But nevertheless, you'll be in a strong position if you arm yourself with scientific knowledge about what interventions really work for people with your condition. This information provides a solid baseline that enables you to move forward with awareness on your digestive health journey.

See Chapter 12 for information on how to identify genuine scientific information and treatments that are shown to be effective.

Identifying the Types of Interventions for Digestive Disorders

Several different categories of interventions for digestive disease exist. Not all of them apply to every condition, of course, but generally your available treatment(s) fall into one of these categories. Sometimes using treatments from more than one category at once is feasible. Your healthcare practitioner can guide you to the most effective ones for your specific situation. The following list is intended to be an overview and a prompt for asking further questions.

Taking medications

Medications are a mainstay of addressing many digestive diseases. Some examples of common medications are as follows:

>> Proton pump inhibitors for GERD

>> Immunosuppressive drugs such as steroids for IBD

>> Metoclopramide to promote motility in the upper gastrointestinal tract

REMEMBER

Drugs are often the most effective intervention for individuals who have a disease and are the most reliable way to relieve yourself of symptoms. Be aware, however, that a drug may not work for every single person. If you try the drug for a while and your condition doesn't show signs of improvement, you're deemed a *drug nonresponder* and your doctor may suggest switching you to another type of drug.

In most countries, the fact that a drug is available to patients on the market means it's already gone through rigorous testing in clinical trials and is judged as appropriately safe and effective. But if your doctor recommends a certain medication, finding out the answers to a few questions around how safe and effective the drug is can't hurt. For example:

>> Does the drug tend to work for certain groups of patients more than others?

>> What are the common side effects?

>> What are the most serious side effects, even if they're rare?

>> Which medications or dietary supplements (including herbal remedies) can't be taken with the drug?

Sometimes you may be offered the opportunity to participate in a *clinical trial* — a rigorous study for the safety and/or efficacy of a new drug. Clinical trials are a necessary part of how drugs are tested, and participation may be an opportunity to try out a promising new drug for your condition. However, you must also accept the possibility that you could end up in the placebo group and not receive the new drug.

Changing what you eat — dietary interventions

Some diets are used therapeutically for diagnosed digestive health conditions — and these various diets have different levels of scientific evidence behind them. A medical professional may recommend that you adopt a certain diet for medical reasons (for example, cutting out gluten when you're diagnosed with celiac disease). Also, a recent study showed that prebiotic fibers (fructo-oligosaccharides) can cause harmful inflammation in some people with IBD who lack the ability to break them down in the colon, so these people shouldn't necessarily follow the advice for healthy people to increase fiber consumption.

On the one hand, the scientific evidence on many therapeutic diets is mixed — with the upshot being that a specific diet may not help everyone. On the other hand, many people with digestive disease experience great success by changing their eating patterns. Typically, a dietary intervention has a relatively low risk of medical harm, but a strict new diet can be challenging to implement and can sometimes be a source of stress. You need to consider all the pros and cons when considering a therapeutic diet.

Here are the main therapeutic diets that your doctor may suggest you follow.

Elimination diets

Elimination diets are typically used when a person with IBS (or simply unexplained digestive symptoms) wants to identify foods that trigger symptoms and know how to optimize their diet. A key feature of an elimination diet is the omission of certain foods. The exact foods excluded and the duration of the exclusion vary depending on the individual's symptoms, age, and medical background.

REMEMBER

Different configurations of elimination diets exist, but a typical one entails three phases:

>> **Food exclusion:** Omitting a food or group of foods believed to trigger the symptom, until the symptom disappears.

>> **Food challenge:** Systematically reintroducing the food or foods to see if the symptom returns.

>> **Maintenance diet:** After *trigger foods* (the items that bring on the symptom) have been identified, going back to a diet that excludes these foods while being nutritionally adequate and having maximum variety.

TIP

An elimination diet is best adopted under the guidance of a registered dietitian who can personalize the diet and reduce the risk of nutritional insufficiencies.

I consider myself a kind of restrictive diet veteran. When I was suffering from unexplained gut symptoms, I cycled through all kinds of restrictive diets: no meat, no dairy or gluten, no caffeine. Once I tried avoiding a long and complicated list of foods given to me by a naturopath, from wheat to soy to black pepper. Cutting out those foods in my daily life became a challenging puzzle. Because of the immense time and effort needed to maintain each kind of elimination diet, inevitably they were temporary. Eventually I found a maintenance diet that allowed me to eat more normally, but during the time when I adopted the diets, I did discover some useful information about the foods that exacerbated my digestive symptoms.

Enteral nutrition

Enteral nutrition, sometimes called *tube feeding*, is a way of delivering nutrition directly to the gut in the form of a nutritionally complete liquid. Enteral nutrition is a remarkably effective treatment to induce remission in individuals (especially children) with Crohn's disease.

REMEMBER

The most effective version of tube feeding is *exclusive enteral nutrition (EEN)*, where no solid foods are consumed at all. Although the science clearly shows the effectiveness of this intervention, tolerating the diet for an extended period can be difficult. Thus, two slightly altered versions of EEN have been developed as follows:

>> The Crohn's disease exclusion diet uses partial enteral nutrition alongside some solid foods. It offers benefits to those with Crohn's disease but isn't quite as effective as EEN.

>> The CD-TREAT diet for Crohn's disease uses a food-based diet that has a similar composition to EEN. The science on this diet is still emerging, but the diet appears to decrease inflammation and effectively treat Crohn's disease.

Gluten-free diet

The gluten-free diet, used as a treatment for celiac disease, strictly prohibits ingestion of gluten. Foods eliminated on this diet are wheat, spelt, barley, and rye. Gluten-free grains and starches such as corn, rice, potatoes, soybeans, and buckwheat, however, are allowed. Oats are only acceptable if they're certified gluten-free because wheat contamination can occur in the process of growing and shipping the oats.

The gluten-free diet is very effective at preventing the intestinal damage of CD. But the diet can also be burdensome over a long term. Refer to the most recent edition of *Living Gluten-Free For Dummies* by Danna Van Noy (John Wiley & Sons, Inc.) for information on implementing a gluten-free diet. The future may bring other treatments — for example, a vaccine is under development that would allow the body to build up resistance to gluten and tolerate small amounts without negative effects.

Low-FODMAP diet

The low fermentable oligosaccharides, disaccharides, monosaccharides, and poly-ols (FODMAP) diet is an eating pattern that excludes specific types of sugars that are poorly absorbed in the small intestine. This diet is meant to be used over a short term and is effective for reducing symptoms in IBS. For this diet, individuals avoid higher FODMAP foods such as:

>> Milk products

>> Wheat products such as cereal, bread, and crackers

>> Beans and lentils

>> Some vegetables such as onions, garlic, and asparagus

>> Some fruits such as apples, cherries, and peaches

Questions remain about how the diet affects the gut microbiota over a long term because it excludes many varied sources of fiber that serve as food for colonic microbes. This fiber restriction means you should only adopt the diet for a short term before returning to a less restrictive diet. For best results, adopt it under the supervision of a registered dietitian.

Mediterranean diet

Even though the Mediterranean diet is the gold-standard diet for people without digestive disease, the diet is also sometimes recommended as an inflammation-reducing diet for people with digestive disease. It entails mostly plant foods (whole grains, fruits, vegetables, legumes, nuts, seeds, and olives) and includes moderate amounts of fish, seafood, poultry, and eggs as well as dairy products. Olive oil is the main source of dietary fats. Chapter 10 discusses this diet in more detail.

Specific carbohydrate diet

The specific carbohydrate diet (SCD) is used for Crohn's disease, ulcerative colitis, and some other digestive diseases. Many anecdotes support its use and a strong community of advocates exists, but the scientific support is still emerging. The diet is based on the theory that eliminating specific complex carbohydrates — thought to be proinflammatory — allows for intestinal healing. The diet is a very strict grain-free, lactose-free, sucrose-free pattern of eating that is intended to dampen inflammation overall.

Other diets

Other diets — including the antifungal diet, ketogenic diet, or low-histamine diet — are sometimes adopted for digestive diseases, but the science on these is relatively skimpy. Further studies may help determine who may benefit from them.

Taking dietary supplements

In a regulatory sense, dietary supplements in most countries fall under the broad category of food rather than drugs, and as such (according to the U.S. Food and Drug Administration) they are "not intended to treat, diagnose, mitigate, prevent, or cure" any disease. They are, rather, meant to supplement the diet in healthy people.

Many *biotics* — probiotics, prebiotics, synbiotics, and postbiotics —fall under the category of dietary supplements. (See Chapter 10 for more information.) Other dietary supplements include the vitamins and minerals that you can buy in grocery stores or pharmacies. Usually dietary supplements are add-on treatments, not main treatments, for digestive diseases.

REMEMBER

If you're considering the use of a dietary supplement, make sure you check if any evidence exists for its effectiveness in your condition. The majority of products on the shelves don't have evidence that they improve digestive diseases. However, some examples of scientifically supported dietary supplements for gut health are as follows:

>> Deglycerized licorice used alongside antacids to help treat ulcers

>> Ginger to quell nausea

>> Peppermint oil to improve symptoms in IBS and to improve functional dyspepsia, functional abdominal pain, and nausea

>> Certain probiotics to reduce symptoms of IBS

The manufacturing quality varies greatly with dietary supplements, so when you choose a product, make sure you pick a reputable company. Ideally the supplement is produced in a facility with high manufacturing standards (adhering to suitable guidelines that cover purity, potency, and so on) and has a *third-party certification*: that is, a company separate from the manufacturer assesses the manufacturing process and independently tests the product to ensure the claims on the label are correct.

WARNING

Supplements can also have serious risks, as shown by the growing incidence of liver injury due to herbal and dietary supplements. Keep your doctor in the loop about any dietary supplements you decide to take.

Exercising

Even though exercise can be made more difficult when living with a digestive disorder, maintaining physical activity to the extent possible is crucial for health. The following digestive conditions are particularly shown to benefit from exercise:

>> **IBS:** Physical activity appears to reduce the severity of symptoms. Yoga in particular improves the digestive symptoms as well as mental health parameters.

>> **Constipation:** Light exercise can help alleviate constipation in some individuals.

>> **GERD:** Vigorous (but not light) physical activity can reduce the number of acid reflux episodes over time, even if initial attempts at exercising trigger heartburn or other symptoms. People with GERD are suggested to pay attention to the timing of exercise and not exercise shortly after a meal.

>> **IBD:** Light exercise can help reduce symptoms in some people with Crohn's disease and ulcerative colitis. A review of studies showed yoga classes in person or on video improves anxiety and quality of life in those with IBD.

Seeking out acupuncture

Acupuncture is a treatment originating from traditional Chinese medicine in which a skilled practitioner inserts thin needles into the skin in precise locations on the body. Little research exists on acupuncture for digestive diseases, but the available evidence suggests the practice may have advantages for treating IBS. Acupuncture may also be effective for treating gastroparesis in the short term, when used alone or in conjunction with other treatments for this condition.

Undergoing the knife — surgery

Although the goal of treating digestive disease is often to delay or avoid surgery as much as possible, specific surgical procedures can be effective treatments for some digestive diseases when medications fail to control the symptoms or when complications develop.

TIP

If your doctor recommends surgery, make sure you fully understand both the benefits and possible risks. Better yet, talk with someone who has gone through the surgery to find out what the procedure was like.

Getting a fecal transplant

Fecal transplants involve taking a stool sample from a healthy person and delivering it to the colon of a person with a digestive illness. The delivery method can vary — often it's by enema (that is, administered directly to the rectum) but it can also be through a series of capsules with fecal matter inside, or through a nasoenteric tube (going from the nose down to the intestines).

Fecal transplants are remarkably effective for resolving recurrent *C. difficile* infections that haven't cleared up with multiple antibiotic treatments.

At the time of writing, two fecal-transplant-based drugs — Rebyota and Vowst — have been approved in the United States for this purpose. Fecal transplants also show some effectiveness for UC, with emerging applications in some other digestive conditions such as IBS. Research on the safest and most effective ways to use fecal transplants is ongoing.

Doctors and researchers who study fecal transplants strongly advise against carrying out this procedure at home because of the risk that the fecal matter from an improperly screened donor could transfer a dangerous infection to a recipient. And even if fecal transplants from appropriate donors appear safe in the short term, their long-term consequences are largely unknown.

Chapter **8**

Empowering Yourself without a Diagnosis

igestive symptoms — bloating, abdominal pain, constipation, diarrhea, and more — are surprisingly common in otherwise healthy people. If you experience digestive symptoms on a regular basis, you need to discuss them with a medical professional (as I outline in Chapter 7). But what happens if you investigate your digestive symptoms from a medical perspective and don't receive an official diagnosis? This situation can occur, for example, if despite your symptoms, you fall within the normal range on diagnostic tests, or if your symptoms aren't frequent enough or severe enough to meet the formal diagnostic criteria.

For individuals who have a digestive disease diagnosis, the standard course of treatment for that condition can begin. But with no diagnosis, you may find yourself with little guidance on how to address your symptoms. You may feel confused or unsupported as you try to cope with the very real inconvenience of your disorderly digestion.

In my era of poor gut health, I was one of the people without a diagnosis: Despite having distressing and debilitating digestive symptoms, the pattern of these symptoms and the medical test results didn't justify an official diagnosis of any condition. My doctor concluded that my symptoms were in the range of normal, which ended any medical help I was offered. Sure, I understood why — no drug or anything else in the medical toolkit was appropriate for me. But that didn't stop me from feeling frustrated that I didn't have a clear solution to my digestive problems. I looked around and saw zillions of products and services that could potentially help me, but I didn't have the ability to tell the sensible ones from the snake oil. Navigating through all these interventions required me to be more active and resourceful, driving my own healing journey.

This chapter is all about giving you some structure and guidance for how to deal with your gut symptoms without a diagnosis. I examine some specific ways to manage your symptoms and how you can decide which one is the best fit. I also offer tips on how to keep increasing your knowledge and progressing toward better gut health step by step while safeguarding your most valuable resources: your time, energy, and money.

Progressing toward Health

The key to progressing toward better health when you don't have a diagnosis is leveraging the power of your lifestyle. All the choices you make in your daily life are powerful means of improving your health. Lifestyle changes may not work as quickly as a drug intervention, but nevertheless they may make a big difference over time.

REMEMBER

Part of focusing on lifestyle factors is ridding yourself of the tendency to get stuck in all-or-nothing patterns: either strenuous exercise every day or no exercise at all. Either a diet of breakfast oatmeal and kale salads or Thai take-out and frozen pizzas. Even though you may feel pure and virtuous when you're in one of the healthy lifestyle phases, the effort it requires is unsustainable, and when you inevitably run out of steam you end up no better off than when you began. Rather, small and systematic lifestyle changes can put you on a trajectory of better health even when you lack a medical condition with specific recommended treatments.

At the same time, with lifestyle changes expect the unexpected. Diet, for example, is where many people look for the answers to a digestive problem. But even when you think you've identified the food that triggers your symptoms and have diligently avoided it, digestive troubles may nevertheless crop up. Gut health is influenced by complex, ever-changing factors, which are, with current technologies, impossible to fully track. Don't blame yourself (as I tended to do) for not being careful enough with your diet or not managing your stress appropriately. Even with unruly symptoms, if you carry on with a gut-supportive lifestyle you can rest assured that you're setting the stage for improvement over time.

MIND THE WELLNESS GAP

Medical interventions (such as drugs) can only do so much. And often they don't have the power to help you feel your absolute best — leaving a big gap between where medical guidance takes you and optimal wellness. And make no mistake, this gap is easily filled by a predatory wellness industry: all kinds of companies and individuals marketing directly to consumers, promising to make you well if you buy or subscribe or take a test or make an appointment. Gut health is an especially trendy area for purveyors of wellness to focus on, so make sure you have your critical thinking cap on when you consider what to do about your digestive symptoms. Chapter 12 provides information you need to know to be a savvy consumer of gut health products.

Here I explain how to move forward confidently in managing your symptoms and how to approach interventions systematically so you can find out what works best for you personally.

Taking symptom management into your own hands

When you decide to adopt interventions to try and manage your digestive symptoms, you have many options, some supported by scientific evidence and others not. The way forward is to experiment with some of these interventions and track results — as long as you're not spending excessive money and effort on interventions that are unproven.

TIP

When looking at all the complex factors of your daily life, pinpointing the factor that improves your gut health can be difficult. To incrementally increase your knowledge about what works for you, I recommend an organized approach to trying out different interventions. Some guidelines for how to gain clarity by testing different interventions are as follows:

>> **On paper, list some interventions/lifestyle changes you think may work for you.** For examples, see the list in the next section.

>> **Prioritize the interventions that are low cost/low commitment and monitor the results.** If you're interested in taking probiotics, for example, rather than signing up for monthly mail-order subscription probiotics, buy a small bottle of probiotics at your local drugstore, take them for a period of time, and evaluate how you then feel.

>> **Start one intervention at a time.** Leave at least one week after starting an intervention to see if you notice an improvement before you switch or add another intervention to the mix.

>> **Keep a written record of your interventions and symptoms.** Figure 8-1 shows an example of how you can track them. Some organizations offer gut health symptom logs or diaries for purchase online.

	Date	Symptom	Notes
Intervention			
GutGlow Probiotic, 1 billion CFU	January 8	Mild diarrhea	Increased stress (work deadline)
	January 9	Fatigue Mild diarrhea	Spicy meal
	January 10	Normal stool	
Intervention			

© John Wiley & Sons, Inc.

FIGURE 8-1: A written record of your gut symptoms and interventions.

GAINING INSPIRATION FROM THE N-OF-1 APPROACH

When interventions are tested scientifically, the number of participants in the study is referred to as *n*. Usually the statistical analysis is stronger when a study has more participants. However, n-of-1 studies have just one participant and aim to find out the best intervention for that exact participant by switching between interventions (or no interventions) for different periods of time.

In managing your own gut health you can take inspiration from this approach to be more scientific and objective about your own symptoms. Here are some ways you can emulate an n-of-1 study:

- Try each intervention for a predetermined amount of time and rate the same digestive symptoms throughout all interventions.

- Be as objective as possible when you record your daily symptoms (perhaps establishing a numerical rating system).

- If you have someone in your household willing to help and you want to compare two different products, ask them to bring you a daily dose of one product the first week and another product the second week, without you knowing which is which. Keep a daily record of your symptoms. After both weeks are complete, look back at your recorded symptoms and see if one product was more effective for you.

Deciding on and implementing interventions

In the realm of gut health, there is no shortage of interventions that promise to cure your ailments. But when you're bombarded with so many gut health products with vague claims, you probably aren't sure which one to choose.

Interventions for gut health fall into several different categories, listed in the following sections alphabetically. I provide a brief summary of each category of interventions and guidance on what symptoms they may relieve, according to the available scientific evidence. (Find more ideas for optimizing digestive health in Chapter 11.)

Acupuncture

Acupuncture, which involves inserting needles into the skin at precise points, is often used to address digestive symptoms. Reasonable evidence exists to show it can improve some symptoms — but in the best-designed scientific studies both real and *placebo* (imitation) acupuncture (for example, for irritable bowel syndrome symptoms) seem to measurably improve people's quality of life. This placebo effect may indicate that something about the experience of receiving acupuncture helps relieve symptoms more reliably than the acupuncture itself.

Biotics

Most products marketed as biotics (probiotics, prebiotics, synbiotics, and postbiotics) don't truly fit the scientific definition, but regardless, they may be appropriate interventions for improving your gut health. A huge variety of formats, doses, and brands exist. You can pick the one with the prettiest bottle or the one promoted by the coolest Instagram influencer, or you can refer to Chapter 12 for how to determine which one has scientific support for its effectiveness.

Body position

Paying attention to your body position after you eat may help ease some digestive symptoms. For heartburn and nausea, lying down or lounging after a meal may cause gastric juices to rise and make your symptoms worse so it's best to remain upright for at least an hour after each meal.

TIP

For heartburn specifically, your body position while sleeping may also affect symptoms; you may want to try elevating your head with extra pillows for sleeping to quell acid reflux.

Cognitive behavioral therapy

Cognitive behavioral therapy (CBT) is a psychological therapy approach that focuses on changing behaviors and dysfunctional thinking patterns to influence mood as well as physiology. It may involve relaxation, cognitive restructuring, problem-solving skills, and/or exposure techniques, and should always be guided by a qualified practitioner. Research consistently shows CBT is effective for improving functional gastrointestinal symptoms and the accompanying psychological factors.

Colonic irrigation

Colonic irrigation is flushing out the colon with water. Although the idea of cleaning out the bowel may seem appealing, the very limited scientific evidence shows no evidence for its benefits, with the potential for side effects that range from vomiting to kidney failure. However, some anecdotal evidence from healthcare practitioners suggests it can relieve constipation in certain people.

Dietary interventions

A wide variety of dietary interventions are available for relieving your gut symptoms. Consider different ones to address the following symptoms:

>> **Constipation:** The classic dietary intervention for digestive health is prunes for the relief of constipation. Indeed, bulking up on fiber and drinking plenty of fluids are usually the first recommendations for improving the ease and frequency of bowel movements.

>> **Diarrhea:** Diet-focused recommendations include avoidance of bowel-stimulating foods such as coffee, fatty or fried foods, and hot spices. Drinking an electrolyte product can help replenish fluids and minerals lost during episodes of diarrhea, helping you recover promptly.

>> **Gas and bloating:** You can try to address these symptoms by eating a balanced diet and avoiding meals high in salt, fat, or hot spices. A low-FODMAP diet for a short term (see Chapter 7) may also bring relief.

>> **Heartburn:** The standard advice for heartburn is to limit your intake of acid-causing foods such as caffeine, alcohol, hot spices, high-fat foods, mint, and highly processed foods. When it comes to the size of meals, eating four or five smaller meals throughout the day rather than two or three larger meals may help with heartburn. In addition, make sure you limit or avoid eating for two to three hours before bed.

I explain other specific types of dietary interventions you can use to relieve digestive symptoms in Chapter 7.

Gut microbiome testing

Several companies now offer gut microbiome testing services directly to consumers along with advice on dietary changes and recommended supplements. Even though the testing itself names the groups of microorganisms in the stool sample provided, scientists and healthcare professionals take issue with the accompanying recommendations. The science to date doesn't support these recommendations; in fact, they may unnecessarily cause you to reduce dietary diversity by cutting out certain nutritious foods from your diet.

Herbal therapies

Herbal therapies are products made from herbs or other plants. These products are typically sold as dietary supplements. A wide range of herbal supplements, such as ginger, fennel, aloe, and licorice, are touted for improvement of digestive symptoms. They may come in different forms: liquid, pill, powder, or tea.

WARNING

The safety of herbal therapies isn't guaranteed. Be careful when trying these interventions because of the risk of side effects, which range from additional gastrointestinal symptoms to possible liver injury.

Hypnotherapy

Hypnotherapy involves a trained therapist guiding an individual to a heightened state of concentration and deep relaxation. Gut-directed hypnosis may not be a go-to treatment, but some emerging evidence suggests it may indeed be effective for taming functional digestive symptoms. If you go this route, make sure you find a qualified and experienced practitioner.

Movement

Gentle movement through stretching exercises or yoga can be effective for relieving gas and bloating as well as constipation. See Chapter 11 for how other forms of exercise can help with optimal gut health.

Over-the-counter medications

Over-the-counter medications are products you can buy without a prescription to treat minor ailments at home. Some of the best ones for addressing digestive symptoms include the following:

» **Pepto Bismol or pink bismuth:** With its main ingredient bismuth subsalicylate, Pepto Bismol is marketed for addressing five symptoms (nausea, heartburn, indigestion, upset stomach, and diarrhea). It may be particularly good for treating food poisoning or traveller's diarrhea.

» **Loperamide:** This medication, sold as Imodium, may work well for relief of diarrhea.

» **Antacids:** These products, which neutralize stomach acidity, can be effective for improving heartburn.

Toileting position

For constipation, changing your sitting posture on the toilet can make a difference to symptoms. Elevating your feet using a specially designed toilet stool can lead to less straining and overall faster bowel movements.

Wardrobe changes

Believe it or not, your wardrobe can be part of how you cope with these digestive symptoms:

» **Gas, bloating, and distension:** Comfortable clothing that's loose or stretchy can make all the difference in how the symptoms affect you throughout the day.

» **Heartburn:** Loose clothing across the stomach and chest can reduce the impact of the symptoms.

Staying Hopeful

When you have ongoing symptoms without clear guidance on how to make them better, staying positive may not be easy. Retaining a sense of hope doesn't mean you repress your feelings — it means you accept the reality of your symptoms and remain committed to striving for better health even when you experience setbacks. This outlook is important because it helps you problem-solve and maintain a sense of control over what you are experiencing.

Furthermore, you do your best critical thinking when you stay positive and avoid choosing interventions out of desperation. (See Chapter 12 to become more savvy about the techniques used to sell you gut health products.) The following sections discuss how to maintain a sense of hope by finding ways to talk about your symptoms, being part of a community, and expressing your thoughts and feelings about your digestive health journey.

Talking about gut health

If you're walking the walk of digestive health, now talk the talk! Maybe not everyone wants to hear the finer details about your bowel movements and gut symptoms. As fascinating as it is, you don't want to be that person who weaves gut health into every conversation. But sharing about digestion can be empowering and can help others in your life understand what you're going through.

REMEMBER

Here are some reasons to normalize talking about gut health and digestive symptoms with friends and family (when appropriate and welcome):

>> You may receive more empathy in dealing with your symptoms.

>> You may help others feel less alone in what they're experiencing.

>> Among family, you may share or discover things relevant to medical history.

>> You help reduce stigma.

>> You may inspire others to seek help for longstanding gut health problems.

Because of the way gut health is trending, opportunities to talk about gut health are everywhere. From advertisements to news articles to popular books, conversation-starters aren't in short supply. Bring one out and see where the conversation leads.

Finding community

Even though it may seem counterintuitive, sometimes talking about gut health and gastrointestinal symptoms may be easier with complete strangers than with your own friends and family. Online or in person, you may find people with common interests or goals in terms of digestive health. Hearing about others' experiences can be immensely helpful and validating and you may even pick up some practical tips for dealing with your own symptoms.

REMEMBER

As part of your gut health journey, you may want to seek out different communities that gather around gut health-related topics. These may include fermented foods enthusiasts, individuals living with digestive disease or supporting someone with digestive disease, parent groups focused on dietary interventions for gut health, and many more. Getting involved may help you feel a sense of belonging and improve your mood — so go ahead and explore different online forums, social media groups, and local organizations to see what appeals to you. Some email lists may help keep you informed about local events.

Keeping a gut health journal

One of the best things you can do for maintaining a positive outlook and reflecting on the state of your gut and overall health is writing a few words every day in a journal specifically dedicated to your gut health. This journal, which is different from the objective record of interventions and symptoms shown in Figure 8-1, can be on paper or on your computer or phone.

REMEMBER

The important part for a gut health journal or diary is that you reflect on what you're feeling and what you think is working and not working, as well as how you're adapting your life to deal with the symptoms. Keeping such a journal specifically for your gut health can serve several purposes:

>> Helping you see patterns in your symptoms over time

>> Clarifying how the symptoms are affecting your daily life and therefore which ones are the highest priority to address

>> Making a link between your symptoms and how you feel

Information from a gut health journal can also be helpful when you visit your doctor. In addition to sharing with your doctor objective details about your symptoms (from a separate record; refer to Figure 8-1 earlier in this chapter), you're more equipped to share important information on how those symptoms are affecting your quality of life on a daily basis.

Chapter **9**

Navigating Life with Digestive Symptoms

G ut symptoms can show up uninvited at terribly inconvenient times, whether or not you have an official diagnosis of digestive disease. Whether they strike while driving, as mine did, during a concert, or on a day at the beach, gut symptoms can put a damper on your daily activities. Symptoms are easier to manage if they adhere to patterns, but sometimes you can't predict when you'll have to deal with them. Gut symptoms can interfere with your day-to-day activities because

» They may create tense situations in your household.

» You may not want to go out in public.

» You may feel uncomfortable or in pain while you're away from home, needing to find a toilet or private space immediately.

» They may impact you socially (for example, when you see the effects of *stigma*, or in other words negative and inaccurate beliefs about those with digestive disorders).

» They may necessitate medical appointments and hospitalizations that cause you to miss work or school, leading to reduced productivity or frequent absences.

Symptoms are no small matter. When your symptoms are part of a diagnosed digestive disease, you have nearly double the risk for anxiety or depression compared to people without digestive disease. Disordered eating is also very common in those with a gastrointestinal diagnosis.

The social impacts of digestive symptoms can be especially challenging because even though you may look well, you don't always feel well. The fear of feeling embarrassed about your symptoms can make you want to stay at home where you can deal with them privately. Worrying about what others might hear (or smell) may cause you to miss out on important and memorable activities: a weekend in a cottage with a shared bathroom; a nature hike with few bathroom facilities along the way; a yoga or exercise class with a friend.

Yet with a little planning and flexibility (and sometimes a pinch of courage), you can tackle a huge range of activities despite your gut symptoms. This chapter is packed with practical advice to manage your symptoms in different settings. Based on my own experiences and those of people who live and thrive with digestive disease, I include the best insider tips for caring for yourself when digestive symptoms are a presence in your daily life.

Managing Your Digestive Symptoms

When I experienced bouts of terrible abdominal pain, I used to daydream about my dream bathroom: soft pink lighting, a toilet with a heated seat, a soft couch where I could curl into the fetal position, a supply of warm blankets, and an ice water dispenser. I felt that managing my symptoms wouldn't be so difficult if I had the luxury of locking myself inside there every time they came upon me. But life goes on outside the bathroom. In the real world, managing digestive symptoms is a tricky game in which you aim to reduce discomfort to yourself while minimizing inconvenience to others, all while being safe and (preferably) discreet.

REMEMBER

Three basic guidelines can help you win at this game and deal with any troubles surrounding the management of your digestive symptoms:

>> Planning ahead to prevent problems

>> Managing your time and monitoring your proximity to bathrooms or other private spaces

>> Equipping yourself with the right items

This section goes through some different settings, from home to restaurants to the workplace, giving you specific ideas for dealing with gut symptoms in each place. Not all of the tips may apply to your unique situation, so pick and choose what works for you or adapt accordingly. Resourcefulness pays off, giving you new strategies for grappling with symptoms on a daily basis.

Coping at home

Home is often the most comfortable place to be if you're dealing with gut symptoms, but being home doesn't mean dealing with them is always easy. Besides trying to care for yourself, you may face challenges in negotiating the space with other household members and balancing everyone's needs.

REMEMBER

One unavoidable fact about gut symptoms is that they require time and space by yourself to deal with properly. Alone time is important not only when you have acute symptoms but also when you have symptom-free times because given the constant communication between the gut and the brain and the potential for your brain to affect gut health (refer to Chapter 3), you need to maintain an element of zen to achieve your best gut health and reduce the chances of symptom occurrence.

TIP

Here are some tips to keep your gut symptoms under control when you're at home:

>> **Schedule time for yourself, especially on busy days when you need to get a lot done.** Your body needs time to rest, relax, and digest. I've found that taking even ten minutes of alone time in a quiet room (without the distraction of screens) can make a stressful day feel more manageable and reduce the impacts on my gut.

>> **Create a daily ritual of toilet time, especially if you suffer from constipation.** Somewhere between 15 and 45 minutes after a meal at a constant time of day, head to the bathroom and sit on the toilet for a fixed number of minutes (for example, 15 minutes). Focus on relaxing your muscles and don't strain. Even if the bowel movement isn't successful on some days, the routine may help you experience more success over time.

>> **Take deep breaths.** If you experience mild or moderate abdominal pain at home and you're not doing anything urgent, stop what you're doing and take a moment to do a breathing exercise or other relaxation technique. Focusing on your breathing may help you get through the pain while preventing you from further exacerbating the symptoms by worrying.

Minimizing digestive issues in public

Choosing to skip an activity and stay home in elastic-waist pants with Pepto Bismol close at hand may be perfectly fine from time to time. But if staying home becomes a long-term habit, you may become isolated and miss out on the joy and variety that life has to offer, ultimately having a reduced quality of life.

TIP

Often with a little planning, you can manage gut symptoms like a pro when you're away from home. The arrangements and accommodations you need to make will depend on your exact symptoms, how often or how unpredictably they occur, and what triggers them. Here are some general tips for when you're out in public places:

>> **Be vigilant.** When you have an important outing planned, pay attention to avoiding any foods or activities that may trigger symptoms in the hours (or even days) beforehand.

>> **Give yourself extra time.** For appointments or meetings in new locations, arrive early the first time and orient yourself to where the bathroom is located, as well as any key or code required to access it.

>> **Be proactive about your bathroom breaks.** When you have an easy opportunity to visit a bathroom, seize the chance so you may be able to delay needing it later on.

REMEMBER

If you carry a purse or backpack, you may want to keep a digestive symptoms kit with you at all times when you're away from home. You can pack any or all of the following items into a small cosmetic bag, so they'll be handy should you need them:

>> **Toilet spray:** Specialty toilet sprays are worth every penny. The good quality sprays work to coat the water in the toilet before you defecate, miraculously reducing or eliminating any smells that could linger. They're ideal for using in public bathrooms.

>> **A clean pair of underwear:** If you've ever experienced incontinence, even on rare occasions, an extra pair of underwear can be a lifesaver. A nonbulky pair of leggings or shorts isn't a bad idea to carry with you, either.

>> **A small plastic bag:** Keep a plastic sealable bag in your kit to contain messes — for example, in case you have to use your clean pair of underwear.

>> **Tissues or a wad of toilet paper:** Nothing induces stress like running into a bathroom stall with an urgent symptom and discovering no toilet paper. But if you carry some with you, a poorly stocked bathroom isn't a problem. Some people may prefer to carry baby wipes as well.

>> **Over-the-counter medications:** Loperamide (Imodium) is good to have on hand if diarrhea may strike. Small quantities of pain relievers or antacids may also be worth carrying.

>> **An extra dose of your prescription medications (if applicable):** You never know when you'll be held up and unable to make it home in time for the next dose of your medication. If you take medications daily, carry a dose with you in case of unforeseen circumstances.

Visiting others' homes

Being a guest in someone else's home — and eating there in particular — may pose some different challenges from being out in public. You may have to juggle the social expectations of the occasion while dealing with your digestive symptoms. Your host is your biggest ally in these cases, so keep the lines of communication open. You can try the following:

>> **Discuss your needs with the host.** Even if the host doesn't specifically ask about dietary requirements, it's good practice to run your dietary needs by them in advance. A host often appreciates if you offer to bring some food you can eat to share with the other guests.

>> **Ask for a more private bathroom.** If you arrive and find out the bathroom is located in a busy place in the house, ask the host if there's a more private bathroom you can use if you need to.

ANUSHA'S ADVICE FOR SOCIAL EVENTS

Anusha Gandhi, patient advocate and founder of Femade women's health clinic in Canada, has lived with abdominal pain and other digestive symptoms for decades. Here are her tips for managing at social events where food is involved:

• Don't be afraid to ask for details about what's in the food and how it's made. If you don't, you're the one who pays for it afterwards.

• Hydrate, hydrate, hydrate — because doing so sets the stage for smooth digestion. You can even bring an electrolyte product (containing essential minerals) to maintain your body's fluid levels.

Eating out and socializing without worry

If you have a digestive disease that requires a special diet, eating out can sometimes be stressful. Restaurants aren't regulated in the same way as food manufacturers, so trust must be established and clear communication with the restaurant staff is important so you feel confident about the meal you receive. Some things that can help you manage your dining out experiences are as follows:

» **Choose wisely when selecting a restaurant.** Call or email in advance to find a place willing to take your dietary requests seriously and make the necessary accommodations.

» **Scope out the menu ahead of time online.** Don't be afraid to contact the restaurant if you have any questions.

» **Communicate with the person who invited you.** If you have very challenging food restrictions, you still don't have to turn down an invitation to meet at a restaurant. Explain to the person inviting you that you prefer to eat before arriving to avoid any issues. When you arrive at the restaurant, order a drink or small snack that you know is safe.

ANUSHA'S ADVICE FOR TRAVELING FOR WORK

Travelling for work — involving not only an unfamiliar place, but also managing various work obligations — can present its own set of challenges. Anusha Gandhi has travelled extensively for work while managing digestive symptoms and adds to the travel advice in this chapter, "Don't feel bad about packing all of the essentials. Heating pads, diapers, pads, or anything else – nobody is in your room, so they won't know what self-care you need to make it through the trip." She also recommends taking short naps where needed, especially if you've travelled across time zones. Chances are that if a nap makes you a few minutes late to a group event, no one will notice and you'll benefit from the much-needed refresher.

Enjoying travel

Travel means you're away from your normal routines and may not have easy access to the comforts of home for helping you manage gut symptoms. Extra planning is required for maintaining a special diet while you travel because bringing a whole suitcase full of your own food is often impractical. Furthermore, the travel itself has the potential to trigger digestive symptoms, with both heartburn and constipation being common occurrences during travel. And that's not to mention acute cases of traveler's diarrhea that can sometimes strike.

TIP

Here are some tips for travel, particularly with a special diet:

>> **Pack some snacks that are safe for you to eat.** If you require certified gluten-free, lactose-free, or allergen-free snacks, they may be hard to find in certain countries or airports. Moreover, language barriers may make it harder to read the labels on the foods you buy.

>> **Bring some over-the-counter medications that you can use for prevention (in the short term) or for treatment of digestive symptoms that arise.** Examples include Pepto Bismol or Imodium. Check with your healthcare practitioner before using these products preventatively, and don't use Imodium if you have blood in your stools.

>> **Do your research ahead of time about food options near where you're staying and keep a list on hand.** Make sure you check on their opening hours, too. If all else fails, locate a convenience store where you can purchase snacks.

>> **If you're in a place where you don't speak the predominant language, learn to say a few key words related to what you may need.** If your phone battery dies and you can't use a translation app, words such as "toilet" and any special dietary words such as "gluten-free" or "dairy-free" can be lifesavers.

TIP

Despite the many upsides of travel, a downside is that it can also expose you to unfamiliar microbes, some of which can make you sick. The most frequent infections that occur during travel are those that affect the gut. For avoiding infections, here are the top tips:

>> **Shore up your health in advance.** Well in advance of your trip, get a travel consultation (available from clinics and some pharmacies) to find out the specific health risks in the place you're going. Follow through with any recommended vaccinations or prescriptions.

>> **Be vigilant about washing your hands thoroughly before you eat.** Sticking to this rule may mean delaying your meals until you find an opportunity to wash your hands, but it will go a long way in helping you avoid illness.

>> **When you're in a different country, err on the side of not drinking the local water.** Stick to beverages that come in bottles or cans. Brush your teeth with bottled water if possible, too.

Managing in the workplace

First and foremost in the workplace, a little education goes a long way. At a new job, make the effort to find out about the policies and rights related to medical issues — sick days, medical appointments, working from home, and so on. Knowing these parameters can help you advocate for what you need and request exceptions where necessary. For example, if your symptoms sometimes make you late in arriving to work, see if you can agree on a way to regularly make up any time you miss.

Day to day, work can be a place where you may want to be discreet about your digestive symptoms. After all, passing gas or doubling over in pain don't exactly lend themselves to a professional image. Depending on the type of job you have, you may be able to make arrangements to deal with your symptoms more comfortably. Here are some tips to make your life a little easier at work:

>> **Wake up early enough to take care of yourself.** Leaving time for a bowel movement in the morning before work may help you avoid inconvenient symptoms later on, for example.

>> **Seek out bathroom privacy.** Find a bathroom in your workplace in a low-traffic area that you can use if you need more privacy. If you must use a busy bathroom, try to choose times when others don't use it as much, such as just before a lunch break.

>> **Take a comb or makeup in your hand as an excuse to head to the bathroom.** If someone else is already in there and you'd prefer privacy, briefly use the item in front of the mirror and then exit the bathroom. Enter again and use the bathroom when the other person has left.

Navigating dating and intimacy

One way to level up the challenge of dating is to have to deal with digestive symptoms at the same time. Because dating often involves dining out or other occasions of eating and drinking, a dietary restriction must be navigated skillfully. One study of those with celiac disease found that dating was associated with feeling uncomfortable explaining their dietary needs and engaging in riskier eating behaviors or even intentionally consuming gluten.

You may have no choice but to communicate with your date early on about any dietary requirements. The good news is that special diets are relatively common nowadays (whether by necessity or by choice), and you may even open a conversation that helps you get to know someone. Here are some ways to manage your diet confidently:

>> **Suggest activities other than dining out in the early phases of getting to know someone.** For example, a walk in the park, a museum visit, or an outdoor live music event may be fun activities you can do without the pressure of navigating a dietary restriction.

>> **If you're dining out, call or email the restaurant in advance and discuss what you need.** Check out the menu online. This preplanning can help avoid awkward situations when you arrive with your date.

>> **Never arrive at a restaurant starving.** If you've had a snack in advance, you may be more likely to make healthy choices.

>> **Let go of the idea that you need to eat or drink specific things to maintain an image or have a good time.** If the conversation is engaging, you can sip a glass of ice water and still enjoy yourself.

People with gut symptoms commonly report negative impacts on their sex life as well. Besides the practicalities of managing your symptoms during sexual encounters, sex can become stressful and less enjoyable if you're constantly worried about symptoms. Mentioning any intimacy issues to your healthcare practitioner is important, so they know your concern and can potentially adjust your treatment plan. If you feel uncomfortable talking with your healthcare practitioner about this aspect of your care, you can seek a referral to a nurse, counselor, gynecologist, or urologist.

Taking Advantage of Technology

Even though pencil and paper are a perfectly acceptable way to track your symptoms and aspects of your lifestyle, technology can provide convenient and enjoyable ways to record your health-related data and support your treatment. Mobile phone apps, devices, and other technologies can assist you in navigating your symptoms appropriately.

Some tech tools may help you see patterns and become smarter about how you manage your gut symptoms. On the other hand, not every technological offering is useful. Some apps or other tools are difficult to understand or don't keep track of information in a helpful format. You may have to try a new tech tool for a week or so before you know if it works for you. If you're spending inordinate time and energy trying to navigate the tool, you may want to try a different one.

A few types of technologies that you may find useful are found in following sections. (I don't endorse any of them in particular. App features may change constantly, so I don't vouch for their usability either — use or purchase them at your own risk.)

Specialized apps

Various mobile apps have been specially developed to help you manage your symptoms and your daily habits that could affect their occurrence. Note the following categories of apps:

» **Symptom tracking and wellness apps:** These tools, which are specific to digestive disease, allow you to track your symptoms over time to find patterns and to navigate wellness interventions such as nutrition and mindfulness techniques. Examples include MyGut and MyHealthyGut for supporting irritable bowel syndrome, and LyfeMD for supporting inflammatory bowel disease and other inflammation-related conditions.

» **Diet and exercise apps:** Several good general apps such as MyFitnessPal or Lifesum (which integrate with Apple Health) can help you track diet and exercise on a daily basis. Be wary of apps that specifically aim to help you lose weight because they may advise you inappropriately and work against your symptoms. Professional, personalized advice is a better bet for guiding what you eat.

» **Bathroom finding apps:** Some apps help you find the nearest public bathrooms and may identify features such as handicap accessibility and baby change tables. Some of them also let users rate cleanliness. Sit or Squat, Bathroom Scout, and Flush Toilet Finder are three of the most popular versions for the general public. Specifically for those with digestive disease, the We Can't Wait app in the United States and the Go Here Washroom Locator in Canada can identify local establishments that are aware of the needs of those with digestive disease who urgently need access to a private bathroom.

» **Special diet apps:** Apps such as Find Me Gluten Free, Gluten-Free Scanner, and Gluten Free 24/7 can help individuals dealing with celiac disease or gluten sensitivity to shop for safe gluten-free foods in their area. Spokin aims to fill a similar role for those with food allergy, providing easier access to safe foods.

Other technology

Other technology products are tailored to digestive disease or special diets. One example is the gluten-testing device that was first released in 2017 to the celiac disease community. The device allows you to test a small piece of your food to check whether it's free of gluten. To use the device, you place a piece of food inside a single-use test capsule and insert the test capsule into a hand-held triangular device. In two to three minutes, the device signals whether or not gluten is detected.

These devices are somewhat controversial in the celiac disease community. On the plus side, they can provide peace of mind for eating out and reduce the chance of becoming sick. On the negative side, the devices seem prone to false positive results — either meaning that the test erroneously identifies gluten when none is present or that gluten is present in miniscule amounts that still meet the criteria for a gluten-free product. The devices are also unable to give valid results for hydrolyzed (malt) or fermented foods (which include alcoholic beverages). Some dietitians caution that the results may lead to hypervigilance and anxiety — and that's not to mention the high cost of the test capsules.

Getting Support

Something I learned from having debilitating gut symptoms is that there's very little glory in going it alone. Even though I tend to be an independent person who doesn't like to ask others for help, I realized I was so much stronger and resilient for the long haul when I had supportive people around me. This section is about finding those supporters in your life. If possible, get a partner or close friend to read this section of the book — it can be the jumping-off point for a discussion about what's helpful in your particular situation.

Disclosing digestive symptoms

You may not feel comfortable telling everyone you've ever known about your digestive troubles. But believe me, when you're ready to disclose, you'll gain benefits from telling certain key people who are able to support you over time.

TIP

Here are some tips for telling someone about your digestive issues:

> » **Ask for discretion.** Before you tell someone, emphasize you want to trust them with some information about your health and you'd appreciate their discretion.

>> **Plan who you're going to tell and plan a short script in advance.** The script can include a calm, matter-of-fact description of what you experience, how it affects your life or work, and what helps you manage the symptoms. Then mention any specific requests you have of them.

>> **Stay upbeat if you can.** A positive conversation makes it easier for the person to hear and be willing to support you. If you're experiencing emotions about your symptoms, wait until you're in an emotional state that allows you to calmly discuss the matter.

In addition to individuals that you tell personally, group supports may be available in your area. For example, if you're someone with a digestive disease, some organizations such as the Crohn's and Colitis Foundation may offer support groups, educational opportunities, services, or free consultations. Don't be afraid to take advantage of these supports.

Providing support

Research shows that when someone has digestive symptoms, social support from partners, friends, or close family members has a powerful role in their health outcomes and in how they feel. As a support person, both your actions and the emotional support you can offer go a long way toward improving the day-to-day life of someone with gut issues.

For example, in high school, I had a close friend who trusted me with the information that she suffered from diarrhea at unpredictable times. One day we were at a pool party and the two of us, along with another friend, were in the host's bathroom getting ready to join the others in the pool. We were chatting and gathering our things when she suddenly turned and gave me a wide-eyed look while gesturing to her belly. I immediately knew that she felt her symptom coming on and that the other friend didn't know about the issue. So I turned to the other friend and suggested the two of us head to the pool right away, asking her to join us when she was ready, which gave her some privacy to deal with her symptom and avoided a socially awkward situation.

REMEMBER

Open communication with trustworthy individuals is key. If someone in your life has told you about their struggles with digestive symptoms, consider yourself privileged and trusted. You can reduce perceived stigma by being a listening ear, reacting calmly and kindly when they share information about their digestive troubles rather than reacting to the ick factor.

These tips can help when offering support:

>> **Set aside a time to talk about how you can make their life easier daily.** You may be able to make small changes that make a big difference to them: For example, support can be something as simple as agreeing to pause the conversation without a grudge if they suddenly need to get up in the middle of dinner. Or if you live with the affected person in a place with one bathroom, you may agree on a particular "I need to go *now*" knock on the bathroom door, so that when you hear it, you'll vacate immediately.

>> **If you spend time in public or social situations with a person who has digestive disease, remember you may need to be flexible.** Some find it helpful to mutually agree on a clear but innocuous gesture (for example, pulling on your ear lobe) that signals you need to leave a social function. That way, you can help cover for the person and make a graceful exit so they can deal with their symptoms.

>> **Err on the side of discretion when it comes to the person's digestive symptoms.** Refrain from telling others — restaurant servers, mutual friends, their coworkers — without their specific permission. While you don't have to fabricate excuses for the person, it's perfectly acceptable to give vague explanations about "feeling ill" or "taking care of something urgent."

ANUSHA'S STORY: DISTINGUISHING THE CAUSE OF ABDOMINAL PAIN

Starting at age 12, Anusha had pain in her abdominal region that was sometimes so severe she would end up in the hospital. But because the pelvic floor as well as the reproductive and digestive organs are so close together, discerning the exact cause of the pain was difficult.

After many medical appointments, she discovered she had bowel endometriosis. When the disease was excised surgically, she assumed her bowel issues would be resolved. Yet the pain persisted, eventually leading her to find out she had ulcerative colitis as well. The endometriosis lesions grew back over time and managing both conditions took some work, but with time and patience she eventually figured out what pangs and twinges were endometriosis as distinct from colitis. She needed to be especially aware of what food and exercise her body could tolerate and what her triggers were for each condition. By avoiding inflammatory and high-fiber foods (as is often recommended for people with ulcerative colitis), she was able to manage her pain for the most part.

3
Optimizing Your Gut Health

IN THIS CHAPTER

» **Understanding essential nutrition knowledge**

» **Discovering the dietary patterns that shape your microbes and your health**

» **Finding out the top five principles for gut-friendly diets that you can put into practice**

» **Navigating scientific facts about fermented foods and biotics**

» **Implementing a gut-friendly diet that works for you**

Chapter **10**

Eating for Good Gut Health

S cientific evidence is beginning to stack up to support the idea that your diet is associated with the sicknesses you may or may not get throughout your lifetime. And researchers now know that the health effects of your foods occur partially through the gut.

Of all the ways you can manipulate the community of microbes living in your gut, the food you eat is the top factor that's under your control. Every bite of food you take is an opportunity to keep your gut microbes fed and thriving — and thus able to carry out the health-supporting functions you need. (Chapter 3 describes those functions.)

In this chapter, I cover what the latest science says about optimizing your gut microbiome through diet in a way that best supports your health. I start with the overall dietary patterns that lead to better health, in part through the gut microbes, and then I examine the main scientifically-backed maxims for a gut-friendly diet.

I help you set the scientific record straight on the biotics (probiotics, prebiotics, synbiotics, and postbiotics) as well as fermented foods, and finally, I give you practical tips for implementing a diet that supports your gut health day in and day out.

Covering the Nutrition Basics

In high school I may have zoned out in health class when my teacher Mrs. Grundy was covering the basics of nutrition, explaining the four food groups (which were current at that time) and how many grams of fat to consume per day. In my defense, the class's nutrition textbook was filled with wholly uninspiring pictures: bunches of unwashed beets, cuts of raw meat, and schematics of the evolution of the wheat plant. I may not have been the only one in the class thinking about the pizza I was planning to buy from the school canteen at lunch time — so much more enticing than whatever sad, effortful diet was being depicted in those photos.

Herein lies the problem: Nutrition education can be a real bore, while diet guides on bookstore shelves tout the latest exciting nutrition hack for weight loss or reduced inflammation or any number of other benefits. Meanwhile, the popular media offers up a steady diet of sensationalized nutrition, much of it contradictory: For example, the fats in butter cause inflammation, but cutting back on butter offers no detectable health benefits. Drink red wine daily for the polyphenols but limit yourself to a maximum of two alcoholic beverages per week. So in the first place you may be unclear on basic nutritional knowledge, and to make matters worse you probably come across a lot of misleading and confusing information about nutrition — all creating a tendency for inflated expectations and unbalanced eating patterns.

Here I explain the nutritional basics in simple terms, including the substances your body needs for nourishment and how they're digested with the help of gut microbes. I present this nutrition information — which I realize now is critically important — with my sincerest apologies to Mrs. Grundy.

Carbs, protein, and fats, oh my

All diets are composed of the same three nutritional building blocks, or *macronutrients*: carbohydrates, protein, and fats. Different foods have different proportions and varieties of these macronutrients, but together they make up the vast majority of the foods you eat. Although you can adjust your diet to manipulate the amounts of each one, all three of these macronutrients are needed for a strong, healthy body.

Here's a brief introduction to each macronutrient, how it's digested, and how your gut microbes contribute to digesting it.

Carbohydrates

Carbohydrates, carbs for short, are sugars, starches, and fibers that are found in foods and that supply most of the body's energy. Carbs get a bad name because most people associate them only with the low-fiber and sugary foods such as white bread and cookies, which are quickly broken down into sugar molecules in the small intestine (with the help of secretions sent from the pancreas and liver) — and they tend to spike your blood sugar. So, eating these foods forces your body to work harder to lower blood sugar effectively and may leave you feeling hungry and lethargic afterwards. But these foods don't account for all carbs.

REMEMBER

The type of carbs called *complex carbohydrates* are fibers that aren't broken down immediately when you ingest them, and instead they pass through most of your digestive tract undigested. These fibers help your body regulate its use of sugar molecules to keep your blood sugar stable, slowing the absorption of sugars in your gut and helping keep hunger and blood sugar under control.

Furthermore, some of the fiber that reaches your colon is broken down by specialist gut microbes, which produce molecules called short-chain fatty acids (SCFAs) that are responsible for numerous health benefits, not just in the gut but all over the body.

Protein

Protein is an essential nutrient that helps you build and maintain body tissues — not just muscle tissues when you work out, but also your vital organs as well as your hair, nails, and bones. Protein in the diet is made up of chemical building blocks called *amino acids.*

Most protein is digested in the stomach and small intestine, but a portion makes it down to the large intestine and gets metabolized by the colonic microbiota. Certain bacteria in the colon can make *enzymes* (substances aiding chemical reactions) that can break down the protein molecules to produce metabolites in the gut.

Generally, the metabolites produced in the colon from protein digestion aren't beneficial for health (and are sometimes toxic), but scientists think the negative effects may be offset by boosting the ratio of complex carbohydrates to protein in the diet.

Fats

Fats are greasy or oily dietary components that are crucial for health, giving you energy and supporting the proper functioning of your cells. They help keep your body warm and maintain your immune system, and they also enable your body to absorb nutrients and produce key hormones.

Fat digestion mainly happens in the small intestine, where bile salts (sent from the liver) grab the large globs of fats and break them down into smaller ones, increasing their surface area so that the enzyme lipase, secreted from the pancreas, can act on them. Then the fats are broken down further into fatty acids.

The microbes in the small intestine help regulate how the body breaks down and absorbs the fats. After this, a small proportion of fats reach the colon, which is capable of digesting fats but with less efficiency than higher up in the digestive tract. Disorders of fat absorption result in greater quantities of fat building up in the colon, leading to loose and particularly smelly stool.

Vitamins and minerals

You also need small quantities of micronutrients — essential vitamins and minerals — to maintain your health. All micronutrients need to be acquired through the diet, except vitamin D, which is produced by the body in response to sunlight. (However, vitamin D can also be ingested. Milk and orange juice, for example, are sometimes fortified with vitamin D.)

REMEMBER

Lack of a micronutrient can result in a deficiency, which causes uncomfortable or severe health conditions. See these examples of five essential micronutrients and what happens when you're deficient in them:

>> **Iron:** A lack of iron means your body doesn't make enough healthy red blood cells, which creates difficulties with oxygen delivery throughout your entire body. This condition of *anemia* may leave you fatigued, short of breath, or with heart problems such as an abnormally fast heartbeat.

>> **Zinc:** A zinc deficiency can affect many different tissues and organs, varying by age. Diarrhea is a common symptom of zinc deficiency in infants, whereas hair loss, delayed growth, and increased susceptibility to infection may show up in older children. Adults may experience skin problems, issues with taste and smell, and slow wound healing. In pregnant individuals, a lack of zinc can cause numerous pregnancy complications and risks to the fetus.

>> **Vitamin A:** Not enough vitamin A primarily causes eye and vision problems such as night blindness, lack of eye moisture, or clouding of your corneas. Further problems that may arise include dry, itchy skin, frequent respiratory

tract infections, and problems with infertility. Children with Vitamin A deficiency may experience delayed growth.

>> **Vitamin D:** Vitamin D shortage is unfortunately common throughout the world. It leads to a decline in calcium levels in your blood, causing your body to take calcium from your bones, which become brittle or misshapen and increase your susceptibility to bone fractures. A lack of vitamin D may also lead to muscle pain or weakness, as well as fatigue or depression. Rickets, which causes bowed or bent bones, can occur in children with Vitamin D deficiency.

>> **Iodine:** Iodine deficiency, which is more common in women than in men, causes your thyroid gland (located at the front of your neck) to work harder so it may become enlarged. Your thyroid also may not be able to produce important hormones that help your body use energy, keep warm, and regulate the function of certain organs. A lack of iodine during pregnancy can cause severe complications for the fetus, ranging from stunted growth to developmental delays.

Your gut microbes produce several micronutrients — primarily B vitamins (see Chapter 3 for more details). Furthermore, some micronutrient levels or deficiency states are associated with alterations in the gut microbiota. The ways in which gut microbes contribute to modulation or absorption of micronutrients is an emerging area of scientific research.

You Are What Your Gut Microbes Eat

For the most part, scientists know what kinds of diets lead to healthier human populations on a large scale. Just look at the official dietary guidelines from any country, and you can find remarkable similarities to those from other countries. Here are some of the common themes:

>> A high vegetable and fruit intake

>> A focus on whole grains

>> A low intake of salt, fat, and sugar

>> A moderate intake of dairy

>> A preference for fish over red meats

>> Adequate water intake

>> An ingestion of a variety of foods

>> A recommendation to be physically active as a complement to a healthy diet

So far, scientists may not know the mechanisms inside your body that are responsible for how these factors help you achieve good health. Microbes, however, are turning up as important players in some of these mechanisms. Because your gut microbes seem to play key roles in turning your food into health benefits, a more specific version of the phrase "you are what you eat" is pertinent: In fact, "you are what your gut microbes eat."

Chapter 4 covers how some dietary patterns and specific substances can deplete or damage your gut microbiome. Here I cover the flip side, explaining how you can eat in a way that affects your gut microbes to benefit your health. Scientists don't yet have criteria for what makes a healthy or optimized gut microbiome, so throughout this chapter the guiding principles for a gut-friendly diet are increased gut microbiome diversity and increased resilience (see Chapter 3 for an explanation of these concepts).

Avoiding the fat-sugar combo

The dietary puzzle pieces — appropriate combinations of macronutrients and micronutrients — can come together in many different configurations to support human health. The proof is that, throughout history, humans have been able to thrive on vastly different diets — from a traditional Polynesian diet dominated by taro, fish, and coconuts, to a traditional Inuit diet consisting of animal-sourced foods (such as meat, fat, and skin) supplemented with berries and some seaweed.

Unfortunately, however, the absolute worst diet for human health is shown to be the diet that many people consume in industrialized countries: lots of sugar and quickly digested carbohydrates, with a high proportion of fats (especially saturated and/or trans fats), and little fiber. Here's an example of what this diet can look like on any given day:

>> **Breakfast:** Plain bagel with cream cheese and a flavored, blended coffee drink

>> **Lunch:** Deli meat sandwich on white bread with soda and a chocolate-dipped granola bar

>> **Dinner:** Steak with french fries and gravy, followed by a dish of ice cream

Not only is the gut microbiota dramatically less diverse when you consume this type of high-fat, high-sugar diet, but also scientists have connected this dietary pattern to disruptions in your gut barrier — meaning the epithelial layer becomes permeable and allows molecules (including lipopolysaccharides, which are toxic) to eke through into the bloodstream, causing inflammation through your whole body. Over the long term this can cause or exacerbate various metabolic problems such as obesity.

TIP

The good news is that you can avoid some of the ill effects of this type of diet by daily addition of more fiber. Just add to the daily diet example a mixed berry smoothie, a bean salad, and a large serving of roasted root vegetables, and you're well on your way to breaking out of this insidious diet pattern, which includes so many tasty foods but seriously impoverishes your gut microbial community and takes away the resources they need to support your health.

Finding a better diet pattern — The Mediterranean diet

Numerous diets with different proportions of nutrients can serve as an alternative to the detrimental high-fat, high-sugar diet. These health-supporting dietary patterns can take different forms: the whole foods diet, vegetarian diet, plant-based diet, and so on. (You need not cut out meat if you balance your nutrients overall and have adequate fiber intake.)

REMEMBER

One diet pattern in particular has been studied in many populations and in many areas of the world and is consistently associated with better health: the *Mediterranean diet pattern*. Here's what characterizes this way of eating:

>> The diet is dominated by plant foods, including whole grains, fruits, vegetables, legumes, nuts, seeds, and olives.

>> Extra-virgin olive oil is the main source of fats.

>> Fruit is typical for dessert; sweets such as cakes and pastries are limited, but when consumed, they tend to be made with olive oil and/or nuts.

>> Fish and seafood are consumed much more often than red meats.

>> Poultry and eggs are consumed in moderate amounts.

>> Dairy products such as yogurt and cheese are consumed in moderate amounts.

>> Consumption of red meat and processed meat is limited overall.

>> A moderate amount of wine is consumed with some meals.

>> A variety of spices, rather than excess salt, are used to flavor meals.

People who eat in a way that resembles the Mediterranean diet pattern tend to have a reduced risk of major chronic diseases and conditions as they grow older: cancer, Alzheimer's disease, metabolic syndrome, type 2 diabetes, heart disease, and depression.

Overall, the Mediterranean diet appears to work by reducing inflammation, lowering cholesterol, and changing nutrient sensing by the body. Scientific clues exist showing that the anti-inflammatory effects are brought about (partially) through the gut microbiota. Because of the high intake of diverse fibers, this diet pattern leads to a gut microbial community enriched in bacteria that fight inflammation and produce SCFAs. Indeed, higher concentrations of SCFAs are found in the stool of people consuming this diet. Scientists also observe decreased markers of a damaged gut barrier.

Being cautious with restrictive diets

A lot of diet and health advice is built around a narrative that you can't optimize your gut health (or overall health, for that matter) unless you strictly avoid certain foods or categories of foods. In the 1990s, the villainization of fat in the diet led to a swathe of new food products, from low-fat sour cream to fat-free cookies, designed to help people cut out fats across the board. More recently, fad diet books caused people to think that wheat and gluten were the enemy. And on a more personalized level, read-outs from microbiome tests and natural health assessments typically generate a long list of foods to avoid, promising you optimal health.

For example, the gluten-free diet is medically necessary in celiac disease. But is it good for generally healthy people to adopt a low- or no-gluten diet? A study from Denmark looked at the effects of a low-gluten diet for 8 weeks in healthy adults and found it altered the gut microbiome, resulting in fewer bacteria associated with fiber intake and health.

REMEMBER

For people who are generally healthy, an overly restrictive diet isn't usually all it's cracked up to be. You may not see any benefits to your health, and you'll also waste a lot of time and effort (and perhaps money) modifying your diet.

Severely restrictive diets can also have negative effects on your gut because they work against the principle of dietary diversity. Instead of embarking on a new restrictive diet, consider focusing on what you can add to your diet, guided by the gut-friendly diet principles that this chapter outlines.

SCIENTIST SAYS

K. Leigh Greathouse, Registered Dietitian and Associate Professor of Nutrition Sciences and Biology at Baylor University in Waco, Texas, says she doesn't generally recommend restricting foods for healthy people. "Restrictions of any kind can lead to unintended nutrient deficiencies and health issues. Food restrictions definitely aren't a good idea if you just think it sounds healthier — often they are part of marketing trends fueled by unclear science."

She notes, however, that if an individual is experiencing a chronic health problem or specific digestive issue that isn't fully managed by either medication and/or adherence to a healthy Mediterranean-style diet, then an elimination diet overseen by a registered dietitian is the possible next step (find out more in Chapter 7).

SUPERFOODS: NOT SO SUPER FOR THE GUT?

Superfoods are nutrient-rich foods such as kale, blueberries, or chia seeds that are said to have special properties or to give powerful health benefits. Yes, superfoods are usually full of great nutrients, but the marketers, rather than the professional dietitians, are the ones who tend to elevate certain foods to this sensational status.

Rest assured that these highly nutritious (and often highly expensive) foods aren't necessary for good gut health. Including some of these foods in your diet is a worthy goal, but if you focus too intently on eating so-called superfoods in a larger quantity, you may compromise diversity in your diet. And diversity is the best way to foster a varied and thriving gut microbiota and support your health.

Discovering the Principles of Gut-Friendly Diets

Given your diet's powerful influence on your gut microbes and overall health, what you eat is a necessary part of maintaining good gut health. Despite the books that claim to offer the one-and-only microbiome diet solution, no specific diet has been scientifically proven to improve your health by giving you a healthy gut microbiome. Therefore, the principles of gut-friendly diets take the form of general rules; the science doesn't back up a recommendation on specific amounts or proportions of different foods. As a result, generally healthy people should be able to implement these diet principles easily, no matter what their current diet looks like.

Here I outline the science-backed principles for supporting your gut health through your diet. As I discuss in the section "Finding a better diet pattern — The Mediterranean diet" earlier in this chapter, scientists have shown across many studies in many populations that the Mediterranean diet pattern benefits health. So, the basis of a gut-friendly diet is to adhere as closely as possible to that dietary pattern.

Layered on top of a Mediterranean diet, the gut-friendly diet principles in this chapter were selected if

>> They're shown to improve health in a measurable way.

>> The health improvement is partially or wholly made possible through the activities of gut microbes.

Thus, you can think of the following five as gut-friendly principles — benefitting health particularly through the community of microbes in your colon. They are applicable to generally healthy people who don't have a medically prescribed diet.

Diet principle No. 1 — Focusing on fiber

A well-established fact in nutrition research is that fiber is good for your health. Studies across large populations show eating more fiber benefits your health in multiple ways — more regular bowel movements, weight reduction, better blood sugar regulation, and a reduced risk of death and chronic disease. This humble substance, obtainable from a myriad of plant foods, seems to work wonders for keeping your body in good repair.

TIP

That brings me to the gut-friendly diet principle No. 1: Every week, aim to consume 30 or more varied plant sources of fiber. This gut-motivated way to consume enough fiber involves counting distinct types of fiber-rich foods, because it's more tangible than the old-fashioned way of measuring how many grams of fiber you consume. Don't worry about whether the fiber is classified as *soluble* (retaining water and developing a gel-like consistency during digestion) or *insoluble* (remaining unchanged during digestion) — all fiber sources count. But if you want to level up on your fiber challenge you may want to specifically incorporate a subcategory of fibers called prebiotics (refer to the section "Prebiotics — Food for beneficial microbes" later in this chapter).

Here I delve deeper into the world of fiber, including where you can get fiber, some obstacles to getting fiber, and how you can increase your fiber intake.

Recognizing fiber sources

Good sources of fiber include the following:

>> Fresh or frozen fruits (such as frozen strawberries or mango chunks)

>> Raw or cooked vegetables (such as steamed broccoli or roasted sweet potatoes)

>> Whole grains (such as whole wheat flour, oatmeal, or quinoa)

>> Nuts (such as almonds or pistachios)

>> Seeds (such as pumpkin seeds or sesame seeds)

>> Legumes (such as chickpeas, lentils, or black beans)

But why do so few people consume the recommended amount of fiber daily? As of 2021, fewer than one in ten Americans were consuming the recommended amount of fiber — around 25 to 30 grams per day. People in industrialized countries, despite usually having many sources of fiber available to them, eat most of their carbohydrates after they've been stripped of their naturally occurring fibers: white flour instead of whole-grain flour, fruit juices instead of whole fruits, and so on.

Overcoming potential obstacles to adding fiber

One barrier to putting fiber recommendations into practice is that the advice eat more fiber can call to mind joyless eating — that is, choosing your foods for their health benefits rather than their taste. A breakfast of bran cereal with a glass of prune juice, all for some vague health benefits in the future? Thanks, but no thanks.

This fiber exhortation, however, has taken on fresh meaning now that scientists have increased people's understanding of exactly how fiber benefits the body through the gut microbes: Some fibers provide a food source for bacteria in the gut, which break it down to produce SCFAs that immediately serve to nourish the gut lining and serve numerous other purposes for health. Moreover, you only need to check a dietitian's Instagram feed to realize that eating more fiber is far from joyless. Fiber-rich foods come in a rainbow of colors and in countless flavors, which can be combined into delicious meals. Examples include lentil salad with creamy avocado dressing on a bed of lettuce, vegetables and bamboo sprouts in a rich curry sauce, or a granola bowl with mango and coconut. Incorporating fiber into varied and colorful dishes can become a fun (and tasty) challenge. You can find some of my favorite fiber-filled dishes in the recipes in Part 4.

REMEMBER

Your gut especially benefits from fiber. Consuming diverse fiber substrates that are undigestible by the human body turns your gut microbiome into a factory for health-promoting SCFA molecules. These magic molecules not only nourish the gut lining, but also make signals that stimulate gut hormones. Like natural forms of popular weight loss drugs, these gut hormones help control blood sugar and regulate your perceptions of hunger.

Data from The American Gut Project showed that people who consumed 30 or more types of plants per week had a highly diverse gut microbiota and more bacteria that produce SCFAs. Other studies show fiber also makes the gut microbiota more stable in the event of perturbations such as antibiotics, increasing its resilience. These studies are the basis for the gut-friendly diet principle No. 1.

Increasing the fiber that you eat

Here are some tips for increasing your fiber intake:

>> **Choose a fiber-packed breakfast.** Start every day with a high-fiber meal that contains at least six to ten plants: for example, multigrain hot cereal topped with nuts and seeds.

>> **Go gradual.** When increasing your fiber intake, add more plants to your diet gradually over time. If you go straight from 10 to 30 plants per week suddenly, you may find you experience unwanted digestive symptoms. Your body may handle the change better if you increase in smaller increments (such as five more plants per week) over a series of weeks, allowing your body and your gut microbiota to adapt to the new substrates.

>> **Do whole-grain swaps.** Try switching out some of the refined carbs in your diet with whole grains. For example, you may choose quinoa over white rice or a whole wheat bagel over a plain white bagel.

>> **Don't let snacks slip through the cracks.** Snacks are a great opportunity to pack a fiber punch — so resist the temptation to reach for sugary, low-fiber snacks such as candy and cake. Instead, a handful of nuts or a piece of cut-up fruit nourishes your gut microbes and adds to your weekly plant count.

Even though most people benefit from increased fiber intake, I should mention that in some diagnosed conditions such as inflammatory bowel disease (IBD), the gut may not be equipped to break down a large quantity of fiber. If you have doubts about how much fiber you should aim to consume, consult with a registered dietitian.

Diet principle No. 2 — Making it fermented

For most of human history, before the existence of refrigerators, an abundance of microbes in foods was normal and expected. The use of certain bacteria to transform foods (whether knowingly or unknowingly) was a way to increase the foods' safety for consumption and to preserve them for a longer period — the original purposes of *food fermentation*. Fermented foods are those that have been changed on purpose through microbial activities.

TIP

That leads me to the gut-friendly diet principle No. 2: Aim to consume fermented foods every day. As for the appropriate number of servings, in a 2021 study in the journal *Cell*, participants consumed six or more servings of fermented foods per day to achieve the health benefits of a diverse gut microbiota and dampened inflammation. A serving of fermented vegetables also counts toward your daily intake of vegetables — and your weekly plant food count, as I discuss in the section "Diet principle No. 1 — Focusing on fiber" earlier in this chapter.

The following sections look at this gut-friendly diet principle to give you examples of fermented foods, explain what you need to know about fermentation, and offer suggestions to add more fermented foods to your diet.

Identifying fermented foods

Fermented foods have a long, rich history as part of the human diet. In fact, every part of the world has its own collection of traditional fermented foods. Delicious, fermented foods can originate from all kinds of substrates, from dairy products to meats and fish, as well as fruits, vegetables, and grains. Some rely on starter cultures (specific microbes added to start the fermentation process) and others rely on spontaneous fermentation (using microbes already in the area).

Some examples of fermented foods are as follows:

>> **Beer:** A fermented beverage produced using water, malt (usually derived from barley), hops, and yeast. Beer is generally filtered and pasteurized before distribution, so it doesn't contain live microorganisms when consumed.

>> **Kefir:** A sour-tasting drink made from milk that's fermented using kefir grains, which contain a combination of bacteria and yeasts.

>> **Kimchi:** A Korean fermented food traditionally made of cabbage and salt, along with red pepper powder, garlic, ginger, onion, and other ingredients. Natural (nonpasteurized) kimchi contains live microbes when consumed.

>> **Kombucha:** A tart fermented beverage made of tea and sugar, which is fermented by adding a jelly-like mat called a SCOBY (symbiotic culture of bacteria and yeasts).

>> **Miso:** A flavorful paste originating in Japan, made from soybeans fermented using salt along with commercial *Aspergillus oryzae* molds, which create enzymes that produce savory compounds.

>> **Sauerkraut:** A fermented vegetable dish made from cabbage and salt. The raw (unpasteurized) version contains a variety of lactobacilli and other bacteria.

>> **Sourdough bread:** A type of bread that's leavened with a fermented mixture of flour and water called a sourdough starter, which contains wild yeasts and lactobacilli. After baking, the live microorganisms are no longer present.

>> **Wine:** A beverage made from grape juice fermented by naturally occurring yeasts, which convert grape sugars into alcohol and carbon dioxide. Many wines contain some live microbes, but the alcohol content reduces the overall numbers.

>> **Yogurt:** The result of milk fermented using two specific bacterial species, *Streptococcus thermophilus* and *Lactobacillus bulgaricus*, along with other bacteria.

Genuine fermented foods are often found in the refrigerator section of a grocery or health foods store. Shelf-stable pickles or sauerkraut made with vinegar, for example, aren't fermented foods and don't contain live microorganisms.

Understanding what happens to food during fermentation

Fermentation causes chemical changes in the original food substrate, resulting in products with altered properties. Think of a crisp cucumber sitting on a countertop. As fresh as the cucumber may be, the microorganisms that attach to its surface are slowly transforming it. If left alone for long enough, the cucumber will eventually shrivel and soften, with visible spots of fungal growth. On the other hand, if the cucumber is immersed in a salt brine calibrated to discourage the growth of rot-inducing microorganisms, lactobacilli can feed on the sugars in the cucumber, producing acid and leaving it slightly less crisp but with a pleasingly sour flavor — creating a tasty, fermented pickle.

Even though microbes are necessary for creating fermented foods, live microbes may or may not be present when you consume the food because sometimes processing steps such as filtering, heating (pasteurization), or canning kill off any live microbes that may have been present.

Fermented foods as a group have been associated with general health benefits such as weight maintenance and a reduced risk of cardiovascular disease, type 2 diabetes, and certain cancers. Several studies have also looked at their link to the gut microbiota. For example:

>> The same 2021 study in *Cell* demonstrated how a diet high in fermented foods leads to increased gut microbiota diversity and modulates the immune system by lowering markers of inflammation.

>> Another study in the journal *Gut Microbiome* showed consumption of fermented vegetables affected the gut microbes in a modest way but led to a much more diverse collection of metabolites in the stool — and higher levels of certain types of SCFAs.

Scientists haven't yet singled out which component of fermented foods is responsible for the observed health benefits. Even though some of the benefits could come from the microbes present in certain fermented foods (see the section "Diet principle No. 3 — The more microbes, the merrier" later in this chapter), for now what scientists can say is that eating a variety of fermented foods appears beneficial for gut health overall.

Adding more fermented foods in your diet

Here are some ways you can include more fermented foods in your diet:

- » **Switch regular dairy products for fermented ones.** Swap regular milk on your cereal with kefir (or if it's too sour, kefir mixed with milk), or use plain yogurt on a baked potato instead of sour cream.

- » **Incorporate miso into your marinades and dressings.** Miso, even in a small quantity, adds a wonderful umami (and salty) flavor to many salad dressings and marinades.

- » **Pile on the fermented condiments.** In addition to (or instead of) your regular condiments for sandwiches, burgers, and hot dogs, add extra zing with fermented condiments such as kimchi, sauerkraut, or fermented pickles.

REMEMBER

Most fermented foods are safe to consume by generally healthy people, but make sure you use your senses. If something tastes or smells wrong, skip it and discard the fermented food. Some individuals are sensitive to a chemical called histamine, possibly resulting from an inability to metabolize histamine in the gut. (Your body also makes histamines naturally in response to allergens.) Because histamine can be present in fermented foods, individuals with this sensitivity may experience symptoms such as digestive problems, headaches, itching, hives, and a runny nose if they consume fermented foods.

NOT ALL FERMENTED FOODS CONTAIN PROBIOTICS

One of the top misconceptions about fermented foods and beverages is that they contain probiotics. Scientifically speaking, probiotics are a very restricted category of live microbes and require that the microbes be listed, quantified, and tested for a health effect. However, the live microbes found naturally in some fermented foods are a wild mix of different microbes that don't meet these criteria.

The beauty of fermented foods is that, unless tightly controlled in a commercial setting, each batch likely has a different collection of live microorganisms, which are dynamic over time. But because these microorganisms vary, they can't be guaranteed to give you a certain health benefit, so they don't qualify as probiotics. The exception to this rule is when bona fide probiotics (with defined strains at a certain dose) are added to the fermented food after it's made. This scenario may apply to some commercial yogurts, which have the probiotic strain(s) listed on the label, and they're in a carefully calibrated quantity to confer a specific health benefit.

Diet principle No. 3 — The more microbes, the merrier

Look around the next time you visit a grocery store: Most of the food offered is packaged, canned, or pasteurized. These features of an industrialized food supply have reduced unwanted microorganisms in foods and greatly increased food safety, preventing many illnesses and deaths. The downside, however, is that these measures have resulted in a nearly sterile food supply — and recent evidence shows this may not be optimal for supporting human health.

TIP

That leads me to the gut-friendly diet principle No. 3: Aim to consume high quantities of live microorganisms — one billion or more — every day.

People of past generations (before industrialization) didn't have refrigerators or freezers to discourage the growth of microorganisms in their foods, so (as I discuss in the section "Diet principle No. 2 — Making it fermented") when they couldn't eat fresh foods, they tended to encourage the growth of beneficial microorganisms that rendered the foods safer and tastier. Thus, they frequently consumed fermented milk products, fermented vegetables, and cured meats — all of them chock-full of safe live microbes.

Most modern diets, by contrast, are relatively low in live microbial intake. One study estimated the quantities of live microbes (also called *live cultures*) in three different typical diets of today:

>> **Balanced diet (according to U.S. dietary recommendations) of fruits and vegetables, lean meat, dairy, and whole grains:** The balanced diet had around 1.3 billion CFU (colony-forming units, a measure of how many viable microbes are present) per day.

>> **Vegan diet that excluded all animal products:** The vegan diet had around 6 million CFU.

>> **Western diet of convenience and fast foods:** The Western diet had only 1.4 million CFU.

All of these diets involve a lower intake of microorganisms than someone would have if their diet included a wide variety of fermented foods, as was typical centuries ago.

These sections identify where you can get live microorganisms, what helps you reach your target intake daily, and tips for eating more of them.

Breaking down which foods provide live microorganisms

The main sources of live microbes in the food supply today are

>> Fermented foods that contain live microbes at the time of consumption

>> Fresh fruits and vegetables, which have safe live microbes adhering to their surface and other parts even after washing

For example, a medium apple contains roughly 100 million bacteria (including the seeds), with the types of microbes — not the amount — being different in organic apples compared to conventionally grown apples.

A good proportion of these safe live microbes in everyday foods are lactobacilli of all sorts, but many other types can be present — from acid-producing bacteria called *Acetobacter* to yeasts such as *Saccharomyces cerevisiae*.

Scientists who examined the dietary habits of more than 46,000 Americans found that people who consumed higher amounts of live microbes in their diets — around one billion per day — showed a range of health advantages: lower blood pressure, reduced blood sugar and insulin, lower markers of inflammation, reduced triglyceride levels, as well as a lower weight and waist circumference. Even though these benefits were small in scale, they show the potential benefits of consuming a diet high in live microbes. This effect may come from the immune cells in the human gut being accustomed to encountering high numbers of live microbes daily and using information from the microbes as inputs to control their activity and prevent inflammation from getting out of control.

Reaching your target intake of live microorganisms

You can consume a billion live microbes per day by generally following healthy diet recommendations, including the following:

>> 2 to 3 servings of fresh fruit

>> 4 to 5 types of raw vegetables

>> 2 to 3 servings of fermented foods with live microbes, such as yogurt or aged cheese

This diet principle overlaps with the principle described in the "Diet principle No. 2 — Making it fermented" section earlier in this chapter — so if you choose fermented foods with high levels of live microorganisms (rather than those without live microorganisms), you'll be checking two boxes for your gut health.

Note that the live microorganisms I'm referring to here aren't the same as probiotics (see the nearby sidebar). In a nutshell, probiotics are taken for more specific purposes, whereas live microbes are consumed for general health benefits. However, a probiotic supplement can contribute to your overall count of live microbes every day.

WARNING

Probiotic supplements can sometimes lead to serious bloodstream infections in immunocompromised people, so if you fit this description, check with your healthcare practitioner before starting to take a probiotic.

One point of clarification: Live microbes in your diet don't quite have the same status as essential micronutrients. In the case of vitamin D or zinc or other micronutrients, consuming too little leads to a deficiency state that can make you very sick. But in the case of live microbes, lacking them in your diet won't necessarily cause illness. On the other hand, if you don't consume them, you may lose out on the associated health benefits. For this reason, some researchers are advocating for including foods rich in live microbes to national dietary guidelines.

Consuming more live microorganisms

Here are some ways you can consume a high number of live microorganisms every day:

>> **Snack on raw vegetables.** Make raw vegetables your go-to snack at least once a day. Stock up on your favorite dip (for example, hummus or sour cream dip) if you find they taste too plain on their own.

>> **Choose cheese wisely.** If you enjoy cheese, skip the processed or pre-sliced cheeses, which typically have few or no live microorganisms. Instead go for aged cheeses or those with a rind — types that likely still contain live microbes when you consume them.

>> **Take the whole-fruit challenge.** Where possible, challenge yourself to eat as many parts of fresh fruits as possible. Although banana and orange peels may be out of the question, you can experiment with eating apple skin, grape seeds, kiwifruit skin, and the brown divots on a mostly peeled pineapple. Lemon, lime, or orange zest can add zing to your yogurt or cereal and may boost the quantity of live microorganisms.

WARNING

Avoid apple seeds, however, because they contain amygdalin, which your digestive system may break down into a poison called hydrogen cyanide.

Live microbes in the diet — the ones associated with fruits, vegetables, or some fermented foods — are safe for most healthy people. Individuals who are severely immunocompromised may want to check with your healthcare professional before attempting to consume more live microbes daily. Furthermore, such individuals may want to choose commercial versions of yogurts or other microbe-containing fermented foods (rather than versions that have been fermented at home) because they're likely to contain quantities and types of microorganisms that are somewhat more consistent and controlled.

Diet principle No. 4 — Balancing fats

Although low-fat diets were once all the rage, now researchers and registered dietitians tend to advise that fats overall aren't the enemy, but rather that certain types of fats should be limited or avoided.

TIP

That leads me to gut-friendly diet principle No. 4: Aim to consume low amounts of omega-6 fats and higher amounts of olive oil and other monounsaturated fats.

These sections examine the types of dietary fats, explain how different fats affect gut health, and offer suggestions for how you can balance fats in your diet.

Breaking down important types of fats

Many foods contain a mixture of fat types, with one type being dominant. Here are the main types of fats:

WARNING

>> **Trans fats:** Also called *trans-unsaturated fats,* trans fats are a form of unsaturated fat that can occur naturally or be produced artificially. Trans fats are made when liquid oils are heated and turned into solid fats such as shortening or margarine, rendering them more stable. Until the 1990s artificial trans fats were commonplace in the American diet in foods such as microwave popcorn and packaged cookies, but after research strongly linked these fats to heart health risks, their use was eliminated.

Reputable dietary professional organizations all around the world agree you should eliminate trans fats or keep them as low as possible in your diet.

>> **Saturated fats:** They're found in foods such as red meat, butter, cheese, and ice cream. Chemically, saturated fats have no double bonds between their carbon atoms. Research has linked excessive saturated fat consumption to cardiovascular disease risk, but consumption in low amounts doesn't seem to have the same effect.

REMEMBER

Most dietary organizations advise that they should account for 10 percent or less of your daily calories from saturated fat.

>> **Monounsaturated fats:** They're unsaturated fats found naturally in foods such as olive oil, nuts, and avocadoes, and chemically they contain one double bond. Research has linked these fats to benefits for heart health and blood lipids, making them well known as "healthy fats."

>> **Polyunsaturated fats:** They're unsaturated fats containing two or more double bonds in their chemical structure, and they're found in soybean oil, corn oil, and sunflower oil, as well as foods such as nuts, seeds (flax or chia), and oily fish such as salmon, herring, sardines, and tuna. Within this broad category are two important types:

- **Omega-3 fats:** For example, in flaxseed, walnuts, and anchovies
- **Omega-6 fats:** For example, in corn oil and sunflower oil

An emphasis on omega-3s over omega-6s is shown to benefit health.

Recognizing how fats affect gut health

Research to date shows that gut microbes react differently to different blends of fat, and that these interactions have consequences for the immune system.

SCIENTIST SAYS

Registered Dietitian Natasha Haskey gave dietary advice to patients with inflamed digestive tracts (that is, individuals with IBD) for many years before deciding to tackle the research question of how different blends of fats impact gut inflammation. Now a researcher with a joint position at the University of British Columbia Okanagan and University of Calgary in Canada, Haskey's work verified the right blend of fats for encouraging the growth of health-associated gut microbes and producing beneficial metabolites that reduce gut inflammation: fewer omega-6 fats in the diet and more monounsaturated fats, such as olive oil. She notes that this combination closely mimics the blend of fats found in a typical Mediterranean diet (see the section "Finding a better diet pattern — The Mediterranean diet" earlier in this chapter).

Haskey says, "In general, we should not be afraid of incorporating fat into our diets." She encourages more focus on the types of fats rather than the specific amounts.

The following is an example of what this entails on a regular basis:

>> Around 3 tablespoons of extra-virgin olive oil per day in your foods

>> Two servings of full-fat dairy per day

>> A 4-ounce serving of oily fish twice per week

You may note that butter and other full-fat dairy is dominated by saturated fats. Even though saturated fats have gotten a bad name in past decades, the research suggests you don't need to completely avoid them if you maintain the right mixture of fats overall. (Basically, go heavy on the olive oil instead.)

Focusing on the right mixture of fats

Here are tips for implementing a health-supportive blend of fats in your diet:

>> **Carefully consider your cooking fats.** Haskey advises not cooking with omega-6-rich oils such as soybean, safflower, corn, or sunflower. Instead, try a miniscule amount of butter along with olive oil.

>> **Ditch the packaged pickings.** Many packaged and ultraprocessed foods such as potato chips and granola bars contain high levels of omega-6 fats, so limit your consumption of these foods overall.

>> **Make your own salad dressings.** Most commercial salad dressings are loaded with omega-6-heavy oils. Whip up your own dressing instead in less than a minute — three parts extra-virgin olive oil, one part vinegar (apple cider vinegar or another kind), a little Dijon mustard, and seasonings to taste.

Years ago, I would have characterized myself as a huge fan of french fries. My cravings led me to consume them three or four times a week — when dining out, between errands at the mall food court, or after a late night of socializing. How bad could they be, I rationalized, if they're made from potatoes, and potatoes are a vegetable? But I hadn't considered the types of fats I was ingesting so regularly with my fry habit: a heavy dose of omega-6s, which are linked to gut inflammation. In my subsequent quest to improve my gut health, I reluctantly decided that that my days as a french fry fangirl were over. I gradually reduced my fry intake until they were only a once-a-month treat — and I was pleased to discover my cravings for them decreased over time, too. Now that my gut health is under control, I eat them occasionally, but I try to balance the fats with an olive-oil-dressed salad at my next meal.

A shift in the proportion of fats in your diet has the potential to affect your metabolism and heart health. So, even though the research so far indicates that implementing this principle should improve your gut and overall health, remember that your healthcare practitioner should regularly monitor related health parameters as they see fit.

Diet principle No. 5 — Saying adios to additives

Diets that are optimized for gut health have more of certain things, such as fiber and safe live microbes, but they also have less of certain other things: the food additives often found in processed or ultraprocessed foods. (See the nearby sidebar about processed and ultraprocessed foods in this chapter.)

TIP

That's why gut-friendly diet principle No. 5 is important: Stay away from foods that contain gut-damaging additives.

These sections identify the main types of additives that are harmful for gut health and explain some ways you can avoid them.

Categorizing the types of additives that damage the gut

I'm as busy as the next person and I'm not entirely against consuming processed foods because some of these items offer enormous convenience and require me to spend less of my time chopping and peeling and baking and cooking. But the science has pinpointed several types of additives typically found in ultraprocessed foods, which seem especially disruptive for gut health and are best avoided. They are as follows:

>> **Emulsifiers:** Food emulsifiers create a smooth texture and give foods such as mayonnaise and ice cream a longer shelf life. The main culprits are

- Polysorbate 80 (PS80)

- Carboxymethylcellulose (CMC)

   They're shown in multiple studies to disrupt the gut microbiota, leading to an increase in flagellated bacteria (which have hairlike structures that help them move around on their own) that activate inflammation. These bacteria then burrow into the mucus layer and damage the gut barrier, allowing bacterial components to enter the bloodstream and supercharge inflammation through the entire body.

- Carrageenan is another emulsifier that may lead to inflammation in the gut by altering the gut microbes and reducing the thickness of the gut barrier's mucus layer.

>> **Noncaloric sweeteners:** Noncaloric or nonsugar sweeteners, which provide a sweet taste with few or no calories, include acesulfame K, aspartame, neotame, saccharin, sucralose, and stevia. The World Health Organization (WHO) released a statement in 2023 recommending against using these sweeteners to control weight because they don't appear to support weight loss over a long term, and they're associated with possible drawbacks such as an increased risk of type 2 diabetes or heart disease.

   Unsurprisingly, noncaloric sweeteners appear to negatively affect gut health as well. One human study asked participants to consume saccharin, sucralose, aspartame, or stevia — and each of these sweeteners altered the gut microbes (in the colon and mouth) in a distinct manner. Saccharin and sucralose led to worse blood sugar responses, which were linked to the gut microbiome disruptions — although some individuals were impervious to these effects. This line of research suggests some of the negative metabolic effects of noncaloric sweeteners can be traced to gut microbiota disruptions but that the effects might differ from person to person.

Avoiding additives: The how-to

Here are some helpful ways you can steer clear of the additives that mess with your gut health:

>> **Add more avocado.** Wherever you'd normally use commercial mayonnaise, use a thin layer of avocado, with its high proportion of healthy monounsaturated fats, instead.

>> **Scream for good quality ice cream.** If you're at the grocery store picking out a tub of ice cream, be sure to read the labels carefully because many varieties of ice cream contain emulsifiers. A good quality variety with no emulsifiers may come in a smaller tub and need to be consumed more quickly before the end of its shelf life. It may also be more expensive, making it a precious treat and giving you a good excuse to savor every spoonful.

>> **Be wise about beverages.** Noncaloric sweeteners are often found in diet sodas and other sweet-tasting beverages. If you're a fan of diet sodas, try to reduce your consumption by replacing one diet soda in your diet with sugar- and sweetener-free bubbly water. To enhance the taste of these waters, you can experiment with adding fruit purees, fruit juices, or herbs such as mint.

TIP

You may need to get out your reading glasses for this one because looking at the fine print on food package labels is important for putting this principle into practice. Skip the products with PS80, CMC, carrageenan, or noncaloric sweeteners (especially saccharin and sucralose). These foods are easier to avoid if you focus on eating fruits, vegetables, and other fresh whole foods — all in line with the Mediterranean diet pattern and the other gut-friendly diet principles in this chapter.

Avoiding emulsifiers and noncaloric sweeteners should be very safe for health but see your healthcare practitioner if you feel that avoiding these foods is making you overly limit the diversity and balance of foods in your diet.

UNDERSTANDING PROCESSED AND ULTRAPROCESSED FOODS

Processing a food, or transforming it from one form to another, can look many ways — from chopping and peeling a carrot in your own kitchen to producing packaged cookies on a factory assembly line. Washing, cutting, pasteurizing, freezing, and even fermenting are all types of food processing.

Food processing isn't a bad thing, but sometimes processing yields foods with greatly diminished nutritional value. Ultraprocessed foods are generally those that are highly altered and typically contain added salt, sugar, fat, or industrial additives; even foods labelled organic or natural can qualify as ultraprocessed. The NOVA food classification system, developed by researchers in Brazil, is the most used system for identifying ultraprocessed foods. Excessive consumption of these foods may have negative effects on overall health.

Navigating the Biotics

The *biotics* — probiotics, prebiotics, synbiotics, and postbiotics — are a group of substances that bring about health benefits. They're most often associated with digestive health and with manipulating the microorganisms in the gut community, although they can potentially target any body site. Importantly, the category of biotics is restricted only to substances whose health effects are proven through scientific studies. So, biotics are an exclusive club, even though many other substances try to imitate them.

The following delves into each biotic substance, including what the science says about its uses and its safety. These sections explain what biotics are and how to use them appropriately.

Clarifying some confusion around biotics

Several decades ago, biotics emerged from the realm of alternative healthcare and were routinely dismissed by scientists and medical professionals because little proof existed for their health benefits. But now the collection of scientific evidence showing that specific biotics benefit specific conditions has grown to the point where biotics are a legitimate and important addition to mainstream medicine. Currently, anyone who dismisses the biotics outright isn't up-to-date on the substantial body of scientific work showing their health benefits for conditions such as antibiotic-associated diarrhea in adults and necrotizing enterocolitis in preterm infants. The key is knowing which biotics are appropriate in which circumstances.

The misinformation that exists on the biotics and on fermented foods, however, can be overwhelming. When you search online for information on probiotics, for example, you'll come across much more fluff and false information than scientifically grounded information. The legitimate science often gets buried underneath glib (and search engine optimized) website posts full of material that would not pass muster with the actual scientists studying these substances.

Food and supplement labels exacerbate the confusion around biotics. The regulations on labeling vary by country, but nevertheless, labels very frequently fall short on the following parameters:

>> The label uses a biotic name (such as probiotic) when the substance inside doesn't meet the scientific criteria for that biotic.

>> The label fails to specify the biotic (for example, the probiotic strain) in enough detail to allow you to search for how effective it is.

>> The label may state the amount of the biotic that is present at the time of manufacture, not at the end of the shelf life. (Live microorganisms in probiotic products, for example, gradually die off throughout the shelf life.)

Defining the biotics and then studying them in a systematic and controlled way is incredibly important for realizing the full potential of their health benefits. A scientific approach takes them out of the realm of vaguely helpful natural health substances and into the realm of substances that people can use in targeted ways to improve their health.

To understand why scientific savvy is important, consider this scenario: You've just started a course of antibiotics and you're suffering from uncomfortable diarrhea. You enter a drugstore and encounter a vast shelf of probiotics — gummies, pills, and powders with dozens of different brands, strains, and doses. Sure, you can pick one at random, spend $20, and attempt to see if it fixes your problem. But if it doesn't help (because you may have picked a probiotic shown to have the ability to prevent the common cold instead), you may need to come back two days later to pick another one at random. You'd have to repeat this over and over until you found one that worked. A better course of action is, in the first place, to be guided by the science and select a product that's been specifically tested and shown to improve antibiotic-associated diarrhea. Scientific knowledge about probiotics and other biotics can ultimately lead you to a faster resolution of your problem and less frustration in the process.

Probiotics — Beneficial live microbes

The most famous biotics are *probiotics*, with more than 65 percent of people reporting that they're familiar with them. Probiotics are widely known as "good bacteria," but the reality is a little more complicated.

Probiotics are the Louis Vuitton handbags of the biotics world: Counterfeit versions are everywhere, making the genuine version hard to spot. Probiotics are live microorganisms that give you health benefits when consumed in proper amounts. In other words, they're a special category of live microbes (or live cultures) that have been scientifically tested to bring you a health benefit.

REMEMBER

A key scientific fact about probiotics is that their health effects are usually strain-specific — so scientific studies must single out a particular strain (or group of strains) to test for effectiveness. In turn, the strain or strains should be listed on the label of any probiotic product that has scientific merit.

In the past two decades, most probiotics have been strains of lactobacilli and bifidobacteria, traditionally associated with foods, which were selected because they confer health benefits and are also relatively easy to manufacture. However, as scientific studies and manufacturing methods become more sophisticated, the field is expanding to include more nontraditional species and strains — for example, those that are isolated from the human gut and administered in supplement format.

Here I explain how to identify probiotic health benefits, what specific benefits probiotics can bring, and frequently misunderstood information about probiotics.

Identifying true probiotic health benefits

Probiotics are known for supporting digestive health and also immune function and metabolism. To be able to navigate what probiotics do scientifically, however, you need to be able to spot the difference between tangible health benefits and health correlates. In general, some examples of tangible health benefits are

>> A reduction in the severity of abdominal pain

>> Fewer occurrences of the common cold in winter

>> Fewer days of experiencing constipation

On the other hand, probiotic marketing materials often use claims based on health correlates (that is, measures that seem to indicate better health but that may not map onto any tangible benefit). Examples of these health correlates are

>> Improving gut barrier function

>> Improving microbial balance

>> Increasing SCFA production

A benefit framed as a health correlate isn't a bad thing, and the vague wording is often motivated by regulatory constraints. But you should view these so-called benefits with skepticism — and you may need to dig deeper to find out whether there is any scientific evidence to back them up. Chapter 12 gives you information on how to tell whether a certain probiotic has any scientific proof for its health benefits.

Don't expect dramatic effects when you consume a probiotic because for the most part, the health benefits offered by probiotics are modest. Typically, they're sold as dietary supplements, not drugs, so even though they aren't as powerful as some drugs for improving health, they are safe and widely accessible.

Understanding specific health benefits from probiotics

Based on the reliable scientific evidence to date, here are the gut health benefits that some strains of probiotics can offer:

>> Preventing antibiotic-associated diarrhea

>> Preventing *pouchitis* (inflammation in a pouch that's created during digestive tract surgery)

>> Preventing necrotizing enterocolitis in preterm infants

>> Reducing the length of time children or adults have infectious diarrhea

>> Reducing symptoms of irritable bowel syndrome (IBS)

>> Improving symptoms of lactose intolerance

>> Improving symptoms in ulcerative colitis (in combination with standard therapies)

>> Reducing crying time in infants with colic

Certain probiotics can also give you benefits unrelated to the gut, such as preventing and reducing the duration of colds and other respiratory tract infections. Additional benefits supported by evidence are lowering cholesterol and other markers of cardiovascular risk and treating urogenital infections. Emerging evidence suggests some probiotic strains may even be effective for weight loss and for reducing depressive symptoms. Probiotic research is a highly active area, with many companies investing in innovation, so additional probiotic applications and health benefits may emerge in the years ahead.

ANTIBIOTICS AND PROBIOTICS: A PERFECT PAIRING?

A common myth about probiotics and antibiotics is that they shouldn't be taken at the same time. According to the common logic, if you're taking antibiotics, which are good at killing bacteria, then any probiotics you take will also be killed. But this begs the question: Can probiotics still give you benefits even if they're at risk of being killed? The scientific studies show, in fact, that when you take antibiotics, certain probiotics can still give you health benefits when taken at the same time.

For maximum benefit (that is, defense against the unpleasant side effect of antibiotic-associated diarrhea), you need to start taking the probiotics at the beginning of a course of antibiotics. Remember that not every probiotic will do the job because some probiotics are shown to prevent recovery of the gut microbiota when disturbed by antibiotics — so you need to choose the right one.

WARNING

Not every probiotic will give you these health effects, so you need to choose a product with a strain (or strains) and dose that matches the health benefit you want to achieve. Several resources exist for helping you choose an appropriate product — for example, the U.S. Probiotic Guide (https://usprobioticguide.com/). Beyond the main consideration of your desired health effect, cost, convenience, and branding may come into play.

Clearing up misunderstandings about probiotics

Here are some answers to frequently asked questions about probiotics, to help you make sense of the marketing hype and distinguish it from the scientific reality:

>> **Do probiotics work better if they're encapsulated (encased in a coating that helps them survive throughout the digestive tract)?** Not necessarily. Some companies want to make you believe that the probiotics must remain alive throughout your entire digestive tract, but in truth, the main question is whether they produce a tangible health benefit. If so, their viability through the digestive tract isn't of concern. In the rare case that a probiotic is specifically designed to act at a certain digestive tract site (such as the colon) to deliver its health benefit, then encapsulation could be necessary.

>> **Are probiotic products with a higher dose (in CFU) better?** No, a higher dose doesn't always mean stronger health effects. The ideal dose of a probiotic is one that has been tested and shown to provide a health benefit on a reliable basis — anywhere from 100 million to 10 billion CFU per day.

>> **Are probiotics more effective when consumed in foods or in supplements?**
For the most part, the *matrix* (or delivery format) of the probiotic makes little difference to its health benefits. So, whether you consume a yogurt drink that has had a particular dose of a probiotic strain added or a pill with the same dose of the same strain, you should receive the same benefits.

>> **Are multi-strain probiotics more effective than single-strain probiotics?**
No, the presence of multiple strains in a product doesn't assure its effectiveness. In some clinical trials single-strain products are tested scientifically and shown to be effective, and in other cases multi-strain products are more effective. However, if you're generally healthy and your goal is simply to increase your intake of live cultures (not bona fide probiotics), you may consider taking a multi-strain product to obtain a variety of microbes that represent different functions.

>> **Should probiotic supplements always be taken with food?** Most studies that test probiotics don't instruct participants to take the probiotics with food, but the health benefits are seen nevertheless. So, in general, taking probiotics with a meal isn't necessary.

>> **Should probiotics be taken at a certain time of day?** Most studies that test probiotics don't require participants to take the probiotics at a certain time of day, yet the probiotics still confer health benefits. So, the time of day you take a probiotic appears not to matter.

Probiotic safety can't be taken for granted and must be verified scientifically. Possible risks of probiotics include the presence of antibiotic resistance genes, or contamination during manufacturing. In general, the evidence shows probiotics have a very low risk of harm for healthy individuals. For immunocompromised people, including those with short bowel syndrome and premature infants, caution is warranted.

Avoiding the probiotic posers

When looking for probiotics to take, be aware of the fakes. The following types of live microbes aren't genuine probiotics:

>> Live microbes already living inside your gut (because probiotics must be consumed)

>> Microorganisms living on fruits and vegetables (because they're present in an unpredictable mix)

>> The wild mix of live microbes present in some fermented foods (because they aren't specifically named and quantified)

Most probiotics are types of bacteria, but they can also be yeasts or other microorganisms. If the microorganism is named (at the strain level), quantified, safe for how it's intended to be used, and supported by at least one study showing a health benefit, it qualifies as a card-carrying probiotic. The quantity of probiotics in a product is typically quantified using either colony-forming units (CFU) or active-fluorescent units (AFU).

REMEMBER

Here's how to interpret some of the phrases you may encounter on the labels of products that masquerade as probiotics:

» **Contains live and active cultures:** The product probably contains live cultures but may not contain genuine probiotics. (However, bona fide probiotics may be added to the finished product, as with some commercial yogurts.)

» **Contains probiotics:** The product may or may not contain genuine probiotics. Sometimes true probiotics really have been added to the finished product, but in many cases the product contains more general live cultures.

» **Supports gut health:** The product may or may not contain probiotics or any other substance that is shown to benefit gut health.

» **Unpasteurized:** The product probably contains live cultures in a wild mixture that doesn't qualify as a probiotic.

» **Fermented:** The product was likely created or transformed through the actions of microbes and may or may not contain live cultures when you consume it. Most likely it doesn't contain probiotics unless the probiotics were added after fermentation was complete.

Prebiotics — Food for beneficial microbes

A *prebiotic* is a substance that a special set of microbes in the gut use to create a health benefit. In other words, prebiotics are food substances for microbes — and not just any microbes, but ones that bring you health benefits. A prebiotic *substrate* (or substance consumed by microbes) can increase any specific group of bacteria, whether it's bifidobacteria or lactobacilli or another group, as long as the microbes that grow are responsible for some kind of health advantage. Most of the currently known prebiotic substances are types of fiber, although the definition doesn't rule out that other substrates such as protein or fats could qualify as prebiotics.

SCIENTIST SAYS

Glenn Gibson, Professor of Food Microbiology and Head of Food Microbial Sciences at University of Reading in the United Kingdom was the first to articulate the concept of prebiotics in a scientific paper in 1995 along with his colleague Marcel Roberfroid. Gibson emphasizes that even though prebiotics often take the form of fiber, not all dietary fibers qualify as prebiotics. He says, "Prebiotics owe their origins to probiotics, not fiber." So, a key point about prebiotics is that they have a special ability to stimulate the microbes necessary for giving you a health benefit.

Prebiotics in both food and supplement form are generally very safe to consume. If you ingest a high amount (or suddenly increase the amount), you can experience temporary digestive symptoms such as flatulence, abdominal pain, bloating, or diarrhea. These typically resolve when you stop taking the prebiotic or reduce the amount.

Here I go over where to find prebiotics, what health benefits they offer, and how to steer clear of misleading information about them.

Understanding where to find prebiotics

Prebiotics take many forms, and here are the main types you may encounter.

GETTING NATURAL PREBIOTICS IN FOOD

Prebiotics occur naturally in some foods, ranging from bananas to onions. According to researchers who analyzed the prebiotics in thousands of foods from the Food and Nutrient Database for Dietary Studies, the top five commonly consumed foods high in prebiotics are as follows:

>> Garlic

>> Leeks

>> Onions

>> Dandelion greens

>> Jerusalem artichokes

These foods have amounts of prebiotics ranging from approximately 100 to 240 milligrams of prebiotics per gram of food — overall, a relatively low concentration that may not be adequate for giving you a specific health benefit. Read more about these foods and how to add them to your diet in Chapter 20.

TAKING PREBIOTIC SUPPLEMENTS

Synthetic prebiotics are also available as supplements, or they're added to foods such as breakfast cereals, granola bars, or breads. Here are important prebiotics that you may see on a food label:

>> Inulin

>> Fructo-oligosaccharides (FOS, pronounced "foss")

>> Galacto-oligosaccharides (GOS, pronounced "goss")

RECOGNIZING SPECIAL TYPES OF PREBIOTICS

Here are three special types of prebiotics that are either found naturally in foods or available in supplements:

>> **Human milk oligosaccharides (HMOs) found in breastmilk:** This is an important prebiotic specifically for infants — find out more about HMOs and how they shape the infant gut microbiota in Chapter 17.

>> **Resistant starch:** This special type of fiber that resists digestion by human enzymes and reaches the colon to be metabolized by microbes is an emerging prebiotic as well. The main outcome of resistant starch fermentation is the production of SCFAs (mainly the one called butyrate), and health effects can be seen in chronic kidney disease, diabetes, and other conditions.

>> **Polyphenols:** Some scientists also consider polyphenols (natural compounds found in plants such as berries and cocoa) prebiotics. Polyphenols are associated with many health benefits, including a reduced risk of heart problems and cancer, and the latest science shows at least some of their health benefits are achieved through the gut microbiota.

Identifying the health benefits from prebiotics

REMEMBER

Gibson says typically four to five grams of prebiotics is a good daily dose to aim for. From the available science, adequate doses of some specific prebiotics are effective for giving you the following health benefits:

>> Improving digestive health, and in particular some symptoms of chronic constipation, such as increased stool frequency

>> Improving mineral absorption, resulting in health benefits such as stronger bones

>> Better cognitive performance

>> Improving cardiometabolic health, including more stable blood sugar and reduced cravings

Gibson adds that emerging evidence suggests prebiotics fortify the gut microbial community so it can better inhibit pathogens, protecting against gut infections.

Being aware of misleading information about prebiotics

The substances identified in this chapter have robust evidence for their prebiotic effects when consumed in high enough doses. However, products purporting to contain prebiotics can be misleading in different ways:

>> A product that has prebiotic on the label may contain a substance that isn't in fact a prebiotic because it doesn't have evidence that it confers its health benefits by stimulating the growth of microorganisms.

>> A product may contain an established prebiotic (inulin, FOS, or GOS), but at a dose that isn't adequate for giving you a health benefit. Food companies often use lower-than-needed doses of prebiotics because higher doses can cause foods to become less appealing to consumers.

Synbiotics — A perfect pairing

Just like socks or salt and pepper shakers, synbiotics are made up of perfect pairs. A *synbiotic* has two parts, live microorganisms and food for live microorganisms, which together bring you health benefits. Scientists see it as more than just a probiotic with a prebiotic. Adhering to the scientific definitions noted in this chapter, combining a probiotic and a prebiotic would mean that each one on its own would need evidence for a health benefit. But the synbiotic definition encompasses both of the following:

>> A product containing live microbes that already qualify as probiotics, along with a substrate that already qualifies as a prebiotic

>> A product containing any live microorganisms paired with a substrate, which show health benefits when taken together — in other words, substances that wouldn't qualify as a probiotic or a prebiotic on their own

TECHNICAL
STUFF

A further scientific distinction exists between types of synbiotics, based on the relationship between the two paired components and how they achieve their health benefits:

>> **Complementary synbiotic:** A combination of an established probiotic and an established prebiotic, where the two parts work independently to bring about health benefits. A good reason may exist for pairing the specific live microbe with its substrate partner, or the pairing may be random.

>> **Synergistic synbiotic:** A power couple synbiotic, in which the substrate specifically feeds the live microbe it's paired with, and together they confer

a health benefit. Taking both substances at once gives the live microbe a competitive advantage in the gut ecosystem by providing its preferred substrate (or food). Scientists can discover synergistic synbiotics by testing different combinations of live microbes and substrates in the lab and see which ones are a good fit for each other.

Of all the so-called synbiotic products on the market, few qualify as genuine synbiotics. Often the prebiotic component is present but not at a high enough dose to ensure a health benefit, either alone or when paired with a live microorganism.

REMEMBER

So far, the best evidence shows specific synbiotics are effective for:

>> Reducing serious infections in infants (shown in developing nations)

>> Improving cardiometabolic health

>> Improving blood glucose levels in type 2 diabetes

Synbiotics appear quite safe to consume, but because they contain live microorganisms, safety parameters similar to those for probiotics apply.

POSTBIOTICS — A TURBULENT SCIENTIFIC TRAJECTORY

Nonliving (in other words, deliberately killed) microbes have been added to many kinds of food products in Japan for more than 100 years. In 1998, a Japanese scientist named Tomotari Mitsuoka articulated the idea of these nonliving microorganisms being administered for health. In the English scientific literature, these substances were called by a variety of different names, including heat-killed probiotics, ghost probiotics, tyndallized probiotics, or nonviable probiotics.

Meanwhile, the term *postbiotics* was being used, perhaps a little carelessly, to refer to something different: the *metabolites* (molecules) produced by microorganisms as the result of their metabolic activities.

Then in 2021, a group of scientists aiming to bring clarity to the concept published a scientific consensus definition of postbiotics: a "preparation of inanimate microorganisms and/or their components that confers a health benefit on the host." This concept required someone to start out with live microorganisms, then apply a process designed specifically to kill them or make them inanimate, and then test the resulting product for a health benefit. At minimum, either the whole (killed) microbial cells or some of their components must be present.

Even though some postbiotic preparations may contain metabolites, the scientists determined postbiotics couldn't refer to the metabolites on their own. They argued the metabolites are better called by their chemical names (for example, butyrate) without needing to specifically reference their relationship with microorganisms.

Some scientists are sticking to the notion that postbiotics should refer to pure metabolites, but they're gradually losing ground. Most scientists seem to be adopting the new definition. Most of the current postbiotics on the market do fit this definition — for example, a preparation of inactivated *Saccharomyces cerevisiae* yeast along with its metabolites.

Postbiotics — Nonliving beneficial microbes

REMEMBER

Postbiotics are substances containing inanimate or nonliving microorganisms, which bring about health benefits. They're a relatively new field of study and applications are still emerging, but may include the following:

>> Reducing gastrointestinal symptoms in IBS

>> Reducing symptoms of colds or seasonal allergies

>> Improving stress responses

Evidence is also emerging to show that some postbiotics change the activity of the immune system in various ways, but researchers don't fully know the benefits of these changes.

BIOTICS GO HEAD-TO-HEAD

Of all the biotics, you may be wondering which one is better. The ultimate reason for deciding to consume a biotic substance is that you're looking for a health benefit — so the best biotic is whichever one is shown to confer the health benefit you're looking for. But if for some reason you want to choose from among the biotics, remember that they each have distinct advantages:

- **Probiotics:** The strength of probiotics is that effectiveness may not depend on the microbes already living in your gut.

(continued)

(continued)

- **Prebiotics:** They may be reliant on certain microbes already being present in your gut, but they have the potential to lead to more powerful effects or longer lasting change in the gut microbiota by providing the substrate that continually nourishes the target microorganisms.

- **Synbiotics:** They may give you the best of both worlds — robust effects with long-lasting change — but few synbiotic products manage to deliver.

- **Postbiotics:** They may be deliverable in many different foods and formats because they don't have to be kept alive, but their specific health benefits are only starting to become clear.

Postbiotics seem to be safe for generally healthy people to consume. Even though they're likely safer than their live microbial counterparts, researchers need to track their safety in individual studies.

Getting Personal with Diet

Dietitians already personalize their food recommendations based on broad categories such as a person's age and sex, while accounting for very personal factors such as a dislike of raisins in baked goods. But the goal in dietetics is to personalize on an individual level — so you'd consume the diet tailored to your optimal health, and I'd consume a slightly different diet tailored to my optimal health.

Some evidence shows your personal collection of gut microbes could partially account for how you and I may respond differently to the same food. Here I explain how gut microbes are starting to lead toward greater diet personalization.

Responding to foods

All the hard and fast rules of nutrition break down on an individual level sometimes. In general, vegetables are good for you, but one of your neighbors lived until 93 with nary a vegetable in sight. In general, excessive saturated fat can harm your heart, but that relative of yours who eats bacon three times a day could outrun a gazelle.

Scientifically, the basis of individual responses to foods isn't entirely known. But one of the most promising avenues of study is how the gut microbes affect your body's response to foods.

One early example of individualized responses to foods in the scientific literature was a study in the journal *Cell Metabolism* looking at blood sugar responses to eating barley-fortified bread. People who had *Prevotella copri* in their fecal samples before eating the bread showed better blood sugar responses than those who didn't.

In another study, researchers from Israel conducted a large-scale experiment on how people's blood sugar responses to the same meal could be vastly different — for example, one person may have stable blood sugar after eating a tomato while another person may experience a blood sugar spike. After closely monitoring 800 people for one week, the researchers developed an algorithm using inputs of gut microbial data and other information, which accurately predicted a person's blood sugar response to a certain food. This study was a preliminary demonstration that gut microbiota could contribute to our bodies' personalized responses to foods. Further research may corroborate gut microbes as key contributors to individuals' unique biological responses to the exact same meal.

Aiming for a diet that protects

Finding a completely personalized diet that shapes your gut microbes in a direction that steers you away from chronic disease seems like science fiction at this point. But taking a systems biology approach, scientists are working on a plan to make this fiction a reality.

Here are some of the scientific steps in this process:

>> Discovering how changes in gut microbes influence the services of the microbial ecosystem (such as which metabolites are produced)

>> Mapping out how these microbial ecosystem outputs affect health (for example, metabolism and immune functioning)

>> Using artificial intelligence to discover connections between microbial ecosystems and health

>> Following up on the connections discovered through artificial intelligence to determine which factors in the microbial ecosystem are the root causes in health and disease

Arming Yourself with Practical Tips for a Gut-Friendly Diet

Put away those fad diet books. The key to a diet that supports your health through your gut is that it's not a fad — it's something you can implement now and keep up for the long term.

But that doesn't mean it's easy to pivot to a gut-friendly diet starting now. You may need a little support and planning to make the transition go smoothly. Here are my general tips for implementing the diet principles in this chapter.

Equipping and organizing your kitchen

You need not buy a lot of new items to make your kitchen gut-friendly. But here are some of the items I find useful to have:

>> Ample small containers for storing cut-up veggies, beans, and more

>> A pair of large kitchen scissors for cutting herbs and greens

>> Basic fermentation equipment such as mason jars and breathable jar covers

TIP

The way you organize your food may also help you implement a diet that's better for your gut. If you have packaged cookies or other ultraprocessed foods in your home, store them away behind closed cupboard doors. Deliberately put more gut-friendly foods in plain sight: a small bowl full of fruit on the counter or a bowl of walnuts or pistachios on the table.

TIP

Also, when you store cooked beans or other legumes in your fridge, keep them in a mason jar or clear glass container at the front of the fridge. You may be more likely to add them to salads, soups, and other dishes.

Planning ahead

Sometimes despite my best intentions, I resort to eating things that don't serve my gut health — a slice of lemon loaf from the coffee shop or a bag of potato chips before dinner. These poor snacks for gut health tend to be consumed especially when I'm in a rush. But the magic of planning ahead is that when the hunger pangs hit, I have something within reach that can help me maintain a gut-friendly diet.

For me, planning has two components (feel free to use these tips):

>> **List snacks and meals for specific days of the week.** At the beginning of every week, I take ten minutes to make a meal list for that week, with four or five different meals. Sometimes coming up with these meals can feel overwhelming, but there's a way around that, too: Take a stack of small sticky notes and on each note write one meal you and your family enjoy. Post these notes (say, 15 to 20 of them) on the inside of a cupboard and go there for inspiration when you're making your weekly meal list. After you choose the meals, you can plan your grocery shopping around them.

>> **Actively prepare for some of these snacks and meals:** When you arrive home with your bundle of groceries, take ten minutes to prepare some of them for the week ahead. That may mean chopping up some veggies or dividing meat or fish into portions. Just a short preparation time can help you eat in a gut-friendly, healthy way all week with minimal fuss.

Being realistic about time and costs

Sometimes I imagine I could be a fermentation goddess, visiting local farmers' markets and bringing home basketfuls of produce, which I'd carefully chop and fit into different sized jars on my kitchen counter. I'd mix up a perfect brine and pour some into each jar, then come back day after day to see the ferments bubble as I added a pinch of this spice or a sprig of that herb.

Most of the time, however, I'm more realistic about what's possible. I pick up a jar of fermented pickles from the local health food store and stick it in the fridge door shelf, next to the mustard.

You don't have to make everything from scratch to eat in a gut-friendly way — you can nourish your gut in plenty of ways that don't take hours and hours of your time. Nor do you have to spend a fortune. Here are some tips for saving on time and/or costs:

>> Find out where the best fermented foods are made locally. For example, you may find a Korean corner store that sells amazing kimchi that you can pick up and add to your noodle bowl at home.

>> If you buy a plain commercial kefir, you may be able to extend it by putting a small amount into a jar with fresh milk. Leave the mixture in the fridge (or on the counter for a few hours) and letting the sour flavor permeate the milk.

>> You can use a few tablespoons of yogurt to create a new batch of yogurt. (Look online for yogurt-making instructions.)

>> A windowsill planter containing three or four kinds of herbs that you can harvest for meals is a great way to increase your intake of diverse plants.

Dealing with picky eating

If you have someone in your household (as I do!) who is very particular about what they eat, this section is for you. My household member isn't into complex flavors and has strong feelings about the textures he finds acceptable, so it can be challenging to make nutritious meals that he finds tasty and that also appeal to the rest of us in the household.

Here are my top tips for mealtimes when picky eating happens:

>> Consistently serve a mini tray of vegetables or fruits you know the eater enjoys. It can be baby carrots, cucumbers, and mandarin oranges; your picky eater can count on it being on the table every night so they won't go hungry.

>> When preparing meals, leave out some of each plain ingredient so the eater can select from the meal components. For example, if I'm making spinach lasagna for the household, I'll set aside separate small dishes of cooked spinach, tomato sauce, noodles, and shredded cheese. The eater can decide which parts to eat separately or combine, and overall, he is sharing the same meal — albeit in a slightly different form.

>> Involve the eater in meal preparation. Sometimes the acts of touching the foods and experiencing their other sensory characteristics may increase familiarity with texture and help them eventually feel safer in tasting it.

Possibly not all your family members will be equally enthusiastic about eating to support their gut microbiomes. But you can start conversations with the younger members of your household, explaining why fiber is important for feeding their gut microbes and keeping them alive and happy. Remember it's not a fad diet, it's a lifestyle — so over time, a gut–friendly way of eating will become more familiar and they may gladly join you on team gut health.

IN THIS CHAPTER

» **Practicing better sleep**

» **Including exercise on a regular basis**

» **Keeping stress under control**

» **Spending time outdoors**

» **Considering other ways to improve or maintain gut health**

Chapter **11**

Adjusting Your Lifestyle For Long-Term Gut Health

I f optimal gut health were as simple as eating fiber and popping a magic probiotic, this book wouldn't need to exist. All the scientific research on the gut microbiome and overall gut health converges to suggest that good gut health requires a holistic approach, meaning you need to manage multiple aspects of your lifestyle at the same time. To achieve your best gut health possible, committing to implementing changes over the long term and persisting with your healthy habits despite the many barriers you may encounter is important.

Managing all the pieces necessary for well-rounded gut health isn't super easy. Potential gut microbial disruptors are everywhere you look, from the donuts on the coffee break table at work, to the bottle of ibuprofen in your medicine cabinet. Gut health is about avoiding those disruptors as best you can while using healthy habits to remediate any damage that's been done. Remaining vigilant will help you hang onto your inner gut health glow.

What you eat, as Chapter 10 covers, is the foundation for optimizing gut health through the gut microbiome. But diet isn't the only thing you have to pay attention to on your gut health journey. Other aspects of your lifestyle are critical for improving and optimizing gut health, too. Whereas Chapter 4 examines the lifestyle factors that influence gut health, this chapter shows how you can leverage this knowledge to improve your health and vitality.

When I suffered from gut health symptoms and realized things had to change, I altered multiple aspects of my lifestyle in a short period of time. I changed my diet to dramatically increase fiber and reduce sugar and fatty foods (goodbye, my dear french fries). I started a regular exercise routine. I trained myself to turn off the TV and computer in the evenings and started making sleep a priority. Today I can't pinpoint one specific thing that made my uncomfortable gut symptoms go away, but I believe, and the research now shows, that multiple lifestyle changes work together to allow gut healing.

This chapter dives into the habits that people without (or with) a digestive diagnosis can establish, in addition to a gut-friendly diet, if they want to optimize gut health over a long term. Many of these habits alter the gut microbes in only a few days, and they may make a tangible difference in your health if you keep them up over a period of many months.

REMEMBER

If you slip back into unhealthy habits, those benefits will be lost. So the name of the game is baby steps — small changes you can adopt permanently. In the same way that regularly depositing a small amount of money in the bank accrues more and more interest over time until you have a substantial sum, small and incremental changes in your lifestyle over time bring you growing and compounding benefits and keep you healthier for a long time to come.

Improving Your Sleep Habits

Restful sleep is essential — not just for gut health, but for overall health. Ample research shows that a lack of adequate sleep increases your risk for lifetime conditions such as type 2 diabetes, heart disease, obesity, and depression. Poor sleep makes you drowsier during your waking hours, raising the chances of mistakes that can cause injury or disability. Furthermore, your memory and cognitive performance also suffer dramatically. According to the U.S. Centers for Disease Control and Prevention, one-third of adults in the United States say they get less sleep than they need.

The following sections explore different aspects of good sleep habits (also called *sleep hygiene*), including:

>> **Sleep duration:** How long you sleep

>> **Sleep quality:** How uninterrupted your sleep is

>> **Sleep timing:** Which periods of the night or day you sleep

These aspects have direct implications for your gut health. Sleep duration, sleep quality, and sleep timing can all affect your gut microbial community, making it less diverse. Poor sleep also makes it harder for you to stick to a nourishing high-fiber diet. Studies associate inadequate sleep with poor dietary choices such as more quick-burning carbohydrate foods, fats, sugar-sweetened beverages, and alcohol — all of which are less than ideal for your gut health, as Chapter 10 outlines.

WARNING

If you have good sleep hygiene and you're still not sleeping well on a regular basis, you may have an undiagnosed sleep disorder, so talk with a healthcare professional. Further, some diagnosed conditions, including obesity, are associated with sleep problems. Talk to your healthcare professional about the available options to address them.

Striving for better sleep duration

Many activities may foil your plans for getting a good night's rest. The Netflix show you're watching segues right into the next episode, for example, at a crucial moment in the plot when you can't stand not knowing what happens. Overall, the blue light emitted by screens (on phones, laptops, or TVs) promotes wakefulness. Sure enough, screen media use in youths is associated with decreased total sleep time or delay of bedtime.

CHILDREN: THE ORIGINAL SLEEP DISRUPTORS

Parents or guardians of small children may find they lack sleep with the constant waking of little ones needing attention or feeding. For infants and young children, waking up several times per night is normal, but parents can feel the effects on health if it happens night after night. And no matter what approach you take as a family — sleep training or no sleep training — the best laid plans for nighttime often go awry. If you're the main caregiver getting up night after night, ask someone to take on the nighttime wake-up duties at least once every few weeks so you can get a full night of uninterrupted sleep.

Furthermore, when you're busy, sleep is often the thing that gets shortchanged. A phenomenon known as *revenge bedtime procrastination* (or perhaps more politely, *behavioral bedtime delay*) occurs when you decide to sacrifice sleep for leisure time because your schedule during the day is lacking in free time. Understandably, when you're busy attending to work and other people all day, you may be tempted to stay up later to have some time to yourself, even though you'll be foreseeably worse off the next day. But unfortunately if you make it a habit, your health will suffer because adequate sleep duration — the simple number of hours — is a crucial part of gut and overall health.

The amount of sleep a person needs to feel rested varies somewhat across the population. An individual needs anywhere from six to ten hours per night, with seven to nine hours being typical. Similarly, a lack of sleep can show up in different ways, but typical manifestations include drowsiness, poor mood, a tendency to overeat, stronger feelings of pain, as well as issues with memory and problem-solving.

Proper sleep duration supports gut health by leading to a nice diversity of gut microbes, while people who are sleep deprived tend to have bacterial groups that are linked with weight gain and inflammation.

For optimal gut health, protect your sleep time. Day in and day out, try to get enough sleep to feel well rested and alert throughout the day — seven to nine hours. Here are some tips for achieving enough sleep:

>> **Aim to go to sleep and wake up at similar times each day, even on the weekends.** Remember that alarms aren't just for waking up; you may want to set a nightly bedtime alarm to remind you when to start preparing for bed.

>> **If you struggle to stay alert through the whole day, experiment with naps.** If your schedule allows, try a 20-minute nap after lunch, which adds valuable minutes to your total sleep duration and may balance out your energy levels.

>> **Limit caffeine in the afternoon and evening.** Caffeine later in the day can interfere with your alertness level and prevent you from getting to sleep on time.

>> **Try to avoid looking at screens such as laptops and phones at least 30 minutes before bed.** According to the National Sleep Foundation, you should try to replace the screen time with activities such as reading a book or magazine, taking a bath, listening to music, or doing a crossword puzzle.

>> **Experiment with techniques to focus your racing mind to get you into sleep mode.** Try a five-minute meditation or relaxation activity such as deep breathing just before you go to bed. Consciously relax your muscles so your brain gets the message it's time to calm down.

>> **Implement a bedtime ritual to signal your body that it's time to wind down.** Be consistent and do these things in the same order, for example:

- Changing into pajamas

- Brushing your teeth

- Putting on calming music and/or a battery-lit candle

- Reading a book in a comfortable chair (rather than in bed) for 15 minutes before getting into bed and turning the lights out

Alcohol may sometimes seem to make you drowsy and ready for sleep but don't rely on alcoholic drinks to wind down at the end of the day because, overall, alcohol is associated with poorer sleep. Avoid it altogether when you're trying to get a good night's rest.

Focusing on better-quality sleep

Interrupted sleep is when you wake up for a prolonged time at least four times a night. For good quality sleep, you'd be awake no more than twice briefly per night. If your sleep is regularly interrupted, your gut health may suffer: You're more likely to have digestive symptoms such as abdominal pain, acid reflux, distension, and belching — or the symptoms may become more severe. Overall, your gut microbial community is less diverse when you have interrupted sleep.

TIP Put the pieces into place for uninterrupted sleep, which may be easier said than done if you tend to be a light sleeper. If you wake up more than twice briefly during the night or find yourself awake at night for prolonged periods of time, try the following:

>> **Make sure your sleeping area is completely dark.** Hide the electronic devices and cover up the small red or blue lights on electronic devices. Light seeping through windows can be blocked with black-out blinds or by fitting towels around the blinds at night. Alternatively, consider wearing an eye mask.

>> **Reduce intake of liquids two hours before bed.** *Nocturia*, which is the need to get up regularly at night to urinate, can be reduced if you focus on hydrating earlier in the day and avoid ingesting liquids in the couple of hours leading up to bedtime.

>> **If you can control the temperature in your room, reduce the temperature by a few degrees overnight.** A cooler room mimics the natural drop in your body temperature during sleep, so your body doesn't have to work as hard to cool you down.

>> **Reduce sources of noise.** A white noise machine can help drown out any noises outside your room. With computers and other devices, either remove them from the room entirely or turn off the sound and vibration so you aren't woken up by sudden buzzes and dings. If you sleep in a room with someone who snores, you can try using earplugs, wearing a soft headband over your ears, or perhaps going to bed earlier than the person who snores.

TIP

If you wake up in the middle of the night and can't get back to sleep, experts recommend getting out of bed after 15 to 30 minutes so that your brain doesn't start to associate lying in bed with long periods of wakefulness. When you get up, avoid turning on bright lights or looking at your phone. Instead try reading with a small light, deep breathing, or meditating. Alternatively, you may want to repeat your normal bedtime ritual. When you feel tired again, return to your bed.

Timing your sleep — a gut in sync

Whether you know it or not, your body's internal biological processes (including digestion, hunger, body temperature, and alertness) are in tune with the day/ night cycle. Light, temperature, and food intake are some of the cues your body responds to in this 24-hour cycle. The implication of this cycle is that certain hours are better for sleeping than other hours. But many people are out of sync with this 24-hour clock and mess with it by ignoring the natural cues.

Your gut operates according to this internal clock as well, meaning that many gut functions — from hormone secretion to nutrient absorption to repair of the gut barrier — operate on a 24-hour cycle. Your gut's internal clock also controls motility, which is not under your conscious control. Even your gut microbes stick to this cycle, although scientists don't yet fully understand the implications of this for health.

THE TRAVELING GUT

When you travel across time zones, you may experience *jet lag* — extreme tiredness and changes in your eating and sleeping patterns. You may feel hungry at odd times because of out-of-whack hunger hormones — namely, increased levels of the appetite regulator ghrelin and decreased levels of the satiety hormone leptin. Jet lag influences the gut by disturbing the normal day-night cycle of your gut microbiota and messing with metabolism and gut function overall.

Here are some tips for adjusting to your new time zone and avoiding the gut disturbances of jet lag:

- As soon as possible when you arrive at your destination, try to shift your meal schedule to that of the new time zone.

- When you arrive at the destination airport, grab a bottle of water and a few snacks (yogurt as well as high-fiber snacks if possible) so you can stay hydrated and stave off hunger between mealtimes in your new time zone.

- For the first few days at your destination, try to eat balanced meals and avoid heavy, fatty foods as well as alcohol.

- Get some sunlight exposure in the morning and throughout the day at your destination to give your body cues it's daytime. Avoid exercising close to bedtime in your new time zone.

Experts advise getting pre-midnight sleep – the 90-minute phase before midnight is especially rejuvenating. Note that adjusting when you eat relative to this 24-hour cycle, too, may affect your health. For more information, refer to the section "Adjusting when you eat" later in this chapter.

Exercising on a Regular Basis

Exercise is physical activity that you purposefully undertake for improving health. With apologies to the couch potatoes, exercise isn't optional if you want a healthy gut and good health overall. It staves off heart disease, cancer, diabetes, depression, and dementia. It promotes a lower body weight. The list goes on. And it helps you feel more vibrant and energetic day to day.

Think of exercise this way: It's the ultimate insurance against health problems. It's better than any drug or supplement in the world for proactively avoiding multiple lifelong health problems. In essence, exercise provides a source of physical stress on your body and forces it to adapt, altering your physiology by lowering inflammatory signals from the immune system. What doesn't kill you makes you stronger, so the saying goes.

REMEMBER

Exercise is specifically important for gut health because it leads to increased gut microbiome diversity. Research also shows that exercise shifts the composition of the gut microbiota and increases the production of short-chain fatty acids (SCFAs).

Despite these incredible benefits of exercise, only about a quarter of Americans get the recommended amount of exercise according to the CDC. The organization recommends at least 150 minutes per week, or slightly more than 20 minutes per day, of moderate-intensity activity, and ideally a mix between aerobic activities (those that make you breathe harder) and muscle-strengthening activities. Adults 65 and older are the least likely to reach this target.

Should you aim to increase your fitness level when you do exercise? Not necessarily. True, better fitness is the result of exercise, but the health benefits come from the exercise itself, not your achievement on a fitness test. Over time when you exercise, you may be inspired to push yourself harder, and your fitness will naturally improve. But what's important above all is that you do the exercise. The following sections walk you through how to decide the amount and type of exercise that work best for you and provide tips for making exercise a part of your normal routine.

Finding the right-sized exercise

When you exercise regularly, your gut microbes will become more diverse, and the community will contain more health-associated species. These changes are accompanied by a reduction in inflammation and intestinal permeability — a green light for gut health.

The ideal amount and type of exercise is highly personal to your body and your lifestyle. The number one sign of a good exercise routine is whether you can stick to it regularly — ideally every single day. Even though you may want to set yourself a goal of running 5K every day, followed by a weights routine and a refreshing lap in the pool, how long can you keep it up until you burn out and stop exercising altogether? Instead, keep your exercise routine achievable. Aim for just over 20 minutes of moderate exercise per day — for example, a 20-minute brisk walk plus a short dumbbell routine. Exercise longer than 20 minutes if you're sticking to light exercise, and you can get away with shorter than 20 minutes if you're doing vigorous exercise. You might be inspired to do more, though, if you're having fun!

According to the CDC, examples of activities with different levels of exercise intensity are as follows:

>> **Light exercise:** Slow walking, stretching, playing table tennis, doing light housework such as washing the dishes, golfing with a cart.

>> **Moderate exercise:** Brisk walking, hiking, bicycling on flat terrain, doing water aerobics, practicing yoga, lifting weights, dancing (ballroom or folk), playing doubles tennis, gardening or doing yard work.

>> **Vigorous exercise:** Running or jogging, wheeling a wheelchair, bicycling on hilly terrain, doing aerobics, jumping rope, weightlifting with intensity, playing singles tennis, squash, or racquetball, swimming laps.

Years ago, I was notorious for going through obsessions with different types of exercise. For a few months it would be pilates, and then I'd go all in on the hot yoga. I'd go to classes every couple of days for a while. But then I'd get out of the routine, stop going, and not exercise at all. When I got serious about my gut health healing journey, I decided to be more realistic and tackle something that I could keep up for a long time. I started doing ten minutes of light running per day, rain or shine. Every day before lunch, I laced up my running shoes and jogged the same few city blocks. I covered a modest distance, but I could easily fit it into my day, every single day. This seemed to be a turning point in my gut health and overall health, showing the power of small but manageable increases in physical activity.

REMEMBER

Even if you have a physically active job, you should exercise recreationally for a couple of reasons:

>> Your work activities may be somewhat repetitive, so exercising for fun gets your body working in different ways, leading to greater health benefits.

>> Recreational exercise may benefit you more because relaxation and enjoyment are part of the benefits.

Creating your exercise regimen

TIP

If you have a diagnosed condition, before you begin any new exercise routine, check with your healthcare practitioner. In general, consider these tips for building your long-term exercise schedule:

>> **Go gradual when you're getting equipped for the type of exercise you want to do.** If you want to start weight training, for example, don't go out right away and buy the top-of-the-line weightlifting equipment. You don't have to get a gym membership right away, either. Buy the $20 set of dumbbells and start with a few minutes of weight exercises a day. Over time you'll figure out if you want to level up with new equipment or access gyms and trainers.

>> **Set a consistent time of day for your exercise.** When this time comes don't overthink it, just grab whatever gear you need and start.

>> **Use a video.** Many qualified fitness instructors offer free instruction online and can guide you through an exercise routine at home. You can choose many different durations or types of exercises. Experiment with a few until you find a style and instructor you like.

>> **If you've never had an exercise routine before, start with walking if your physical capabilities allow.** Find a destination around ten minutes from home and walk there and back daily. As you get used to this routine, you can try a brisker pace for one or more minutes during your walk, until you can walk the entire distance at a brisk pace.

Managing Stress

Stress is worry or mental tension caused by a difficult situation. The Vienna-born physician Hans Selye, who spent his working life at McGill University in Canada, is known as the founder of the stress theory. Selye advanced this theory in his 1956 book, *The Stress of Life*, and defined stress as the "nonspecific response of the body to any demand." (By *nonspecific*, he meant the response looked the same no matter what particular stressor was reported.) Thus, both in its origin and the way researchers currently understand it, the stress that people feel mentally is strongly connected to biological impacts.

Stress is a normal part of life — it's what happens when people engage meaningfully with life, pushing themselves to interact and succeed and grow. But stress over time can cause inflammation and lead to lasting physical consequences such as heart disease, stroke, obesity, or diabetes.

REMEMBER

If you don't manage your stress, you may tend to slip into maladaptive habits such as impulsive eating, excessive alcohol consumption, procrastination, or avoidance. The goal of managing stress is to flip the script so you replace these with adaptive habits that demonstrate your resilience. The sections that follow explain the impacts of short-term and chronic stress and offer tips for reducing their impacts.

Dealing with brief stressful moments

Fleeting daily moments of stress are part of the human condition — whether it's the nerves before public speaking or being late for an important appointment because of traffic. These moments trigger the body's fight-or-flight response. A flood of three main chemicals enters your bloodstream: epinephrine (adrenaline), norepinephrine, and cortisol. Your digestive system becomes less active to conserve energy. You may experience gut pain or diarrhea. But when the stressful moment passes, your body functions and chemical levels normalize. The gut symptoms and the mental vexation may go away, or they may linger for a short time after you're no longer in the stressful situation.

To cope with these moments of stress, you can do one of the following:

>> **Reduce the number of stressful situations you experience.** You can save yourself from having to experience traffic stress by leaving extra early for your appointment, for example. But then again, you can't control the traffic all the time.

>> **Develop adaptive ways of dealing with the situations when they arise.** You can adapt in a positive way that makes you stronger — otherwise known as *resilience*. This stress bounce-back skill can be developed over a lifetime. For example, you can control your body's reactions to the stress of heavy traffic and problem-solve to figure out the best way of dealing with the situation.

Here are some ways to increase your resilience to stressful moments:

>> **Become aware of how your body reacts in a stressful moment.** Does your jaw clench? Does your face feel hot? You can find easy ways to counteract these — for example, consciously relaxing your jaw muscle or stepping outside (if possible) for some fresh air.

>> **Establish a go-to deep breathing exercise that you can do when you feel stressed out.** Step into a bathroom stall or go for a brief walk, giving yourself two minutes to go through the exercise.

>> **Establish and stick to your exercise routine.** Exercise is an excellent stress reliever. Refer to the section "Exercising on a Regular Basis" earlier in this chapter.

>> **Regularly practice mindfulness meditation.** These include any one of a range of techniques that promote awareness of the present moment and calm acceptance of thoughts and feelings. Meditation practices help you feel more at peace and diminish your stress response.

To meditate, find an environment that works for you, whether it's sitting in a quiet room or sitting on a park bench with a favorite view. You can either sit quietly and focus on the present moment, or use a video or app (for example, Calm or Headspace) to guide your meditation. Yoga classes can also be meditative, encouraging you to pay attention to your body in the moment.

If you're interested in finding out more, check out the recent editions of books ranging from *Mindfulness For Dummies* by Shamash Alidina, *Meditation For Dummies* by Stephan Bodian, and *Yoga For Dummies* by Larry Payne, Brenda Feuerstein, and Georg Feuerstein (all by John Wiley & Sons, Inc.).

>> **Set aside time in your schedule for an activity that relaxes you mentally.** Examples include listening to music, playing a musical instrument, working on a jigsaw puzzle, knitting, or getting lost in a good mystery novel. Plan when you know you have a demanding day, and make sure you schedule time for one of these activities before bed.

TIP

USING THE GUT TO CALM THE BRAIN

Deep breathing is a simple and highly effective way to trick your brain into feeling calmer. When you take a belly breath, your *vagus nerve* (a collection of neurons running between your gut and the base of your brain) sends a signal up to your brain that all is well, relaxing you from the belly up.

Here's an example of a breathing exercise you can use to calm your brain any time you have two minutes to spare:

1. **Sit or stand in a place where you'll be undisturbed.**

   Close your eyes or keep them open and fixed on a single point.

2. **Slowly inhale air through your nose as you count to 10, letting your belly gently rise as you do so.**

3. **Exhale the air rapidly through your mouth while pushing your belly flat.**

4. **Pause for a few seconds to feel the sensation in your body.**

   Repeat several times.

   To level up, you may also want to incorporate gentle humming or vocalizing on the exhale (like the "om" in some yoga classes) because the vocal cord vibration may have a further calming effect on your nervous system.

Practice increasing your resilience before stressful moments happen, so you'll have a strategy ready to implement when you do experience one of these moments. You may not be able to implement the strategy right away in the moment, but shortly after you experience stress, you can undertake an activity that will help you feel relaxed and alert again.

Coping with chronic stress

Chronic stress is a consistent feeling that you're pressured and overwhelmed, experienced over a long period of time. This type of stress is especially dangerous when it comes to your health because it activates your stress response system and gives you regular exposure to cortisol and other hormones that disrupt normal body functioning. People who report greater chronic stress are at an increased risk for heart disease, obesity and metabolic syndrome, type 2 diabetes, arthritis, and mental health conditions such as anxiety and depression and problems with memory and focus.

Digestive problems also go hand in hand with chronic, low-level stress because digestive tract function can be overactive. This type of stress can trigger or worsen digestive diseases such as irritable bowel syndrome (IBS), inflammatory bowel disease, or acid reflux. In fact, IBS is said to be a stress-sensitive disorder, meaning that the symptoms are highly dependent on the level of stress someone experiences. Stress also directly affects the gut microbiota, reducing bacteria associated with better health. They may even be involved in the mechanisms of how stress affects the body; for example, they may contribute to increased inflammation and impaired cognitive performance under conditions of chronic stress.

Avoiding the negative health effects of chronic stress is like dealing with acute stress, which I discuss in the preceding section, and comes down to these two things simultaneously.

Managing sources of chronic stress

Managing the origins of chronic stress in your life is highly personal and comes down to your unique circumstances. If you're stressed out with no relief in sight, it may be worth considering some big-picture adjustments in your life. These steps can help you:

1. Pinpoint the source(s) of stress.

Some places to look include work demands, a specific person, or a part of your schedule.

2. After you identify the source, you can brainstorm strategies for reducing this source of stress.

I'm not advocating impulsively quitting your job. Think through any big decisions because for example, if you leave your job suddenly, the work-related chronic sources of stress may be replaced by financial ones. But maybe you can come up with creative solutions that reduce your chronic stress while allowing you to thrive and move forward. You don't have to entirely remove your exposure to the stressor, but reducing exposure may be helpful.

3. Pick a strategy to implement.

Discuss the strategies with trusted people in your life and decide which one to put into practice. You may want to implement the strategy that's the easiest or has the least impact on the rest of your life. See if it makes a noticeable difference in how you feel.

In the period when I experienced difficult gut health issues, I had a stressful job with constantly shifting demands and a relentless schedule. As part of my plan to manage stress, I negotiated with my employer to transition to four days a week rather than full time. There was only a slight decrease in salary and my chronic stress was much lower because I had more recovery time in my week.

Increasing your resilience so you cope in a positive manner

To become more resilient in the face of chronic stress, try the following:

>> **Invest time in developing strong relationships with family and friends.** These people provide the foundation for getting through stressful times. Meet a friend for lunch, join a support group or club, or offer to accompany a neighbor while walking their dog.

>> **Write several pages in a journal daily.** Writing whatever comes to your mind forces you to put your muddled thoughts into clear words. After they're on the page in a linear organization, they become easier to manage. After you write, you may decide to keep your thoughts for later or immediately crumple up the page and throw it away.

>> **Practice mindful eating.** The concept of mindful eating involves taking your meals without distractions, allowing you to pay attention to the present moment and the flavors and textures of your food. Remember when you're chronically stressed, your digestive system doesn't work optimally, so eating mindfully can make all the difference in getting proper nourishment from your food physically as well as mentally. It also helps you tune into how your body feels so you'll be more likely to stop eating when you feel full and less likely to turn to excessive eating to cope with stress.

Going Outside

Spending time outdoors in natural environments through activities such as hiking, camping, or sitting in the park, is a way to gain exposure to a diverse collection of microbes that are associated with the outdoors. For gut health, certain microbes from the outdoors may increase diversity and provide beneficial effects.

SCIENTIST SAYS

They may even be the microbial "old friends" that evolved in tandem with humans, as proposed by Graham Rook, a professor of medical microbiology at University College London in the United Kingdom. In his recent writings, Rook points out that traditional homes were built with products such as timber, mud, and thatch, so that the microbes residing in the homes would have resembled the microbes of the natural environment. Modern homes in industrialized countries, built with an abundance of plastic, glass, concrete, and metal, separate individuals from the natural environment and drastically reduce facetime with the outdoor microbes.

But getting your fill of outdoor microbes isn't to say you should get careless about hygiene. (See the section "Taking precautions against infection" later in this chapter for more information.) Nor should you deliberately let your indoor environment become dirty. It does mean the microbial exposures in nature are desirable and you should adjust your lifestyle to maximize exposure to the natural environment wherever possible. The following sections provide details on spending time outdoors and doing specific activities that bring you into contact with diverse microbes.

Bathing in nature

Is there a spot in nature where you feel completely relaxed and at peace? Maybe it's feeling a breeze on a rocky beach? Or deep in a mossy forest with the spongy ground underneath you? This sensation of peace in nature can arise from something called *forest bathing* — a form of deliberate relaxation involving time spent in a forest or another outdoor setting, focusing on the sensory experience of being in nature. Even though the research in this area is just starting to emerge, some studies show spending time among diverse outdoor microbes may change the diversity of microbes in your gut or on your skin, thereby influencing your immune system.

REMEMBER

Get exposure to the outdoors every day for 15 minutes or more. Here are some ideas to implement this recommendation safely and enjoyably:

>> If you have a minor outdoor chore, such as taking out the garbage, take a few extra minutes outside after you complete the chore. Find a place to sit or stand and notice everything around you, or just close your eyes and relax.

>> Don't let a little inclement weather stop you from enjoying the outdoors. Equip yourself with weather-appropriate clothing and get out into the elements.

>> If you live in a very cold or very hot climate and don't relish the thought of going outside, open a window for a short period of time daily and enjoy the fresh air.

WARNING

When you're out enjoying nature while hiking or camping, never drink water from a stream or lake *unless* it's been filtered. As pure and refreshing as it may look, the water can carry bacteria or parasites that can make you ill for a short (or even a long) time.

Getting your hands dirty

Soil contains beneficial microbes — some that have been isolated and are currently sold as probiotic supplements. So, when you get your hands dirty by working in the garden, you're giving yourself exposure to a diverse mix that may include these specifically beneficial microbes. Some scientists have even hypothesized that soil microbes help calm your immune system, so it doesn't overreact to harmless substances.

Animal-related chores can also give you exposure to a diversity of microorganisms — the origin of the *farm effect* hypothesis, after all, was the observation that children who lived on farms and had exposure to farm animals were protected against certain immune-related diseases. (Chapter 18 discusses this further.) Whether this protection comes from spending time in the barn or microbes carried into the house isn't certain. But the upshot is that the children experienced a health benefit from living in this environment. Even if you don't live on a farm there may be specific activities you can do to come into contact with potentially beneficial microbes.

Here are some ideas for getting your hands dirty:

>> Keep a garden and tend to it regularly during the growing season. If you lack an appropriate outdoor space, have a small planter indoors where you can grow herbs or other plants.

>> Spend time with pets. After you spend time touching pets, always wash your hands.

>> Volunteer for a community or school gardening project where you can get your hands dirty while you socialize with others.

>> During the growing season, shop at farmers' markets where you can pick a bundle of organic vegetables with dirt still attached. Brush off the dirt and eat the vegetables raw.

Looking at Other Lifestyle Factors

Some additional lifestyle factors can play a supporting role in your gut health, which the following sections discuss. By implementing these suggestions over the long term, you can set yourself up for a scientifically solid lifetime of gut health.

Adjusting when you eat

Chapter 10 covers what types of foods you should eat for a gut-friendly diet. However, it's not just what you eat, but when you eat that can affect gut health.

Time-restricted eating (TRE) is a pattern of eating that limits the hours during which you ingest your food. Different TRE plans use different windows of time for ingesting food, which can be anywhere from 4 to 12 hours per day. You may or may not consume fewer calories this way, but research suggests that eating the same number of calories in a more restricted window of time leads to a healthier weight, better blood sugar levels, and lower levels of inflammation. Scientists think this has to do with the body's circadian clock, which regulates aspects of metabolism and immunity on a 24-hour cycle.

A specific connection to gut health exists in that TRE noticeably alters the gut microbiota, leading to greater microbial diversity. Because your gut microbes are attuned to the day-night cycle as well, TRE may be giving your gut a needed break when your gut microbiota can do their housekeeping. The microbes' prolonged break from contact with food may even contribute to the metabolic benefits of TRE.

REMEMBER

The optimal number of hours to restrict eating has yet to be determined. But in the meantime, you can try to limit the hours in which you ingest food. Try the following science-backed tips:

>> Eat breakfast first thing in the morning and aim to have your last bite of food for the day no more than 12 hours later. For example, if you ate breakfast at 7:30 a.m., you'd finish your dinner no later than 7:30 p.m. and avoid snacks after this time.

>> If you're tempted to snack late at night, drink clear fluids such as water or herbal tea.

Taking precautions against infection

Exposure to microbes can be good — except to certain ones that cause disease. Infections are triggered by disease-causing bacteria, viruses, fungi, or parasites, which enter the body, multiply, and interfere with normal functioning. On many occasions the infection goes away after a short time, but sometimes longer-term consequences affect gut or overall health — for example, in post-infectious IBS or infection with the Epstein-Barr virus, which may predispose specific individuals to develop multiple sclerosis many years later. Infections can also have collateral damage on the gut microbiota.

REMEMBER

Good hygiene is essential for reducing your risk of infections because when you're exposed to an adequate dose of a pathogen, your immune system doesn't have a fighting chance and you're very likely to get sick. Pay special attention to hygiene in crowded areas or spaces used by a lot of people. Here are some best practices for reducing your risk of infection:

>> **In public places, avoid touching your face.** You may accidentally touch a mucous membrane such as the corner of your eye, where a pathogen can take hold.

>> **Wash your hands at every opportunity.** Do so not just after using the bathroom or before preparing food or eating, but also when coming in from outdoors, after blowing your nose, and after spending time with a pet. Thorough handwashing (and I mean really getting in there and scrubbing those paws – back, front, between the fingers, under the fingernails) is an incredibly effective way to stop the spread of pathogens.

>> **Don't share dishes, glasses, or cutlery with other people without washing them.** Saliva can spread pathogens from one person to another, so reduce the chances of disease spread by not sharing dishes and cutlery. Soap and hot water is adequate for washing dishes between users.

>> **Wash all cuts and cover them with a bandage.** This protects them against infection from microbes and discourages you from picking at or touching them.

>> **Stay current on your vaccinations.** As a public health measure, vaccinations have been incredibly effective at reducing life-threatening infections across the globe. Follow the advice in your area for which vaccinations to get.

>> **Avoid contact with wild animals.** Not only is it better for the animals if you leave them alone, but you also reduce the chances of acquiring a *zoonotic* infection, which is a pathogen that jumps from an animal to a human.

Knowing the impact of medical interventions

Medical interventions are usually recommended to you for very good reasons. But awareness is key — you can follow the guidance of your healthcare professionals while being alert to how certain interventions may impact your gut microbes and overall gut health. When you know the effects of medical treatments on your gut microbiota, you can take steps to mitigate any impacts. For example, if you have an infection that requires antibiotics, you can eat more fiber or ingest certain probiotics. Refer to Chapter 4 for which medications and other interventions tend to impact the gut microbiota negatively.

The best strategy is prevention, though. If you implement the tips in Chapter 10 and this chapter, you may be able to avoid some microbiota-disturbing medical treatments in the first place, keeping your gut community healthy and thriving.

Chapter **12**

Becoming Savvy with Gut Health Science

nformation related to gut health appears in countless advertisements, books, blog posts, media articles, and social media posts (including those with the hashtag #guttok, which frequently trends on TikTok). Celebrities have jumped on board, too. Whereas in 2007 the actress Jamie Lee Curtis was viewed as brave for endorsing Activia yogurt for digestive health, today a whole parade of celebrities, from Kate Hudson to Gwyneth Paltrow, endorse various probiotic products.

Hype (or exaggerated statements about importance and benefits) is rampant in the area of gut health, as it is in any popular area of health and wellness. Gut microbiome testing companies assert that they'll "make chronic illness optional" and probiotic sellers tout their products' singlehanded ability to balance the immune system. Influencers share the surprising fact that around 90 percent of the body's *serotonin* (known as a feel-good hormone) is produced in the gut, without mentioning the fact that this serotonin doesn't reach the brain. Even though some of this hype is shared by individuals who simply don't know better, it's more often disseminated by those who have a financial motivation.

WARNING

Rina Raphael, journalist and author of *The Gospel of Wellness*, explains that companies often use words from emerging scientific areas to create a sheen of scientific legitimacy and market products that are unproven. She says this phenomenon amounts to *science-washing,* or "exaggerating benefits by invoking scientific jargon, distorting research studies, or oversimplifying the nuances of biological chemistry" — similar to the classic phenomenon of blinding with science, when people who want an air of credibility use technical-sounding words to cause confusion.

Raphael says that besides the time and money that people waste when they fall for this type of misinformation, there can be real medical consequences. She says, "These products and protocols potentially replace actual science-backed interventions and rob consumers of real therapeutic opportunities. What if someone depends on a useless supplement instead of getting the legitimate medical diagnosis or treatment?"

Science-washing is all too common in the area of gut health. But in this environment where scientific language is used regardless of whether any actual evidence exists, legitimate information can be difficult to identify. This chapter gives you some clues on how to spot misinformation and how to look at gut health products with a critical eye so you select the one(s) that have the best chance of improving your gut health. My hope is that you'll take the basic information in this chapter and apply it in the real world when you encounter new information about gut health. Stay curious — and also critical!

Seeking Science-Based Information on Gut Health

In the landscape of online information, people who create digital content aren't always incentivized to tell scientifically credible truths. It's a shameful little secret known by social media influencers: Saying something surprising and untrue often gets rewarded with more likes and engagement than sharing a boring truth.

Addressing the veracity of every piece of gut health information shared online would take many more pages than the ones in this book. So instead of doing that, here I give you some basic principles for identifying credible science-based information in the digital world.

Evaluating online information

You're scrolling on your phone one evening and you come across an article on melatonin (a hormone associated with sleep) and the gut. You're a bit surprised by the information and you want to know if it's backed up by evidence. Look for these positive signs that the information you're reading is scientifically credible:

>> A person, preferably one with medical or scientific knowledge/credentials, is listed as the author or social media account owner.

Someone should be standing behind the information, so be wary of what you read on faceless company accounts or unnamed individuals with nicknames such as "The Gut Explorer."

>> A published scientific study is linked or cited for the key points of the article or post. Some social media platforms are set up to easily share links, but others don't allow clickable links so they may have a citation that helps you find the supporting scientific study.

>> The article or post mentions the limitations of the study or product. An unequivocally positive post may not provide a proper perspective on what a study does and doesn't show.

>> The information isn't directly linked to an online space where you can buy something. If the sole purpose of the online information is to drive you to purchase something, you may not be able to trust it. Seek information instead from online sources that don't link you directly to the product or category of products that's being discussed.

Looking to AI for answers

Artificial intelligence (AI) language models have many exciting applications and are undoubtedly changing how people create and consume online information. The question is whether you should use them to find information about gut health online.

Unfortunately, the current publicly available AI language models aren't suitable for finding accurate health information. Some models are trained on information online, and when it comes to gut health, online information largely doesn't match what scientists consider to be evidence-based truths. Thus, the models are highly likely to give inaccurate answers. Even if the language model is trained on a body of scientific articles, the output may lack the necessary language nuance that would ensure its accuracy in scientific circles.

The answers given by AI chatbots lack context. Given a choice between finding information using a traditional online search versus an AI chatbot, an online search is more reliable because you're able to evaluate the source and cross-check the facts more easily.

Scrutinizing the science

If you're looking for credible information on gut health and a scientific study is presented as evidence, make sure the study shows what it's supposed to show. Furthermore, not all published science is of the same quality — some studies are more rigorous or provide stronger evidence than others.

For example, in 2016 the comedian and late-night talk show host John Oliver did a segment on the hyping of scientific studies. He gave the example of a study reported as evidence that drinking champagne reduced the risk of dementia, which in a news report was accompanied by pictures of people sipping from champagne flutes. The news item never mentioned the study was done only in rats, so it had questionable applicability to humans. Oliver demanded the news coverage provide pictures of the rats sipping from small champagne flutes for the sake of accuracy.

His point was that, even though all science is valuable as a report on what someone has observed about the world, not all science has direct relevance to humans.

Here are ways to ensure a scientific study related to gut health is relevant to humans and provides high-quality evidence:

>> Check if the study involved human participants. Research involving animals or cells are useful for laying the groundwork and helping scientists know what to study in humans, but they don't give a complete picture of what happens in people. For example, studies in which a gut microbiome from a person is transferred to a mouse can be informative but aren't directly translatable to humans. A *randomized, controlled trial* (in which a group of similar participants are randomly assigned to receive either the intervention or a look-alike intervention that's ineffective) typically produces high-quality evidence.

>> Check the year of the study's publication. If it was published ten or more years ago, more up-to-date observations may exist.

>> Verify that the study was *peer-reviewed* (evaluated by scientific experts in the field) and published in a credible journal. Each journal has an *impact factor* (a metric of how often the articles tend to be cited in other places), with good journals having an impact factor of 3 or more.

>> If possible, find a *meta-analysis* that pulls together the results from multiple individual studies. These analyses provide much stronger evidence than single studies.

Understanding science news

As the topic of gut health garners more interest, the media responds and reports on gut health and microbiome studies more frequently. But not all science news reporting is equally rigorous, so you should maintain a healthy skepticism when you see a new headline.

After an important scientific study is published, the normal process for science news reporting is that the university or research center produces a press release highlighting the results of that study. The press release often has a positive spin because its purpose is to make the results seem exciting and relevant; but all too often, a press release veers toward hype or even misleading information about the study.

Some media outlets then take the press release and publish it with few or no changes, parroting the headline and thereby perpetuating the hype. Because of time constraints or a lack of knowledge about the topic, the reporter may not even read the original study. However, the better media outlets get the reporter to dig deeper, using the press release as a starting point but not reproducing it outright.

REMEMBER

When you come across an interesting gut health–related science news article, don't immediately assume it has been reported in a balanced manner. Here are some signs of a better-quality science news article:

>> Rather than only reporting on one new study, the article mentions multiple studies that give context and either support or refute its conclusions.

>> The article includes details about how the scientists reached a certain conclusion — at minimum, whether the study was done in humans or animals and how many participants were included. (A larger number of participants may increase the certainty of the conclusion.)

>> The article mentions limitations of the study — not only what it showed, but what it didn't show.

>> The article includes a comment from researchers not involved in the published study. Such comments can help put the study into context.

Making Sure You Don't Waste Your Money on Bogus Products and Tests

A huge number of products and tests sold directly to consumers are touted as solutions for better gut health. Probiotics are the best known, but they're only the beginning — other offerings include prebiotics, synbiotics, postbiotics, and special forms of fiber such as potato starch. You can have your gut microbiome tested, and then receive not only dietary advice but also supplement recommendations based on the results.

The significant commercial activity in this area is exciting. After all, no gut health product can reach customers without a company bringing it to them. And often companies put significant risk and investment into making a product or service safe and suitable for delivery to consumers.

Unfortunately, however, the quality of these products and services varies. And very few of them have rigorous scientific evidence that they actually do anything for gut health — so they rely on slick Instagram images and white-coat-clad actors to convince unwitting consumers to hand over their money. The problem is that the process that companies follow for discovering, formulating, manufacturing, and marketing biotics and other gut health dietary supplements isn't set up for consumer transparency, so it can be difficult to judge the quality of a product and the evidence behind it.

When I suffered from gut symptoms and didn't have a medical diagnosis, I was willing to try almost anything for relief. This helpless position made me vulnerable to the marketing messages of the companies selling gut health products. Hence, I spent hundreds of dollars on digestive enzymes, herbal supplements, tinctures, and probiotics of questionable quality, none of which gave me relief.

But now I realize that finding products that are science-backed and high-quality (that is, manufactured to a high standard by a reputable company) is possible with a little know-how. The ground rules that follow can steer you toward better, more effective products and avoid wasting your money.

Understanding the basic principles

Three foundational principles can help set your expectations when you look to purchase a gut-focused product or service:

>> **Principle No. 1:** No miracle product exists. Usually to improve or optimize gut health you need to address multiple factors at once: your stress levels, sleep

patterns, diet, and more. Perhaps a specific product will help you along in your journey, but it's unlikely to change your gut health overnight.

>> **Principle No. 2:** The vast majority of products sold directly to consumers are relatively safe substances that have been formulated based on some plausible theory of why they should work, but they haven't been specifically tested in humans to ensure they work. Likewise, current gut microbiome consumer tests give you accurate information about your gut microbes, but their dietary advice is based on theory rather than hard science. Finding the products with scientific evidence behind them is the best way to ensure you don't waste your money.

>> **Principle No. 3:** For probiotics and the other biotics, countless studies have shown that in a general population of humans, some people tend to respond well to the intervention and others don't respond at all. Scientists don't yet know what creates the right context for them to work, but further research on individual responses is currently addressing this question. Thus, keep in mind that your response to a product may be different from others.

TIP

To make the most of your time and money, choose a gut health product that's shown to work for the issue you want to address. For example, different probiotic products have been shown to work for reducing antibiotic-associated diarrhea, for alleviating symptoms of irritable bowel syndrome, and so on. In the United States, one easy way to find a probiotic product that works for your symptom is to check out the Clinical Guide to Probiotic Products Available in USA at https://usprobioticguide.com/. This free online tool links probiotic evidence to specific products you can purchase. A similar tool exists in Canada: the Clinical Guide to Probiotic Products Available in Canada at www.probioticchart.ca/.

Approaching anecdotes with caution

Social media influencers are great for sharing what's new in hairstyles, makeup, and fashion. They can also give you great ideas on what to make for dinner. But when it comes to products to improve your health, a fatal flaw exists with the influencer model: They rely on anecdote.

An influencer may show convincing before and after photos of how a probiotic reduced their distended belly, or they may recount how their mood improved dramatically after taking a gut health supplement. Yet, a single person's experience with the product is in the realm of anecdote, so it's not good evidence that the product works. If the product has been scientifically tested and shown to work across a group of people, then the influencer doesn't need to tell you how the product affected them personally. Not to mention that an influencer's financial reward almost guarantees they give a positive report rather than tell the truth.

Anecdotes from doctors or other medical professionals, describing how a product has worked for one of their patients or multiple patients over time, may be slightly more convincing. But even these reported experiences don't carry the same weight as a scientific study.

Ultimately, no personal story in the world is as powerful for showing something works as scientific data. So, if an influencer makes you aware of a product or test for gut health and you're interested to try it, dig deeper and find out if any evidence exists for how effective it is.

Looking for clues on the label

REMEMBER

The label is the first thing you should examine on a gut health product such as a probiotic. What follows are some important components of a label and the clues that indicate a good quality product:

>> **A clear description of the product:** The label should describe exactly what substance is contained in the product. For probiotics, the label should list the genus, species, and strain of each microorganism. (It shouldn't have just the species *Lacticaseibacillus rhamnosus*, for example, but *Lacticaseibacillus rhamnosus* GG — the last numbers or letters being the all-important strain designation.)

>> **The dose or serving size:** For high-quality biotics that have been tested, the amount or dose matters to how effective they are. Probiotic quantity should be shown on the label as colony-forming units (CFU) or active-fluorescent units (AFU), and other substances are generally shown as grams or milligrams. There's no set dose that you should be looking for because it depends on what has been tested and shown to be effective for a specific symptom.

>> **Storage instructions:** For probiotics, high-quality products usually specify a temperature range for storing the product. Not all probiotics need to be refrigerated, but some stores keep them refrigerated anyhow to increase the chances of maintaining their quality.

>> **Expiration or best before date:** Products have a shelf life, for the duration of which their quality is guaranteed. After the best before date, the quality may vary — for example, after expiration the quantity of live microorganisms in each pill may be less than what's specified on the label, leaving you with an ineffective dose.

>> **Company name and contact information:** The label should have information that directs you to where you can find out more about the product.

>> **Third-party certification(s):** Various types of third-party (outside the company) certifications are available for gut health products. These certifications are voluntary, and if present, they can increase your confidence in the product. They

show, for example, that the product contains what it says it contains, is consistent from batch to batch, is free of contamination, and so on. IPRO (International Probiotic Standards) is an example of a third-party certification.

Finding the supporting evidence

When you consider purchasing a gut health product, don't settle for blanket assurances in a company's marketing materials that they value science. Try to find the science for yourself. No matter where you hear about a product — an ad, a website, a friend, a store employee, a healthcare professional — your main question should be: Where is the evidence that this product works?

TIP

Here's how to find the scientific evidence that backs up the safety and effectiveness of a probiotic product before you buy it:

>> **Look on the label for the strain or group of strains.** If the label has only one strain, type it into the search bar of PubMed (a database of published scientific articles from the most reputable journals). If the label has multiple strains with a formulation name such as "Gut Restore," you can try typing in the formulation name. If nothing comes up, type several of the strain names in the search bar and see if the results feature the whole formulation.

>> **Limit the search to studies in humans by checking off the "Clinical Trial" box under the article type.** This action ensures you get only studies with results that apply to human populations.

>> **Look through the articles in the results list.** Pick an article and scan through the *abstract* (the brief summary that precedes a scientific article) to find out what health effects the strain(s) had on the participants. If this is similar to the effects you're looking for, the product may be a good fit. Check whether the other articles in the search results list have similar findings.

TIP

You can use the same approach to find the science behind other biotics — just make sure you search for the main ingredient in the product. Pay attention to the amount or dose used in the study, because if you want the same health effect, it should be the same amount that's in your product.

TIP

If no results come up in PubMed, evidence still may exist, but you'll have to dig a little further. Try the following:

>> **Search for the strain or ingredient on** `www.clinicaltrials.gov`. This website is a record of human studies that are currently underway but not yet published. One or more studies focused on the ingredient can indicate an ongoing interest and willingness to invest in proving its effectiveness.

>> **Look on the company's website for specific evidence on its product.** You may need to click through a disclaimer or download a document to find the studies.

WARNING

Rina Raphael notes that wellness companies sometimes pad their website's science section with links to scientific studies that have little to do with the product. Some of the research they include may be a summary of emerging science or an animal study with indirect relevance.

>> **Contact the company and ask for a summary of scientific evidence on their product.** Someone may be able to send you a slide deck or share internal data (not published in a scientific journal) showing evidence of its efficacy. Occasionally a healthcare professional needs to request this information on your behalf.

These tips apply when you have a specific issue you're looking to address with a gut health product. If you aren't experiencing any specific symptom, but you still want to generally improve or optimize your gut health, then you may still want to look up whether or not the product has been tested for any health effects. Sometimes products are shown to have a beneficial effect in healthy people, such as reducing sugar cravings.

However, if you just want to increase your intake of live cultures (see Chapter 10) to impart general health benefits, you may not need evidence that a product works for a specific symptom. Instead, look for a high-quality product that gives you a high dose of live cultures.

Also pay attention to the evidence on the safety of gut health products. Every study should mention detrimental health effects that the participants experienced while they were taking the product to give a clear picture of the risks versus the benefits.

CONSIDERING WHETHER THE SCIENCE FROM COMPANIES IS CREDIBLE

Often, studies showing the effectiveness of a product or ingredient are carried out by the same company that sells it. Even though at first glance this appears to be a conflict of interest, with reputable and well-resourced companies the science remains credible and can still be taken as good evidence that the product works.

Here are some guardrails that ensure the science done by companies has value:

- Some studies are done with collaborators at respected medical centers or universities whose reputation depends on leading and publishing well-conducted studies.

- Studies are often outsourced to clinical trials companies, which have protocols for conducting high-quality research.

- All studies involving humans need to be reviewed and monitored by an Institutional Review Board (IRB) to protect the welfare of participants. Best practices dictate an IRB should include a variety of experts and not just people who work at the company or have a financial interest.

- The company may need to provide regulators with evidence for certain claims, so they need to adhere to regulatory guidelines when they carry out their research.

Yes, some of these studies end up being biased and scientists sometimes criticize the way they were conducted. But in most cases, if the company selling the product doesn't run the study, then no one will. Investing in the science is a mark of a credible company that wants to give its product an edge by providing consumers with evidence that it works.

Hearing from experts

A good indicator of a high-quality, effective product is when experts are willing to recommend the product or mention it without financial motivation — either privately in a clinic visit or publicly in the media. The type of expert matters, however. The title "doctor" is no guarantee of expertise or credibility because the range of professionals and practitioners that go by this title can vary widely on how strongly they value scientific evidence. Some alternative medicine practitioners may not use scientific studies to inform their recommendations at all, for example.

Medical doctors (including specialists) and registered dietitians are trained to value scientific evidence and need to adhere to strict guidelines to retain their ability to practice, so they're among the most credible experts for recommending gut health products. On the other hand, if they're selling a product themselves, you may want to seek other experts' advice on that product. Furthermore, an expert with longtime clinical experience in gut health (as with a gastroenterologist) or someone who has published research in the area is more likely to provide a valuable opinion on a product.

Scrutinizing the company

In the competitive marketplace of gut health products, each time you buy a product you're voting with your dollars for the survival of the company that makes it. So another factor in your purchasing decisions should be whether you want to support that specific company.

The following are some markers of a credible science-based company:

>> **The company isn't newly established.** Although every company has to start somewhere, ones that have been around for more than a few years show they have some traction with consumers and/or healthcare professionals.

>> **The founders and executives have previous experience in health or life sciences companies.** Some gut health company founders have boasted that they'll disrupt the food and medical industries by coming with no experience and thinking outside the box. This bravado may be effective in the tech world, but it doesn't work in health-related fields. The food and drug industries have defined regulatory frameworks and best practices that have been established and adapted over time to protect people from harm. So knowledge and experience in health-related industries (including dealing with applicable regulations) is essential for those at the helm of a reputable company.

>> **Scientific advisors are listed on the company website.** Normally a science-based company will have a scientific advisory board made up of experts who agree to help guide the company's scientific direction but who don't benefit financially from the company's success. A website listing only the company cofounders and paid employees is a reason for caution. On the other hand, an extensive list of scientific advisors is also a red flag — a long list may be a public relations stunt because a company usually has a hard time engaging in a meaningful way with a large number of scientific advisors.

Judging how well a product or test works

Science can help you choose a product that's likely to work for a specific gut health issue, but the question is how it works when thrown into the mix of your unique physiology and lifestyle. Try to determine how well a product or test works for you as an individual.

When you adopt a new diet regime recommended by a test or start taking a new product, decide in advance how long you're willing to wait for the product to work. If a product is indeed effective, you should see results anywhere between two weeks and two months (or alternatively, however long it took to show results in a relevant scientific study). You may want to mark your calendar for a set period of time, or simply complete one bottle or package of the product, to remind yourself to evaluate how the product worked for you. Keeping a gut health journal (see Chapter 8) can be useful for this purpose.

If you're not taking the product for a specific reason, then you may not actually feel a difference after taking it for a period of time. However, if the product fits within your budget and you enjoy taking it, you may decide to continue as long as you haven't noticed any negative effects on your health and well-being.

4

Nourishing Yourself and Your Gut

Put into practice your gut health knowledge by creating meals and snacks that support the community of microorganisms living in your digestive tract.

Discover tips for making gut-nourishing meals quickly and easily.

Experiment with new flavors in tasty and colorful dishes.

Chapter **13**

Nourishing Soups & Salads

Here's a meal hack for eating in a way that nourishes your gut: Give yourself permission to make a meal of soup or salad. The traditional place of soups and salads may have been before the main meal, but it's time to think outside that box. Soups and salads can be hearty and satisfying — and they're a great way to mix multiple plant foods to get your 30 per week for gut microbiome diversity. And they need never get boring because you can make endless variations of soups and salads, depending on what's in the crisper drawer of your fridge.

This chapter gives you a variety of soup and salad recipes designed to boost your intake of plants, especially the gut-feeding fiber they contain. You can enjoy any one of them as a meal in itself.

Making Gut-Healthy Soups

Soups are one of the most flexible meals you can possibly make. All you need is a few minutes to put the basic ingredients together and get the base of the soup simmering, and then you can come back here and there to add ingredients and check how it tastes. I love making a soup on a lazy Sunday afternoon and sitting down to a simple dinner of soup and biscuits as the last meal before another busy week begins.

The following section features some of my favorite soup recipes that have a tasty mix of fiber sources, giving your gut the fuel it needs to do its important jobs. You can find these soup recipes:

» **Italian White Bean Soup:** This soup has a creamy texture from pureed beans that makes it comforting as well as filling.

» **Chicken Barley Soup:** This chicken barley soup is a higher fiber version of a classic chicken noodle soup. The added spinach makes it visually appealing and extra nourishing.

» **Kale Sausage Soup:** This is a frequently requested soup in my household, perfect for cold winter nights.

» **Buckwheat Noodle Miso Soup:** The buckwheat noodles cook quickly, making this easy, nourishing soup a great lunch at home. Try making it instead of instant ramen.

» **Double Pea Soup:** In this soup, dried peas add depth and fresh/frozen peas add brightness. It's delicious either hot or chilled.

Italian White Bean Soup

PREP TIME: 15 MIN	COOK TIME: 40 MIN	YIELD: 4 SERVINGS

INGREDIENTS

1 tablespoon (15 mL) extra-virgin olive oil

½ tablespoon (7 mL) butter

3 cloves garlic, peeled and chopped

1 cup (250 mL) sliced leek, well washed

1½ teaspoons (7 mL) ground thyme

2 teaspoons (10 mL) salt

Pinch of black pepper

2 cups (500 mL) chopped green kale, stems removed

1 cup (250 mL) celery, chopped

1 medium tomato, chopped

½ cup (125 mL) carrot, peeled and chopped

One 19-ounce (540 mL) can cannellini beans (white kidney beans), including liquid

2½ cups (625 mL) chicken broth

2½ (625 mL) cups water

1 cup (250 mL) additional cannellini beans (white kidney beans), drained

Balsamic vinegar and grated Parmesan cheese (optional)

DIRECTIONS

1 Heat the olive oil and butter in a large pot over medium heat. Add the garlic and leek and cook until soft, about 5 minutes. Add the thyme, salt, pepper, kale, celery, tomato, and carrot. Continue to cook for about 5 minutes or until the kale has softened slightly.

2 Meanwhile, put 1 can of beans (including liquid) in a blender (or a medium bowl, if using an immersion blender) and blend until smooth. Set aside.

3 Add the broth and water as well as the reserved cannellini bean puree to the pot. Cover and bring to a boil over medium-high heat, and then reduce the heat to medium.

4 Add the 1 cup (250 mL) of remaining beans and simmer for 30 minutes or more, until carrots and other vegetables are fork tender.

5 Serve hot, garnished optionally with Parmesan cheese or a few drops of balsamic vinegar.

VARY IT: Use vegetable broth to make this soup vegetarian.

PER SERVING: *Calories 282 (From Fat 70); Fat 8g (Saturated 2g); Cholesterol 71mg; Sodium 1575mg; Carbohydrate 24g (Dietary Fiber 7g); Protein 32g.*

Chicken Barley Soup

PREP TIME: 5 MIN | COOK TIME: 50 MIN | YIELD: 4 SERVINGS

INGREDIENTS

1 tablespoon (15 mL) extra-virgin olive oil

½ tablespoon (7 mL) butter

1 medium onion, chopped

5 cups (1.25 L) chicken or vegetable broth

2 cups (500 mL) water

2 teaspoons (10 mL) salt

Pinch of black pepper

½ teaspoon (2.5 mL) apple cider vinegar

⅓ cup (60 g) dry barley

3 medium carrots, peeled and chopped

1 teaspoon (5 mL) ground sage

½ teaspoon (2.5 mL) ground thyme

2 cups (500 mL) cooked, chopped chicken

5 ounces (150 mL) chopped frozen spinach (approximately half of a frozen package)

DIRECTIONS

1 Heat the olive oil and butter in a large pot on medium heat. Add the onion and sauté until softened, approximately 5 minutes.

2 Increase the heat to medium–high. Add the broth, water, salt, pepper, apple cider vinegar, barley, carrots, sage, and thyme. Bring to a boil.

3 Reduce the heat and add the chicken and frozen spinach. Simmer for 40 minutes or until the barley is tender.

NOTE: This recipe is the perfect use for leftover cooked chicken.

VARY IT: After a Thanksgiving meal, you can substitute the chicken with leftover turkey for equally tasty results.

PER SERVING: *Calories 290 (From Fat 84); Fat 9g (Saturated 3g); Cholesterol 58mg; Sodium 2237mg; Carbohydrate 21g (Dietary Fiber 5g); Protein 30g.*

Kale Sausage Soup

INGREDIENTS

3 mild pork or turkey sausages, frozen

1 tablespoon (15 mL) extra-virgin olive oil

1 medium onion, chopped

1 medium green pepper, chopped

5 cups (1.25 L) vegetable or chicken broth

1 teaspoon (5 mL) salt

Pinch of black pepper

Pinch of hot pepper flakes, optional

1 teaspoon (5 mL) apple cider vinegar

2 cups chopped green kale, stems removed

One 16-ounce (470 mL) can black beans, drained

DIRECTIONS

1 Thaw the sausages at room temperature for about 10 minutes and then slice into thin rounds while partially frozen.

2 Over medium–high heat, add the olive oil to a large pot. Then add the sausage, onion, and green pepper and cook, stirring constantly, until the sausage looks slightly brown, about 5 minutes.

3 Add the broth, salt, pepper, hot pepper flakes (if desired), apple cider vinegar, and kale. Bring to a boil and then reduce the heat to medium.

4 Add the black beans and simmer over medium heat until heated through, approximately 10 minutes.

TIP: Vegetable or chicken broth from a carton works well for this soup, but you can really bring it up a notch with homemade chicken broth.

PER SERVING: *Calories 381 (From Fat 121); Fat 14g (Saturated 3g); Cholesterol 49mg; Sodium 1983mg; Carbohydrate 40g (Dietary Fiber 9g); Protein 28g.*

☁ Buckwheat Noodle Miso Soup

INGREDIENTS

2 cups (500 mL) vegetable broth

1 cup (250 mL) water

½ teaspoon (2.5 mL) salt

Pinch of black pepper

1 teaspoon (5 mL) rice vinegar

One 1-inch (2.5 cm) piece of fresh ginger, peeled

1 bundle (1-inch or 2.5 cm in diameter) soba

2 cups (500 mL) raw broccoli florets, chopped

1 tablespoon (15 mL) red miso

2 tablespoons (30 mL) additional cold water

Kimchi to garnish (optional)

DIRECTIONS

1 Combine the broth, water, salt, pepper, rice vinegar, and ginger in a medium pot over medium–high heat and bring to a boil.

2 Remove the ginger with a slotted spoon and discard. Add the soba and vegetables and boil for 5 to 6 minutes or until vegetables are lightly cooked.

3 Remove from the heat and cool for 2 to 3 minutes. Meanwhile, combine the miso with the additional 2 tablespoons water in a small dish and mix with a fork to make a smooth paste.

4 Add the miso paste to the soup and stir gently to combine. Ladle into serving bowls and top with kimchi.

NOTE: *Soba* are thin Japanese noodles made with between 40 percent and 100 percent buckwheat flour. You're likely to find them at an Asian grocer or the Asian section of the grocery store, and they're often packaged in serving-size bundles.

NOTE: Red miso is recommended here, but white miso works equally well.

VARY IT: Substitute chopped cauliflower, asparagus, or other firm vegetables for the broccoli.

VARY IT: Optional added toppings, depending on your taste, include a fried egg, half a hard-boiled egg, fresh spinach, pickled radishes, pepper flakes, and/or sriracha.

PER SERVING: *Calories 398 (From Fat 26); Fat 3g (Saturated 1g); Cholesterol 0mg; Sodium 2421mg; Carbohydrate 78g (Dietary Fiber 3g); Protein 22g.*

Double Pea Soup

PREP TIME: 5 MIN	COOK TIME: 55 MIN	YIELD: 4 SERVINGS

INGREDIENTS

½ tablespoon (7 mL) butter

1 tablespoon (15 mL) extra-virgin olive oil

1 medium onion, chopped

1 cup (250 mL) sliced leek, well washed

1¾ teaspoons (9 mL) salt

Pinch of black pepper

5 cups (1.25 L) vegetable broth

1½ cups (375 mL) water

⅓ cup (75 g) dried split peas, green

2 cups (500 mL) frozen peas

Fresh parsley, chopped (optional)

DIRECTIONS

1   Melt the butter and olive oil in a large pot over medium heat. Add the onion and leek and cook until softened, approximately 5 minutes.

2   Add the salt, pepper, broth, water, and split peas. Increase heat to medium–high and bring to a boil. Reduce heat and simmer covered for 40 minutes or until the split peas are tender.

3   Add the frozen peas and simmer for 5 to 10 minutes until heated through. Remove from heat and cool slightly.

4   Pour into a blender or use an immersion blender to puree the soup. Serve garnished with fresh parsley.

TIP: Use fresh peas in place of frozen if they happen to be in season or readily available.

PER SERVING: *Calories 234 (From Fat 63); Fat 7g (Saturated 2g); Cholesterol 4mg; Sodium 2052mg; Carbohydrate 28g (Dietary Fiber 9g); Protein 15g.*

Assembling Salads for a Well-Fed Gut

Stereotypical salad has a reputation for being a little dull: iceberg lettuce, shredded carrot, and a mealy tomato. Luckily, salad has come a long way. Walk into any supermarket and you can find multiple types of lettuce, bite-sized veggies and cheese to throw on top, and croutons and other crunchy toppings. The diversity of salads you can make is only limited by your imagination.

TIP

The most important gut-saving tip about salads, though, is to always make your own dressing. Most commercial dressings have emulsifiers or other ingredients that aren't so good for the gut. So instead of reaching for that bottle of Italian dressing in the store, do what the real Italians do and pick up some olive oil, vinegar, and some regular or Dijon mustard. Those three ingredients are the basis of a tasty dressing that goes with almost any salad.

This section features a variety of inventive salads that will fill your belly while increasing your weekly plant count without the sneaky emulsifiers — helping you live your best gut life:

>> **Tangy Tuna and White Bean Salad:** Who knew tuna and white beans were such a perfect match? These hearty ingredients are offset by crunchy cucumber in this satisfying salad.

>> **Mexican Lentil Salad:** The dressing is the star of the show in this flavorful salad. For best results, eat the salad fresh.

>> **Summer Watermelon Salad:** This juicy and flavorful salad makes a great accompaniment to burgers, hot dogs, or other grilled foods.

>> **Greek Quinoa Salad:** Turn Greek salad into an entire meal by rounding it out with quinoa. This recipe is great to make for a potluck or summer picnic.

Tangy Tuna and White Bean Salad

PREP TIME: 10 MIN   YIELD: 6 SERVINGS

INGREDIENTS

2 cups (500 mL) English cucumber, chopped (approximately 1 medium cucumber)

One 19-ounce (540 mL) can cannellini beans (white kidney beans), drained

Two 6-ounce (170 g) cans chunk light tuna in water, drained

1 tablespoon (15 mL) chopped scallion

2 tablespoons (30 mL) capers, drained

2 tablespoons (30 mL) chopped parsley

DIRECTIONS

1 Combine the cucumber, beans, tuna, onion, capers, and parsley in a large salad bowl.

Dijon Dressing

INGREDIENTS

2 tablespoons (30 mL) extra-virgin olive oil

½ tablespoon (7 mL) Dijon mustard

2 tablespoons (30 mL) rice vinegar

1 tablespoon (15 mL) maple syrup

¼ (1.25 mL) teaspoon salt

Pinch of black pepper

DIRECTIONS

1 In a jar or small bowl, combine the olive oil, Dijon, rice vinegar, maple syrup, salt, and pepper. Mix well.

2 Pour the dressing over the ingredients in the bowl and mix until coated.

NOTE: This protein-packed salad makes a great lunch. Serve by itself or on a bed of chopped lettuce.

PER SERVING (USING 2 CANS): *Calories 240 (From Fat); Fat 5g (Saturated 1g); Cholesterol 60mg; Sodium 806mg; Carbohydrate 19g (Dietary Fiber 6g); Protein 28g.*

Mexican Lentil Salad

INGREDIENTS

1 cup (250 mL) cherry tomatoes, halved

½ cup (125 mL) canned black beans, drained

One 15-ounce (440 mL) can of lentils

One 12-ounce (350 mL) can of corn, drained

1 medium red pepper, chopped

2 tablespoons (30 mL) cilantro, chopped

DIRECTIONS

1 Combine the cherry tomatoes, black beans, lentils, corn, red pepper, and cilantro in a medium salad bowl.

Avocado Dressing

INGREDIENTS

½ medium avocado

¼ teaspoon (1.25 mL) lime zest

Juice of 1 lime

¼ cup (60 mL) plain kefir

1 teaspoon (5 mL) honey

Pinch of salt

Pinch of black pepper

DIRECTIONS

1 In a jar or small bowl, combine the avocado, lime zest and juice, kefir, honey, salt, and pepper. Pour into a blender and pulse to blend or use an immersion blender.

2 Pour the dressing over the ingredients in the bowl and mix until coated. Serve immediately.

NOTE: You can also cook your own lentils from dried ones. An advantage of home-cooked lentils is their nicer flavor, and you can also adjust the level of salt according to your preference.

PER SERVING: Calories 290 (From Fat 45); Fat 5g (Saturated 1g); Cholesterol 2mg; Sodium 25 mg; Carbohydrate 45g (Dietary Fiber 14g); Protein 16g.

Summer Watermelon Salad

INGREDIENTS

4 cups (1 L) seedless watermelon, cubed and with rind removed (approximately ¼ of a medium watermelon)

2 cups (500 mL) English cucumber, chopped (approximately 1 medium cucumber)

¼ cup (60 mL) mint, finely chopped

1 tablespoon (15 mL) scallion, chopped

½ cup (125 mL) feta cheese, crumbled

DIRECTIONS

1 Combine the watermelon, cucumber, mint, onion, and feta in a large salad bowl.

Dressing

INGREDIENTS

2 tablespoons (30 mL) extra-virgin olive oil

2 tablespoons (30 mL) apple cider vinegar

1 tablespoon (15 mL) Dijon mustard

½ teaspoon (2.5 mL) salt

Pinch of black pepper

2 teaspoons (10 mL) maple syrup

DIRECTIONS

1 In a jar or small bowl, combine the olive oil, vinegar, Dijon, salt, pepper, and maple syrup and stir until well mixed.

2 Pour the dressing over the ingredients in the bowl and mix gently. Refrigerate for approximately 1 hour before serving.

PER SERVING: *Calories 179 (From Fat 103); Fat 12g (Saturated 4g); Cholesterol 17mg; Sodium 550mg; Carbohydrate 17g (Dietary Fiber 1g); Protein 4g.*

🍅 Greek Quinoa Salad

INGREDIENTS

2 cups (500 mL) quinoa, cooked

1 medium red pepper, chopped

1 medium green or orange pepper, chopped

2 cups (500 mL) English cucumber, chopped (approximately 1 medium cucumber)

1 cup (250 mL) cherry tomatoes, halved

1 cup (250 mL) feta cheese, crumbled

½ cup (125 mL) kalamata olives, pitted and chopped

DIRECTIONS

1 Combine the quinoa, peppers, cucumber, cherry tomatoes, feta, and olives in a large salad bowl.

Dressing

INGREDIENTS

¼ cup (60 mL) extra-virgin olive oil

2 tablespoons (30 mL) balsamic vinegar

2 tablespoons (30 mL) Dijon mustard

1 teaspoon (5 mL) dried oregano

1 teaspoon (5 mL) salt

Pinch of black pepper

DIRECTIONS

1 In a jar or small bowl, blend the olive oil, balsamic vinegar, Dijon, oregano, salt, and pepper.

2 Pour the dressing over the ingredients in the bowl and mix until coated. Serve at room temperature or chilled.

NOTE: This potluck-sized salad works well with leftover quinoa, but you can also prepare fresh quinoa right before you make the salad.

TIP: To cook quinoa from dried, follow the package directions. To make fluffy quinoa you typically use slightly less than a 2:1 ratio of water to quinoa: say 1¾ cups water for every cup of dried quinoa.

VARY IT: Add a handful of diced red onion if you like stronger flavors.

PER SERVING: *Calories 196 (From Fat 119); Fat 13g (Saturated 4g); Cholesterol 17 mg; Sodium 623mg; Carbohydrate 16g (Dietary Fiber 3g); Protein 6g.*

Chapter **14**

Gut-Friendly Main Courses

D espite the vast array of foods available to many people at the supermarket and local grocery store and an endless supply of recipes online and on social media, the decision of what to make for dinner is surprisingly difficult. It's easy to feel overwhelmed — how can you pick one single dish from among the thousands of possibilities, while managing your shopping and meal prep time, your budget, as well as your taste preferences?

The good news is that letting your gut lead the way can make dinner planning easier. Equipped with guidelines for what to eat to nourish your digestive health, you'll zero in on some great possibilities that are as tasty as they are healthy.

This chapter gives you dinner ideas that are easy and delicious — and designed to support your digestive health. Enjoy these meals with the knowledge that you're prioritizing your digestive health and, in doing so, you're giving a gift to your future self.

Satisfying Your Gut with Plant-Based Meals

The way to get adequate amounts of gut-nourishing fiber is to base your meals around plants; the research shows consuming 30 or more types of plants per week is associated with the highest gut microbiome diversity. You don't necessarily need to cut out meat altogether in a gut-friendly diet, but it's beneficial to put plants front and center in your meals where possible, so your gut microbes have enough fiber for a proper feast.

You can find the following recipes in this section:

» **Roasted Vegetable Ratatouille:** Roasting veggies brings out their rich, full flavors, which blend together perfectly in this dish.

» **Butternut Cheesy Mac:** This nourishing dish is perfect for fall. Round out the meal with a green salad topped with pumpkin seeds.

» **Fantastic Veggie Frittata:** Make yourself popular at your next potluck by bringing this versatile dish, which can be served warm or cold. Or make it for yourself and enjoy it for breakfast or lunch.

» **Quick 'n Tasty Veggie Curry:** This meal is ideal for warming you up on a cold evening. Make extra because it tastes even better the next day.

» **Easy Chickpea Feta Bake:** This tasty meal is a variation on a sheet pan dinner, which involves putting all your dinner ingredients into one pan or dish and leaving it in the oven to bake.

» **Savory Miso Noodle Bowls:** An easy, well-rounded meal for when you're craving the rich, salty flavor of miso.

Roasted Vegetable Ratatouille

PREP TIME: 15 MIN	COOK TIME: 60 MIN	YIELD: 4 SERVINGS

INGREDIENTS

4 cups (1L) eggplant, peeled and cubed

3 tablespoons (45 mL) extra-virgin olive oil, divided

2 teaspoons (10 mL) salt, divided

2 cups (500 mL) zucchini, diced

2 cups (500 mL) uncooked butternut squash, peeled and cubed

1 tablespoon (15 mL) butter

1 cup (250 mL) onion, chopped

1 medium red bell pepper, seeded and chopped

4 medium vine-ripened tomatoes

2 tablespoons (30 mL) tomato paste

½ teaspoon (2.5 mL) dried oregano

1 tablespoon (15 mL) fresh basil, chopped

DIRECTIONS

1 Preheat the oven to 350 degrees F. Line two cookie sheets with parchment paper. On the first cookie sheet, spread out the eggplant and drizzle it with 1 tablespoon of the olive oil. Sprinkle ½ teaspoon (2.5 mL) of the salt over top.

2 On the second cookie sheet, spread out the squash and zucchini and drizzle them with 1 tablespoon of the olive oil. Sprinkle ½ teaspoon (2.5 mL) of the salt over top. Place the cookie sheets in the oven side by side and bake for 15 minutes.

3 Remove the eggplant from the oven (it should be tender). Stir the squash and zucchini and return them to the oven for an additional 10 minutes or until fork-tender. Set aside.

4 Meanwhile, over medium heat in a large pot, heat 1 tablespoon of the olive oil with the butter. Add the onion, red bell pepper, and 1 teaspoon of the salt. Sauté for 8 to 10 minutes, or until both the peppers and the onions are tender.

5 While the onion and peppers are cooking, prepare the tomatoes by grating them into a large bowl and chopping the remaining skin to add to the bowl.

6 Add the tomatoes (including their juice) to the cooked mixture. Add the eggplant, squash, and zucchini to the pot as well. Add the tomato paste and oregano, and then simmer on medium heat for 20 minutes to gently soften all the vegetables.

7 Increase the heat to high and simmer for 10 minutes, stirring frequently, until some of the liquid evaporates. Turn the heat to medium-low and simmer for an additional 5 minutes, or until the ratatouille reaches the desired consistency. Stir in the fresh basil and serve.

NOTE: Freshly shaved Parmesan cheese makes a great garnish for this flavorful ratatouille.

PER SERVING: *Calories 227 (From Fat 127); Fat 14g (Saturated 3g); Cholesterol 8mg; Sodium 1209mg; Carbohydrate 8g (Dietary Fiber 8g); Protein 4g.*

Butternut Cheesy Mac

INGREDIENTS

½ small butternut squash

1½ teaspoons (7.5 mL) salt, divided

3½ cups (700 g) uncooked high-fiber rotini pasta

1 cup (250 mL) 2% milk

1 tablespoon (15 mL) butter

½ teaspoon (2.5 mL) ground sage

2 cups (165 g) medium cheddar cheese, grated

2 tablespoons (30 mL) kefir

⅓ cup (50 g) panko breadcrumbs (whole wheat if available)

DIRECTIONS

1 Preheat the oven to 300 degrees F.

2 Slice the butternut squash lengthwise and scoop out the seeds. Place the squash face down on a parchment-lined baking sheet. Bake for about one hour, or until fork-tender. Remove from the oven and cool slightly. Adjust the oven to 350 degrees F.

3 Meanwhile, bring a large pot of water to a boil. Add ½ teaspoon (2.5 mL) of the salt, along with the uncooked pasta. Cook the pasta *al dente*, and then drain and set aside in a large bowl.

4 Peel the cooked squash and cut it into cubes. Add 2 cups (500 mL) of the cubed squash and the milk to a blender (or a medium bowl, if using an immersion blender). Blend until smooth.

5 In a medium pot over medium-low heat, melt the butter. Add the blended squash along with 1 teaspoon of the salt. Add the sage, grated cheese, and kefir. Whisk until all the cheese is melted in, approximately five to seven minutes.

6 Pour the sauce mixture over the pasta and mix until the pasta is coated. Transfer to a 9x9 baking dish and sprinkle the panko over top. Bake at 350 degrees F for 15 to 20 minutes, or until the top is slightly browned.

NOTE: *Al dente* means to cook the pasta until it's tender but slightly firm when bitten.

VARY IT: To make this dish vegan, use unsweetened oat or coconut milk instead of dairy milk, olive oil instead of butter, vegan cheese instead of dairy cheese, and plain vegan yogurt or cream cheese instead of kefir.

PER SERVING: *Calories 354 (From Fat 93); Fat 10g (Saturated 6g); Cholesterol 30mg; Sodium 1046mg; Carbohydrate 53g (Dietary Fiber 9g); Protein 14g.*

🍅 Fantastic Veggie Frittata

PREP TIME: 15 MIN	COOK TIME: 55 MIN	YIELD: 8 SERVINGS

INGREDIENTS

1 teaspoon (5 mL) butter

1 teaspoon (5 mL) extra-virgin olive oil

½ medium onion, chopped

1 teaspoon (5 mL) salt

2 cups (500 mL) assorted raw vegetables, chopped (broccoli, cauliflower, bell peppers, mushrooms, zucchini)

½ cup (5 oz or 140 g) frozen spinach, thawed, with liquid pressed out through a sieve

2½ cups (210 g) medium cheddar cheese, shredded

5 eggs

DIRECTIONS

1 Preheat the oven to 350 degrees F.

2 In a large saucepan, heat the butter and olive oil over medium heat. Add the onion and sauté for 2 to 3 minutes until the onion is soft.

3 Add the salt and assorted vegetables, and sauté 4 to 5 more minutes, until the vegetables are slightly tender. Add the spinach and cook for about another minute while stirring to break up the spinach.

4 Remove from the heat and let the mixture cool for 10 minutes.

5 Crack the eggs into a large bowl and beat slightly with a fork until combined. Add the cheese and the slightly cooled vegetable mixture.

6 Pour into a greased 9x9 baking pan or oven-proof skillet. Bake for around 30-45 minutes, or until the middle rises and the edges are slightly browned.

NOTE: This frittata can be served hot or cold and makes a great main dish for brunch.

PER SERVING: Calories 205 (From Fat 141); Fat 16g (Saturated 9g); Cholesterol 141mg; Sodium 574mg; Carbohydrate 4g (Dietary Fiber 1g); Protein 14g.

Quick 'n Tasty Veggie Curry

PREP TIME: 10 MIN	COOK TIME: 15 MIN	YIELD: 2 SERVINGS

INGREDIENTS

½ tablespoon (7.5 mL) butter

1 tablespoon (15 mL) extra-virgin olive oil

½ medium onion, chopped

2 medium cloves garlic, chopped

3 tablespoons (45 mL) tomato paste

1 cup (250 mL) canned crushed tomatoes with juice

1⅓ cups (330 mL) water

1 teaspoon (5 mL) salt

2½ teaspoons (12.5 mL) curry powder

1 teaspoon (5 mL) ground cumin

1 teaspoon (5 mL) lemon juice

1 teaspoon (5 mL) sugar

Pinch of black pepper

Pinch of ground cloves

3 cups (750 mL) assorted vegetables, chopped (broccoli, bell peppers, green peas, zucchini)

½ cup (125 mL) light cream

DIRECTIONS

1 In a large saucepan, melt the butter and olive oil over medium heat. Add the onion and sauté for 3 to 4 minutes, or until the onion is tender. Add the garlic and sauté an additional minute, or until the garlic is slightly softened but not browned.

2 Add the tomato paste, crushed tomatoes, water, salt, curry powder, cumin, lemon juice, sugar, pepper, and cloves. Simmer for 2 to 3 minutes until well combined.

3 Remove the saucepan from the heat and pour the contents of the saucepan into a blender (or a medium bowl, if using an immersion blender). Blend until smooth.

4 Return the sauce to the saucepan. Over medium heat, add the vegetables and simmer for 7 to 8 minutes, or until the vegetables are tender.

5 Add the cream to the saucepan and heat through, about 1 to 2 minutes.

NOTE: This versatile curry works well with almost any raw vegetables you have on hand. Serve this dish over your favorite grain with a dab of yogurt on top.

VARY IT: Add ⅛ to ¼ teaspoon of cayenne if you want a little heat.

PER SERVING: *Calories 291 (From Fat 200); Fat 22g (Saturated 10g); Cholesterol 49mg; Sodium 1273mg; Carbohydrate 22g (Dietary Fiber 6g); Protein 7g.*

Easy Chickpea Feta Bake

PREP TIME: 5 MIN	COOK TIME: 40 MIN	YIELD: 2 SERVINGS

INGREDIENTS

½ medium onion, sliced into half moons

2 cups (500 mL) whole cherry tomatoes

1½ cups (375 mL) canned chickpeas, drained

1 cup (250 mL) feta cheese, crumbled

1 tablespoon (15 mL) extra-virgin olive oil

2 teaspoons (10 mL) dried oregano

DIRECTIONS

1 Preheat the oven to 350 degrees F.

2 Use parchment to line a 9x9 baking dish or cookie sheet with edges. Combine the onion, cherry tomatoes, chickpeas, and feta cheese in the dish and mix loosely.

3 Drizzle the ingredients in the dish with the olive oil and sprinkle the oregano over top.

4 Bake for 20 minutes, and then remove and stir the ingredients briefly. Return to the oven for another 10 to 20 minutes and bake until the tomatoes are soft and wrinkled.

NOTE: This incredibly easy dish makes a perfect meal when paired with hummus and pita.

PER SERVING: *Calories 531 (From Fat 227); Fat 25g (Saturated 13g); Cholesterol 67mg; Sodium 1403mg; Carbohydrate 57g (Dietary Fiber 11g); Protein 22g.*

Savory Miso Noodle Bowls

PREP TIME: 5 MIN	COOK TIME: 15 MIN	YIELD: 2 SERVINGS

INGREDIENTS

1 tablespoon (15 mL) butter

1 medium clove garlic, minced

1 teaspoon (5 mL) ginger, minced

⅓ cup (80 mL) vegetable broth

3 tablespoons (45 mL) miso paste, divided

½ block firm tofu (12 oz or 175 g), cubed

2 cups (500 mL) broccoli florets

1 tablespoon (15 mL) warm (not hot) water

2 bundles (1-inch or 2.5 cm diameter) soba

Kimchi, to garnish

DIRECTIONS

1 In a large saucepan over medium heat, melt the butter and add the garlic. Sauté for about a minute, or until the garlic is slightly tender.

2 Add the ginger, broth, and 2 tablespoons (30 mL) of the miso paste. Simmer until no lumps of miso remain, about 2 minutes.

3 Add the tofu and broccoli. Simmer until the broccoli is tender and some water has evaporated, approximately 5 to 8 minutes.

4 Meanwhile, bring a pot of water to a boil. Add the soba and cook several minutes until tender. Drain and set aside.

5 In a small dish, combine the water with the remaining tablespoon (15 mL) of miso and stir with a fork to create a paste.

6 Remove the tofu-broccoli mixture from the heat and cool for two to three minutes. Add the noodles and the miso paste and mix. Transfer into serving bowls, garnish with kimchi, and serve.

TIP: If you're using a very salty commercial miso, you may want to use half the specified amount.

PER SERVING: Calories 376 (From Fat 99); Fat 11g (Saturated 5g); Cholesterol 15mg; Sodium 1163mg; Carbohydrate 53g (Dietary Fiber 6g); Protein 18g.

Enjoying Meat and Fish in a Gut-Happy Dish

A happy gut diet can definitely include meat and fish in moderate amounts. If you're in the habit of eating these sources of protein, you're in luck. These three delicious recipes provide you with ideas for satisfying meals that don't compromise your gut health:

>> **Mediterranean Tomato Almond Chicken:** This dish brings together the contrasting textures of roasted tomatoes and crunchy almonds to create something that tastes truly decadent.

>> **Crispy-Topped Halibut:** This recipe is a great way to prepare fish, with a flavorful topping that adds color and crunch.

>> **Rustic Noodles and Cabbage:** If you weren't already a big fan of cabbage, this simple, comforting meal may inspire you to eat it more regularly.

ARE RAW FOODS OR COOKED FOODS BETTER FOR THE GUT?

Many people are accustomed to cooking their meals — but a small proportion of people adhere to a diet made up of mainly raw (uncooked) foods. Does a raw food diet lead to better outcomes for gut health?

Few researchers have studied the gut effects of a completely raw food diet. However, consuming some amount of raw foods is indeed beneficial because they contain more live microorganisms and a greater intake of these microorganisms is associated with better health.

One mouse study found that raw versus cooked meat made no difference to the gut microbiota, but raw versus cooked sweet potato had differing effects. The raw version led to lower diversity and a spike in bacteria that break down carbohydrates. All in all, cooking made the food more digestible. For humans, no compelling evidence points to the need for a diet of all raw foods, but including some proportion of raw foods (namely, raw fruits and vegetables) may be beneficial for gut and overall health.

Mediterranean Tomato Almond Chicken

PREP TIME: 5 MIN	COOK TIME: 25 MIN	YIELD: 2 SERVINGS

INGREDIENTS

1 medium red bell pepper, seeded and chopped

2 cups (500 mL) cherry tomatoes

¼ cup (60 mL) extra-virgin olive oil, plus 2 tablespoons (30 mL)

½ teaspoon (2.5 mL) garlic powder

1½ teaspoons (7.5 mL) salt plus a pinch more

1 cup (250 mL) sliced almonds

2 chicken breasts, cut into 1-inch (2.5 cm) strips

½ teaspoon (2.5 mL) oregano

DIRECTIONS

1 Line a medium oven-safe dish with foil (not parchment). Add the red pepper, cherry tomatoes, ¼ cup (60 mL) olive oil as well as the garlic powder, and ½ teaspoon (2.5 mL) salt.

2 Position the dish around 8 inches from the oven's broiler element, and then broil on high for 10 to 15 minutes. Remove the dish and stir the ingredients every 5 minutes as some of the tomatoes start to blacken.

3 Meanwhile, put 1 tablespoon (15 mL) of the olive oil in a small saucepan over medium-high heat. Add the almonds and a pinch of salt and stir frequently for 3 minutes, or until browned.

4 After the tomato mixture is done, remove it from the oven and set aside. Turn the oven to bake and adjust the temperature to 425 degrees F. Put the chicken breasts on a foil-lined pan and sprinkle with 1 teaspoon (5 mL) of the salt. Rub the salt on both sides of the chicken, and then drizzle the top with the remaining 1 tablespoon (15 mL) of the olive oil and sprinkle the oregano on top.

5 Bake the chicken at 425 degrees F for 12 minutes, or until the chicken is slightly browned. Serve the tomato mixture topped with almonds and chicken.

NOTE: This delicious Mediterranean-style dish can be served on a bed of rice or couscous.

PER SERVING: *Calories 489 (From Fat 343); Fat 38g (Saturated 5g); Cholesterol 64mg; Sodium 1806mg; Carbohydrate 15g (Dietary Fiber 5g); Protein 27g.*

Crispy-Topped Halibut

INGREDIENTS

12-ounce (340 g) raw halibut fillet

1 tablespoon (15 mL) butter, melted

½ cup (60 g) panko breadcrumbs (whole wheat if available)

1 tablespoon (15 mL) fresh chopped parsley

¼ teaspoon (1.25 mL) garlic powder

¼ (1.25 mL) teaspoon salt

1 teaspoon (5 mL) Dijon mustard

DIRECTIONS

1 Preheat the oven to 350 degrees F.

2 Place the halibut on a parchment-lined baking sheet, skin side down.

3 In a small bowl, combine the melted butter, panko, parsley, garlic powder, and salt. Mix well.

4 Spread the Dijon mustard in a thin layer on top of the halibut fillet. Spoon the crumb mixture over and press it into the fish.

5 Bake for 20 to 30 minutes, or until the internal temperature of the fish reaches 125 to 130 degrees.

TIP: Your cooking time varies depending on the thickness of the halibut, so have a meat thermometer on hand to check the inside temperature of the fish during the final stages of cooking. Avoid overcooking the halibut.

PER SERVING: *Calories 306 (From Fat 96); Fat 11g (Saturated 5g); Cholesterol 60mg; Sodium 635mg; Carbohydrate 20g (Dietary Fiber 2g); Protein 33g.*

Rustic Noodles and Cabbage

PREP TIME: 10 MIN | COOK TIME: 15 MIN | YIELD: 4 SERVINGS

INGREDIENTS

2½ tablespoons (37 mL) butter, divided

1½ cups (375 mL) onion, chopped

3 strips of pancetta or raw bacon, diced

2 teaspoons (10 mL) salt

4 cups (1 L) green cabbage, chopped

2 tablespoons (30 mL) extra-virgin olive oil, divided

Black pepper, several pinches

6 cups (170 g) uncooked egg noodles

DIRECTIONS

1 In a large saucepan, melt 1½ tablespoons (22 mL) of the butter over medium heat. Add the onion and pancetta or bacon and sauté for about 5 minutes, or until the onions soften.

2 Add 1 teaspoon (5 mL) of the salt to the saucepan along with the cabbage, 1 tablespoon (15 mL) of the olive oil, and the remaining tablespoon (15 mL) of butter. Add a pinch of black pepper. Fry for 8 to 10 minutes, or until the cabbage is slightly tender.

3 Meanwhile, bring a large pot of water to a boil and add the egg noodles along with the remaining 1 teaspoon (5 mL) of salt. Cook the noodles *al dente* and drain. Toss with the remaining 1 tablespoon (15 mL) of olive oil.

4 Combine the cabbage mixture with the cooked pasta in a large serving dish. Garnish with additional black pepper.

NOTE: This dish can also be made with thin whole wheat noodles. Serve with a dab of whipped cream and garnish heavily with pepper.

PER SERVING: *Calories 537 (From Fat 195); Fat 22g (Saturated 8g); Cholesterol 104mg; Sodium 1569mg; Carbohydrate 69g (Dietary Fiber 6g); Protein 18g.*

Chapter **15**

Sustaining Sides & Snacks

Side dishes and snacks can seem like afterthoughts in your daily diet, but the foods you choose for these can play a strong supporting role for your gut health. With a little effort, you can leverage your sides and snacks to boost the overall amount of fiber in your diet while making your taste buds happy.

This chapter provides a sampling of recipes for side dishes and snacks that both you and your gut microbes will love. Vegetables are the stars of the show, with fermented foods incorporated into some of the recipes. Even though some of the fermented foods are heated, killing off the live microbes, they still retain ample nutritional (and taste) benefits.

Supporting Gut Microbes with Sides

Yes, you could simply steam some spinach to go along with your main dish at dinner. But vegetables are so much more fun when you dress them up and bring out their best qualities. The following easy recipes are great fiber-rich side dishes that'll please your palate:

» **Balsamic Glazed Mushrooms:** These mushrooms make a great side dish for meat or fish — or use whole mini button mushrooms and serve them cold as part of a Mediterranean appetizer platter.

» **Classic Creamed Spinach:** Frozen spinach is great to keep on hand in your kitchen because of its great versatility. This recipe shows you how to turn it into creamed spinach, a retro classic that's due for a comeback.

» **Zucchini with Parmesan:** This side dish is so flavorful you might even want to make it as your main course. Serve it with a green salad and crusty bread for a light summer meal.

» **Mediterranean Baked Rice:** Forget plain rice, this baked rice has sundried tomatoes and a mild tomato flavor that turns it into a satisfying comfort food.

» **Tangy Jicama Sticks:** Look for jicama in a health food store or greengrocer. These jicama sticks make a nice accompaniment to tacos, and they can also serve as taco fillings.

Balsamic Glazed Mushrooms

PREP TIME: 5 MIN	COOK TIME: 15 MIN	YIELD: 4 SERVINGS

INGREDIENTS

1 teaspoon (5 mL) butter

¼ cup (60 mL) extra-virgin olive oil

4 cups (or 2 8-ounce boxes) (1L) whole white button mushrooms, cleaned and sliced

¼ teaspoon (1.25 mL) salt

1 garlic clove, chopped

2 tablespoons (30 mL) brown sugar

3 tablespoons (45 mL) balsamic vinegar

1 tablespoon (15 mL) water

Pinch of black pepper

2 teaspoons (10 mL) fresh thyme, chopped (or 1 teaspoon (5 mL) dried thyme)

DIRECTIONS

1 Melt the butter and olive oil in a medium saucepan over medium–high heat.

2 Add the mushrooms and salt, cooking for about 5 minutes until the mushrooms begin to soften. Add the garlic and cook for an additional 1 to 2 minutes, until the garlic is soft but not browned.

3 Add the brown sugar, balsamic vinegar, water, and black pepper. Continue cooking for about 5 minutes or until the sauce is slightly thickened.

4 Transfer the mushrooms to a small serving bowl, drizzling the remaining sauce from the pan over the top. Add the thyme and toss. Serve hot or cold.

PER SERVING: *Calories 159 (From Fat125); Fat 14g (Saturated 2g); Cholesterol 3mg; Sodium 162mg; Carbohydrate 8g (Dietary Fiber 1g); Protein 3g.*

Classic Creamed Spinach

INGREDIENTS

1 teaspoon (5 mL) butter

1 clove garlic, chopped

One 10-ounce (285 g) package of frozen spinach, thawed, with the liquid pressed out through a sieve

⅛ teaspoon (0.6 mL) ground nutmeg

¼ teaspoon (1.25 mL) salt

⅔ cup (160 mL) light cream

1 teaspoon (5 mL) Parmesan cheese

DIRECTIONS

1 Melt the butter in a medium saucepan over medium heat. Add the garlic and cook for about a minute or until slightly soft-ened but not browned.

2 Add the spinach, nutmeg, salt, and cream. Stir with a whisk to break up the spinach.

3 Cook for 5 to 7 minutes or until the mixture starts to bubble slightly. Remove from the heat and transfer to a serving bowl. Garnish with the Parmesan cheese and serve.

VARY IT: For a vegan dish, use extra-virgin olive oil instead of butter, substitute coconut milk for the cream, and use nutritional yeast in place of the Parmesan cheese.

PER SERVING: *Calories 218 (From Fat 168); Fat 19g (Saturated 11g); Cholesterol 59mg; Sodium 463mg; Carbohydrate 9g (Dietary Fiber 4g); Protein 7g.*

Zucchini with Parmesan

INGREDIENTS

1 teaspoon (5 mL) butter

1 teaspoon (5 mL) extra-virgin olive oil

½ medium onion, sliced into half moons

3 cups (750 mL) zucchini, sliced into half moons

1 teaspoon (5 mL) salt

½ tablespoon (7 mL) sugar

1 cup (250 mL) canned crushed tomatoes

1 teaspoon (5 mL) oregano

Pinch of dried thyme

⅓ cup (80 mL) water

⅓ cup (80 mL) Parmesan cheese, grated

DIRECTIONS

1 Melt the butter and olive oil in a medium saucepan over medium heat. Add the onions and cook for 7 to 8 minutes or until the onions are soft and golden brown.

2 Turn the heat up to medium–high. Add the zucchini and salt, cooking for about 3 minutes, stirring constantly, until slightly browned.

3 Reduce the heat to medium, add the sugar, tomatoes, oregano, thyme, and water, and simmer for about 5 minutes.

4 Reduce the heat to low and simmer for 5 to 10 minutes, until the zucchini skin is tender. Remove from the heat.

5 Add the Parmesan cheese and mix well. Transfer to a serving dish and serve.

NOTE: This recipe is a tasty way to use your garden zucchini at the end of the summer.

PER SERVING: *Calories 107 (From Fat 41); Fat 5g (Saturated 2g); Cholesterol 10mg; Sodium 823mg; Carbohydrate 11g (Dietary Fiber 3g); Protein 6g.*

Mediterranean Baked Rice

PREP TIME: 5 MIN	COOK TIME: 35 TO 40 MIN	YIELD: 4 SERVINGS

INGREDIENTS

3 cups (750 mL) water

1½ cups (275 g) rice, uncooked

1 teaspoon (5 mL) extra-virgin olive oil

1¼ (6.25 mL) teaspoon salt

1 teaspoon (5 mL) oregano

1 tablespoon (15 mL) tomato paste

1 tablespoon (15 mL) lemon juice

2 tablespoons (30 mL) chopped sundried tomatoes

DIRECTIONS

1 Set your oven to 350 degrees F.

2 In a 6-cup baking dish (loaf pan), combine the water, rice, olive oil, salt, oregano, tomato paste, lemon juice, and sun-dried tomatoes. Stir gently and tightly cover the top of the pan with foil.

3 Bake for 20 minutes or until the rice starts to absorb the water. Remove from the oven and stir.

4 Return the rice to the oven for 15 to 20 more minutes or until the rice is completely cooked. Transfer to a serving dish and fluff the rice with a fork before serving.

TIP: You can add more Mediterranean flavors to this comforting rice dish — try diced olives or chopped fresh herbs for added zing.

PER SERVING: *Calories 273 (From Fat); Fat 2g (Saturated 0g); Cholesterol 0mg; Sodium 778mg; Carbohydrate 58g (Dietary Fiber 2g); Protein 5g.*

🍅 Tangy Jicama Sticks

PREP TIME: 7 MIN   YIELD: 6 SERVINGS

INGREDIENTS

1 tablespoon (15 mL) lime juice

½ teaspoon (2.5 mL) dried chili flakes

1 teaspoon (5 mL) Mexican chili powder

1 tablespoon (15 mL) fresh cilantro, chopped

2 cups (500 mL) raw jicama, peeled and cut into matchsticks (about ¼ inch or 0.6 cm thick and 2 inches or 5 cm long)

DIRECTIONS

1 In a small bowl, combine the lime juice, dried chili flakes, chili powder, and cilantro, and mix well.

2 Place the jicama sticks in a medium bowl and pour the mixture over top. Toss well to coat all the sticks. Serve right away.

NOTE: Jicama (see Figure 15-1) is a large root vegetable with thick brown skin that's in the pea family. It has a mild, refreshing flavor and a crunchy texture that resembles a water chestnut or a pear.

PER SERVING: *Calories 17 (From Fat 0); Fat 0g (Saturated 0g); Cholesterol 0mg; Sodium 6mg; Carbohydrate 4g (Dietary Fiber 2g); Protein 0g.*

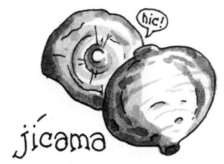

hic!

jícama

FIGURE 15-1:
A jicama.

Illustration by Liz Kurtzman

Making Some Gut-Lovin' Snacks

When it comes to snacks, many convenient options exist that are less than ideal for your gut health. But you can fortify yourself against vending machine temptation by having gut-friendly snacks ready and available. Try the following snack recipes to make sure you get a boost of fiber between meals:

>> **Miso Snack Mix:** When you're in the mood for something salty, this snack mix can tide you over with a mix of richly flavored nuts and cereal.

>> **Cannellini and Parsley Dip:** This dip makes an instant lunch when served with pita bread and raw vegetables. Or if you bring it to a potluck you're sure to be asked for the recipe.

>> **Kimchi Pancakes:** These pancakes score high on taste as well as simplicity. Hot or cold, they make a good afternoon snack.

>> **Spiced Chickpeas:** You may find these chickpeas a little bit addictive. They taste great on their own, or they can be added as a topping to salads or soups.

Miso Snack Mix

PREP TIME: 5 MIN | COOK TIME: 25 MIN | YIELD: 6 SERVINGS

INGREDIENTS

½ tablespoon (7 mL) butter

1 teaspoon (5 mL) olive oil

1½ tablespoons (22 mL) honey

½ teaspoon (2.5 mL) garlic powder

1 tablespoon (15 mL) white miso paste

2 cups (85 g) cereal squares (Chex or similar)

2 cups (260 g) mixed nuts (peanuts, cashews, pecans, and so on)

1 teaspoon (5 mL) sesame seeds

Pinch of dried chili flakes (optional)

DIRECTIONS

1 Set your oven to 250 degrees F.

2 Combine the butter, olive oil, honey, garlic powder, and miso in a small saucepan over medium heat. Heat, stirring constantly, until slightly bubbling. Add the sesame seeds and mix.

3 In a large bowl, mix together the cereal and nuts.

4 Remove the saucepan from the heat. Pour the hot mixture over the dry ingredients, mixing well to coat. Sprinkle with the dried chili flakes if desired.

5 Spread the mixture onto a parchment-lined cookie sheet. Bake for 15 minutes.

6 Remove the mixture from the oven and stir well. Return to the oven for an additional 10 minutes.

7 Cool the mixture, stirring occasionally. Serve right away, or store in an airtight container when completely cooled.

VARY IT: You can change up the dry ingredients for countless snack mix possibilities: Use peanuts rather than mixed nuts or add pretzels or different types of cereal such as Cheerios.

PER SERVING: *Calories 376 (From Fat 264); Fat 29g (Saturated 5g); Cholesterol 3mg; Sodium 448mg; Carbohydrate 25g (Dietary Fiber 3g); Protein 9g.*

Cannellini and Parsley Dip

INGREDIENTS

2 cups (500 mL) cooked cannellini beans, drained

⅓ cup (80 mL) feta cheese, crumbled

⅓ cup (80 mL) fresh parsley, chopped

¼ teaspoon (1.25 mL) minced garlic

2 tablespoons (30 mL) lemon juice

1 teaspoon (5 mL) lemon zest

2 tablespoons (30 mL) extra-virgin olive oil

¼ teaspoon (1.25 mL) salt

DIRECTIONS

1 Combine the beans, feta cheese, parsley, garlic, lemon juice and zest, olive oil, and salt in a blender (or a medium bowl, if using an immersion blender). Blend until smooth.

2 Transfer to a small serving dish. Garnish with additional parsley and serve.

TIP: Serve this tangy dip with mini pitas or crackers. You can adjust the amount of garlic according to your taste.

PER SERVING: *Calories 205 (From Fat 95); Fat 11g (Saturated 3g); Cholesterol 11mg; Sodium 670mg; Carbohydrate 20g (Dietary Fiber 7g); Protein 9g.*

☙ Kimchi Pancakes

PREP TIME: 5 MIN | COOK TIME: 15 MIN | YIELD: 2 SERVINGS

INGREDIENTS

1 cup (250 mL) fermented kimchi, finely chopped

2 scallions, chopped

½ cup (125 mL) flour

1 teaspoon (5 mL) sugar

¼ cup (60 mL) water

1 teaspoon (5 mL) butter

DIRECTIONS

1 Combine the kimchi, scallions, flour, sugar, and water in a medium-sized bowl.

2 In a small frying pan, melt the butter over medium-high heat. Place about ¼ cup of the kimchi mixture into the pan and flatten gently.

3 Cook the pancake for about 2 to 3 minutes on each side, or until slightly browned.

4 Repeat with the additional kimchi mixture.

NOTE: These pancakes make a great party food — but make extras because they'll be eaten quickly!

PER SERVING: *Calories 158 (From Fat 21); Fat 2g (Saturated 1g); Cholesterol 5mg; Sodium 307mg; Carbohydrate 29g (Dietary Fiber 2g); Protein 5g.*

Spiced Chickpeas

PREP TIME: 2 MIN	COOK TIME: 35 MIN	YIELD: 4 SERVINGS

INGREDIENTS

3 cups (Two 15-ounce or 425g cans) cooked chickpeas, drained

2 tablespoons (30 mL) extra-virgin olive oil

¼ teaspoon (1.25 mL) lemon zest

1 teaspoon (5 mL) smoked paprika

¼ teaspoon (1.25 mL) salt

¼ teaspoon (1.25 mL) garlic powder

Pinch of black pepper

Pinch of cayenne (optional)

DIRECTIONS

1 Set your oven at 450 degrees F.

2 Place the chickpeas into a foil-lined 9x9 baking dish. Drizzle with the olive oil and shake the dish slightly to coat.

3 Bake the chickpeas for 10 minutes. Remove from the oven and stir, and then return to the oven for 10 more minutes or until slightly browned.

4 Meanwhile, in a small dish mix the lemon zest, smoked paprika, salt, garlic powder, black pepper, and cayenne (if desired).

5 Remove the chickpeas from the oven, sprinkle the spice mix over top, and stir to coat. Return to the oven for 10 to 14 more minutes, removing once to stir during this time. Remove from the oven when the chickpeas look slightly browned.

NOTE: These chickpeas can be eaten warm or cold as a snack or they make a great topping for carrot or squash soup. Store them in an airtight container overnight.

PER SERVING: *Calories 205 (From Fat 76); Fat 8g (Saturated 1g); Cholesterol 0mg; Sodium 506mg; Carbohydrate 28g (Dietary Fiber 6g); Protein 6g.*

Chapter **16**

Digestive-Friendly Desserts

Yes, you can have your higher-fiber cake and eat it too. Occasional sweets can be part of a balanced diet pattern that you're able to stick to without feeling deprived. The key to satisfying your sweet tooth while adhering to the gut-friendly diet principles is supercharging your sweets with extra fiber so your gut microbes have something to eat while you indulge. Forget the impulse purchases of coffee counter muffins and loaves — you can whip up tasty treats at home that satisfy your cravings while providing more substantial nutritional value.

This chapter presents an array of sweets that are easy to make, while upping your sweet tooth game with gut-approved ingredients.

Baking Muffins and Cakes to Feed Your Gut Microbes

Typical cakes and muffins are made with lots of sugar and white flour that your digestive tract quickly absorbs, leaving nothing to nourish your gut microbes and help your body create the all-important short-chain fatty acid molecules. The recipes here, however, are bolstered with extra fiber and often use olive oil to help you balance out the different types of fats in your diet. Try one of these cake or muffin recipes on a quiet weekend morning — and don't forget to put some of the baked goods aside in the freezer for a day when you need a quick breakfast to go.

This section includes the following recipes:

>> **Banana Oat Muffins:** These hearty muffins, which freeze well, are a great way to make use of ripe bananas.

>> **Orange Kefir Cake:** This is an excellent brunch cake that tastes great with a dollop of yogurt (plain or fruit flavored) and berries on top.

>> **Rhubarb Cake:** Rhubarb is a tangy treat that's also a great source of fiber. This cake is a stand-out for coffee hour and is delicious topped with whipped cream.

>> **Cranberry Breakfast Cake:** Sour cranberries (fresh or frozen) add both flavor and fiber to this delicious cake.

BEST FLOURS FOR GUT-FRIENDLY BAKING

If you're a generally healthy person, increasing your fiber intake is one of the key tenets of eating for good gut health. Whole-grain flours are better for gut health (and for stabilizing blood sugar) than white flour, but some whole-grain flours create very dense baked goods that are less appealing to eat. Sometimes recipes that involve mixing different types of flours (for example, white flour and spelt flour) lead to the most satisfying results. For the recipes in this chapter, I've tried to strike a balance between boosting fiber content and maintaining good texture and taste.

When baking, you can experiment with replacing a small portion (say, one quarter) of the white flour in a recipe with any of the following flours, which can amp up the fiber content:

- Medium rye flour
- Oat flour
- Spelt flour
- Whole wheat flour

🍅 Banana Oat Muffins

PREP TIME: 10 MIN	COOK TIME: 25 MIN	YIELD: 12 MUFFINS

INGREDIENTS

3 ripe medium bananas, mashed

½ cup (125 mL) white sugar

⅓ cup (80 mL) applesauce

⅓ cup (80 mL) quick oats

1 egg

½ cup (125 mL) spelt or whole wheat flour

1 cup (250 mL) white flour

1 teaspoon (5 mL) baking soda

1 teaspoon (5 mL) baking powder

½ teaspoon (2.5 mL) salt

⅓ cup (80 mL) butter, melted

DIRECTIONS

1 Preheat the oven to 350 degrees F.

2 In a large bowl, combine the bananas, sugar, applesauce, quick oats, and egg. Mix well.

3 In a medium bowl, combine the flours, baking soda, baking powder, and salt. Stir to combine.

4 Add the dry ingredients to the wet ingredients and mix gently. Add the melted butter and mix until no large lumps remain.

5 Pour the batter into greased or papered muffin tins and bake for 20 to 25 minutes, or until a toothpick inserted in the center of a muffin comes out clean.

NOTE: Feel free to jazz up these muffins by adding a handful of nuts, dried fruit pieces, chocolate chips, or carob chips before baking.

PER SERVING: *Calories 180 (From Fat 54); Fat 6g (Saturated 3g); Cholesterol 27mg; Sodium 244mg; Carbohydrate 30g (Dietary Fiber 2g); Protein 3g.*

Orange Kefir Cake

INGREDIENTS

1 cup (250 mL) white sugar

3 eggs

¾ cup (180 mL) plain kefir

2 teaspoons (10 mL) orange zest

¼ cup (60 mL) orange juice

1 teaspoon (5 mL) vanilla extract

1 teaspoon (5 mL) baking powder

½ teaspoon (2.5 mL) salt

2 cups (500 mL) flour

⅔ cup (160 mL) extra-virgin olive oil

DIRECTIONS

1 Preheat the oven to 325 degrees F.

2 Combine the sugar with the eggs in a large mixing bowl and whip using a hand mixer on medium speed until light and frothy, about 1 minute.

3 Add the kefir, orange zest and juice, vanilla extract, baking powder, and salt. Using the hand mixer, blend on low until combined.

4 Add the flour and olive oil, and then use the hand mixer to blend on low until the batter is smooth.

5 Pour the batter into a greased 9-inch round pan and bake for 40 to 45 minutes, or until a toothpick inserted in the center of the cake comes out clean.

PER SERVING: *Calories 392 (From Fat 171); Fat 19g (Saturated 3g); Cholesterol 51mg; Sodium 183mg; Carbohydrate 51g (Dietary Fiber 1g); Protein 6g.*

Rhubarb Cake

PREP TIME: 15 MIN | COOK TIME: 55 TO 60 MIN | YIELD: 8 SERVINGS

INGREDIENTS

½ cup (125 mL) butter, melted

¾ cup (180 mL) brown sugar, packed

¾ cup (180 mL) white sugar, divided

1 egg

1 teaspoon (5 mL) vanilla extract

1 cup (250 mL) plain kefir

1 cup (250 mL) spelt or whole wheat flour

1 cup (250 mL) white flour

1 teaspoon (5 mL) salt

1 teaspoon (5 mL) baking powder

1 teaspoon (5 mL) baking soda

2 cups (500 mL) chopped fresh or frozen rhubarb

1 teaspoon (5 mL) cinnamon

DIRECTIONS

1 Preheat the oven to 350 degrees F.

2 In a large bowl, combine the butter, brown sugar, ½ cup (125 mL) of the white sugar, egg, vanilla extract, and kefir. Mix well.

3 In a medium bowl, combine the flours, salt, baking powder, and baking soda. Add the dry ingredients to the wet ingredients and mix well.

4 Add the chopped rhubarb and stir to combine.

5 Pour the batter into a greased 9x9 baking dish and bake for 55 to 60 minutes, or until a toothpick inserted in the center of the cake comes out clean.

6 As soon as the cake comes out of the oven, combine the remaining ¼ cup (60 mL) of white sugar with the cinnamon and immediately sprinkle over the cake as it cools.

PER SERVING: *Calories 379 (From Fat 120); Fat 13g (Saturated 8g); Cholesterol 53mg; Sodium 558mg; Carbohydrate 60g (Dietary Fiber 3g); Protein 6g.*

Cranberry Breakfast Cake

INGREDIENTS

½ cup (125 mL) white sugar

¼ cup (60 mL) extra-virgin olive oil

1 cup (250 mL) plain kefir or yogurt

2 eggs

2 teaspoons (10 mL) orange zest

1 teaspoon (5 mL) orange or lemon juice

1 cup (250 mL) spelt or whole wheat flour

1 cup (250 mL) white flour

½ cup (125 mL) quick oats

½ teaspoon (2.5 mL) salt

1 tablespoon (15 mL) baking powder

3 tablespoons (45 mL) butter, melted

1 cup (250 mL) fresh or frozen cranberries

DIRECTIONS

1 Preheat the oven to 350 degrees F.

2 In a large bowl, combine the white sugar, olive oil, kefir, eggs, orange zest, and juice. Mix well.

3 In a medium bowl, combine the flours, oats, salt, and baking powder.

4 Add the dry ingredients to the wet ingredients and stir to combine. Gently stir in the melted butter.

5 Add the cranberries and mix.

6 Pour the batter into a greased 9x9 baking dish and bake for 40 minutes, or until a toothpick inserted in the center of the cake comes out clean.

VARY IT: This cranberry cake is equally good in muffin form: pour the batter into muffin tins instead and adjust baking time to 20 to 25 minutes.

PER SERVING: *Calories 324 (From Fat 118); Fat 13g (Saturated 4g); Cholesterol 54mg; Sodium 217mg; Carbohydrate 44g (Dietary Fiber 3g); Protein 8g.*

Creating Cookies and Other Treats for Delightful Digestion

The reason I love baking isn't only about the treats themselves, as tasty as they are. Baking is about more than the finished products: It's about someone in your household sneaking a taste of the batter. It's about the smell of baking cookies permeating your living space. It's about licking the spatula when you're all done.

With that said, these recipes make appealing desserts — and your gut will thank you for the extra nourishment that's packed into them. They're some of my favorite treats to have on hand when I want to satisfy my sweet tooth:

>> **Cardamom Oat Cookies:** Cardamom gives these chewy cookies a unique and addicting flavor.

>> **Beanie Brownies with Chocolate Kefir Icing:** Chocolaty and rich, these brownies secretly pack a big fiber punch.

>> **Peanut Butter Oat Cookies:** These flourless cookies make a great after-school treat.

>> **Pumpkin Spice Baked Apples:** Try this recipe for an ultra-quick dessert that's perfect when you're craving fall vibes.

🍅 Cardamom Oat Cookies

INGREDIENTS

¾ cup (180 mL) butter, softened

½ cup (125 mL) brown sugar, packed

½ cup (125 mL) white sugar

1 egg

1 egg yolk

¼ teaspoon (1.25 mL) salt

2 teaspoons (10 mL) vanilla extract

2 teaspoons (10 mL) lemon zest

1 cup (250 mL) quick oats

1 cup (250 mL) white flour

2 teaspoons (10 mL) ground cardamom

1 teaspoon (5 mL) baking powder

⅓ cup (50 g) shelled pistachios, coarsely chopped

DIRECTIONS

1 Preheat the oven to 350 degrees F.

2 In a large bowl, combine the butter, brown sugar, and white sugar. Mix well. Add the egg, egg yolk, salt, vanilla extract, and lemon zest. Stir.

3 In a medium bowl, combine the oats, flour, ground cardamom, and baking powder.

4 Add the dry ingredients to the wet ingredients and stir well. Add the pistachios and stir to combine.

5 Form into small balls and place on a parchment-covered cookie sheet. Bake each batch for 15 minutes, or until slightly browned.

PER SERVING (1 COOKIE): *Calories 136 (From Fat 70); Fat 8g (Saturated 4g); Cholesterol 24mg; Sodium 87mg; Carbohydrate 15g (Dietary Fiber 1g); Protein 2g.*

Beanie Brownies with Chocolate Kefir Icing

PREP TIME: 10 MIN | COOK TIME: 45 MIN | YIELD: 24 SQUARES

INGREDIENTS

2 cups (500 mL) cooked black beans, rinsed and drained

2 eggs

½ cup (125 mL) cocoa powder

½ cup (125 mL) plain yogurt

¼ cup (60 mL) maple syrup

¼ cup (60 mL) brown sugar

½ teaspoon (2.5 mL) salt

1 teaspoon (5 mL) baking powder

1 teaspoon (5 mL) vanilla extract

2 tablespoons (30 mL) olive oil

½ cup (90 g) semisweet chocolate chips

2 tablespoons (30 mL) butter, softened

¼ teaspoon (1.25 mL) salt

1 cup (250 mL) icing sugar

2 tablespoons (30 mL) plain kefir

DIRECTIONS

1 Preheat the oven to 350 degrees F.

2 In a large blender (or a medium bowl, if using an immersion blender), mix the black beans, eggs, cocoa powder, yogurt, maple syrup, brown sugar, salt, vanilla extract, baking powder, and olive oil. Blend all the ingredients until smooth.

3 Pour the batter into a greased 9x9 baking dish. Bake for 45 minutes or until cracks form all over the top of the brownies.

Chocolate Kefir Icing

1 To make the icing, combine the chocolate chips and the butter in a small saucepan and heat on medium, stirring constantly until smooth.

2 Remove the mixture from the heat and add the icing sugar and kefir. Mix well. Spread over the slightly cooled brownies.

TIP: If you want even more chocolaty flavor in your brownies or if you want to add sweetness without the icing, you can add half a cup of semisweet chocolate chips to the batter before pouring it into the baking pan.

PER SERVING: *Calories 133 (From Fat 41); Fat 5g (Saturated 2g); Cholesterol 17mg; Sodium 98mg; Carbohydrate 20g (Dietary Fiber 3g); Protein 5g.*

Peanut Butter Oat Cookies

PREP TIME: 15 MIN | COOK TIME: 15 MIN | YIELD: 48 COOKIES

INGREDIENTS

1 cup (250 mL) white sugar

1 cup (250 mL) brown sugar, packed

2 cups (500 mL) natural peanut butter

4 eggs

1 ripe medium banana, mashed

¼ cup (60 mL) honey

2½ teaspoons (12.5 mL) baking soda

1 teaspoon (5 mL) salt

1 teaspoon (5 mL) vanilla extract

⅔ cup (160 mL) butter, melted

1 cup (175 g) semisweet chocolate chips

DIRECTIONS

1 Preheat the oven to 350 degrees F.

2 In a very large bowl, combine the white sugar, brown sugar, peanut butter, eggs, banana, and honey. Mix well (using either a wooden spoon or a hand mixer).

3 Add the baking soda, salt, vanilla extract, and melted butter. Stir to combine.

4 Add the chocolate chips and stir to combine.

5 Form into small balls and place on a parchment-covered cookie sheet. Bake each batch for 13 to 15 minutes, or until slightly browned.

PER SERVING: *Calories 153 (From Fat 86); Fat 10g (Saturated 4g); Cholesterol 20mg; Sodium 142mg; Carbohydrate 14g (Dietary Fiber 1g); Protein 4g.*

🍅 Pumpkin Spice Baked Apples

PREP TIME: 15 MIN | **COOK TIME: 30 MIN** | **YIELD: 4 SERVINGS**

INGREDIENTS

3 large apples

½ cup (125 mL) cream cheese, softened

½ cup (125 mL) canned pumpkin puree

1 teaspoon (5 mL) cinnamon

½ teaspoon (2.5 mL) ground nutmeg

¼ teaspoon (1.25 mL) ground cloves

1 tablespoon (15 mL) plain kefir or whole milk

1 teaspoon (5 mL) vanilla extract

¼ cup (60 mL) white sugar

⅓ cup (40 g) walnuts, coarsely chopped (optional)

DIRECTIONS

1 Preheat the oven to 350 degrees F.

2 Quarter the apples and cut out the cores. Chop the apples into bite-sized chunks, leaving the skin on. Arrange the apple pieces on the bottom of a 9x9 baking dish.

3 Using a hand blender, combine the cream cheese, pumpkin puree, cinnamon, nutmeg, cloves, kefir, vanilla extract, and sugar. Blend until smooth.

4 Pour the mixture evenly over the apples in the baking dish. Sprinkle with the chopped walnuts if desired.

5 Bake for approximately 30 minutes, or until the apples are fork-tender and the pumpkin cream cheese mixture is bubbling. Serve warm.

NOTE: The baking time for this apple treat depends on the variety and freshness of the apples, so keep an eye on them in the oven and test them for tenderness. Leftovers from this dish make a great topping for hot oatmeal.

TIP: Regular cream cheese makes this dessert creamy and satisfying and can be part of a healthy mix of fats in your diet. But low-fat or fat-free cream cheese also work in this recipe if you have them on hand.

TIP: The best type of apples for this dish are those that stay relatively firm when cooked: Fuji, Gala, Granny Smith, and Braeburn are the most well-known varieties.

PER SERVING: *Calories 318 (From Fat 152); Fat 17g (Saturated 7g); Cholesterol 32mg; Sodium 91mg; Carbohydrate 41g (Dietary Fiber 6g); Protein 6g.*

LOW-FODMAP BAKING

For those with functional gastrointestinal symptoms, doctors or dietitians sometimes recommend a diet low in FODMAPs (fermentable oligosaccharides, disaccharides, monosaccharides, and polyols), which are types of carbohydrates that are poorly absorbed in the small intestine. During digestion FODMAPs move into the colon, where they can cause uncomfortable symptoms such as gas, diarrhea, and abdominal pain in sensitive individuals.

Ample evidence backs up the low-FODMAP diet as a way to relieve gastrointestinal symptoms in the short term, but sticking to the diet can be difficult because many products in grocery stores and restaurants have a high FODMAP content. Baked goods are particularly challenging because they are predominantly made with wheat flour, which is not low-FODMAP.

If you're on a low-FODMAP diet, it's okay to indulge in sweets a few times a week as long as they're made with low-FODMAP ingredients. Making them yourself can give you confidence that they don't contain any gut-irritating ingredients.

When doing low-FODMAP baking, I recommend using a recipe someone else has already tested because substituting low-FODMAP ingredients in a regular recipe can have unpredictable results. Some irritable bowel syndrome specialist dietitians on social media regularly share low-FODMAP recipes.

Some low-FODMAP flours you can consider using in your baked goods are as follows:

- Buckwheat flour
- Maize or corn flour
- Millet flour
- Oat flour
- Quinoa flour

Honey isn't low-FODMAP, but most sugar is okay to use as long as it's not a specific trigger for your gut symptoms. Types of sugar that are allowed (in moderate amounts) on a low-FODMAP diet are as follows:

- Brown sugar
- Icing sugar
- Maple syrup
- White sugar

5

Supporting Health through the Gut at Times in Life

Find out how gut health shapes fetal growth and development during pregnancy.

Become aware of how the events surrounding birth can shape the baby's gut, with possible consequences for health in the long term.

Discover how the baby's diet in the first three months of life helps shape gut health.

Explore the factors that impact gut health during childhood and adolescence and find tips for promoting gut health during these important years of development.

Recognize the importance of gut health in older age and how to support health through the gut at this stage of life.

Chapter **17**

Paying Attention to Gut Health in Pregnancy, Birth, and Infancy

The great span of a human lifetime is spent living in symbiosis with microorganisms — but the level of microbial influence on the body doesn't remain constant during all this time. During certain critical windows of development, humans' symbiotic microbes have an increased influence on health.

Even though some microbial influences occur in the womb, as this chapter describes, the most important phase of influence extends from birth through the first few months of a human's life. Observations in germ-free animals, which are born using a sterile procedure and spend their first weeks in a microbe-free environment, reveal distinct abnormalities in their physical development — namely:

» Reduced levels of specific gut immune cells and increased susceptibility to infections

>> Neurodevelopmental differences that include disrupted communication between brain cells, different patterns of cell pruning in the hippocampus and hypothalamus, and a larger forebrain

If these germ-free animals are exposed to microbes again later in life, some of these abnormalities resolve but others (such as the gut immune system alterations) never fully normalize after the early-life microbial signals are missed. Humans, too, seem to require microbial instruction at birth and shortly thereafter to ensure optimal development and lifelong health. The microbe-human conversations begin in early life — and although they're far from the only factor determining health throughout the lifespan, evidence clearly shows they're a contributing factor.

The digestive tract, which harbors an important site of immune activity called *the gut-associated lymphoid tissues (GALT),* is control central for microbial influence on the body in early life. Because the gut is a classroom where the microbes instruct the body on proper development of the immune system as well as the brain, gut health and optimal microbial influences are especially important at birth and shortly afterward.

In this chapter, I discuss the importance of gut health in pregnancy, birth, and early life, as well as its consequences for health later on. I specifically cover what alters the gut microbiota at these various stages — and what scientists have discovered about how to support gut health in utero, at birth, and through the first three months of life.

Supporting Gut Health during Pregnancy

When someone becomes pregnant, no changes may be immediately apparent on the outside. But the body is starting to undergo massive changes that set the stage for supporting fetal growth and development. Changes that occur overall in the body during pregnancy include the following:

>> The placenta produces a flood of hormones.

>> The blood vessels widen and the heart pumps more blood, with heart rate increasing.

>> The lungs breathe more air overall, although they can handle less capacity.

>> The body retains water and the kidneys have increased throughput.

>> Metabolic changes occur that somewhat resemble metabolic syndrome in nonpregnant people, such as:

- Weight gain

- Higher fasting blood sugar

- Insulin resistance

- Low-grade inflammation

- Changes in metabolism-related hormones

>> The immune system changes rapidly; contrary to common belief it isn't suppressed overall, but it responds differently depending on the stage of pregnancy and the specific microorganisms shaping immunity. This means at certain times the pregnant individual is more at risk for certain infections or may experience more severe infections.

Understanding how the gut changes during pregnancy

The overall function of the gut, too, changes in pregnancy. In fact, gut-related symptoms such as nausea or vomiting, which affect 50 to 80 percent of pregnant women, are some of the notorious first signs of pregnancy. Here are typical digestive-related changes that occur in pregnancy:

>> Progesterone-triggered relaxation of the digestive tract muscles, slowing the transit time of food through the stomach, small intestine, and large intestine

>> Delayed emptying of the gallbladder

>> Nausea, vomiting, constipation, or heartburn, related to the slowed action and reduced resting muscle tone in the digestive system

>> Appetite changes — either increased or decreased hunger and either cravings or aversions for specific foods

>> More pressure on certain parts of the digestive system because of the growing uterus

REMEMBER

The gut microbes exhibit dramatic changes, which are dependent on the phase of the pregnancy. Generally, pregnancy is characterized by a higher quantity of bacteria in the gut as well as shifts in composition. In the first trimester the gut microbiota may look similar to that of nonpregnant individuals, but the changes really emerge in the second and third trimesters. During this time, the gut microbiota becomes more eclectic, with reduced diversity and a reduced proportion of some anti-inflammatory groups of bacteria — a pattern not unlike that seen in people with metabolic syndrome.

Experiments that have transferred a pregnant person's gut microbes to animals show that gut microbes are at least partially responsible for the metabolic abnormalities in the body — but that these changes are beneficial in the context of pregnancy because the fetus requires lots of energy to develop appropriately. In fact, women who gain more weight than the average during a pregnancy have a distinct microbiota composition, which may drive weight gain. Overall this shows how the microbes play an active role in the metabolic changes and huge energy needs that support the developing fetus.

Even though these changes occur in the mother's gut during pregnancy, an important caveat is that these gut microbes don't reach the baby directly (refer to the nearby sidebar for more information). Nevertheless, the microbes have ways of signaling to the fetus to help shape its growth and development. Some metabolites produced by gut microbes and circulating in the blood can cross into the placenta, creating a mode of communication with the fetus. Recent research also shows particles secreted by bacteria in the mother's gut in a healthy pregnancy may migrate to the amniotic fluid and, in doing so, convey messages to the fetus.

Scientists still have a lot to learn about how to support gut health during pregnancy. Yet throughout all the changes that occur in this complex physiological state, several factors, which I introduce in the sections that follow, can affect the mother's gut microbiota and overall gut health, ultimately supporting both her own state of health and proper development of the fetus.

THE DEBATE OVER A STERILE PLACENTA

The issue of whether the placenta is sterile has been the topic of much scientific debate in the past decade. Before microbiome sequencing techniques were widely used, scientists assumed that the placenta was devoid of living microorganisms and that detection of microbes in the placenta was a sign of infection. But in 2014 one scientific group in the United States published a study, backed up by several subsequent studies, showing the apparent presence of a community of living microorganisms in the placenta. This work prompted a skeptical response from some other scientists in the field, who contended that the so-called placental microorganisms must have originated from contamination when the samples were obtained from pregnant individuals or analyzed in the laboratory.

In 2023, a large group of scientists from all over the world published a definitive paper analyzing all the available evidence and cross-referencing it with basic knowledge about immunology, microbiology, and the study of germ-free animals. The scientists concluded that healthy fetal tissues don't harbor live microbial communities after all, backing up the original idea of a sterile placenta. Even though the debate over the evidence will likely continue in the years to come, the prevailing scientific opinion at present is that the fetus lacks direct exposure to live microorganisms before birth.

Managing digestive symptoms

Digestive symptoms that emerge during pregnancy may be uncomfortable and may also affect the mother's ability to get adequate intake of nutrients and fluids. A healthcare professional should guide the management of these symptoms because certain medications, including some over-the-counter products, aren't recommended during pregnancy. However, some simple changes in habits may help alleviate digestive symptoms that may occur.

For nausea and vomiting during pregnancy, the following approaches may be effective:

» Eating smaller, more frequent meals

» Avoiding high-fat foods

» Consuming small amounts of ginger (up to one gram per day) or ginger tea

» On a daily basis, drinking around one and a half quarts (or 1.5 liters) of water or electrolyte drinks such as coconut water, nutrient-added water, or electrolyte solution

TIP

Gastroesophageal reflux disease (GERD) is especially common in pregnancy. Here are some tips for helping reduce heartburn:

» Finish eating early in the evening, several hours before bedtime

» When sleeping, elevating your head by 4 or more inches (10 or more centimeters)

» Lying on your left side in bed

» Subject to your doctor's recommendation, taking occasional doses of antacids containing calcium carbonate and magnesium hydroxide

An existing digestive disease may require special management in pregnancy and sometimes a new digestive disease may emerge. I discuss management of symptoms in the following sections.

Managing digestive disease symptoms during pregnancy

Symptom management is an entirely different ball game when a pregnant individual has a digestive disease. A disease of the gastrointestinal tract must be medically well-managed to maintain good outcomes for both the mother and the baby — and even then, changes in the disease may occur throughout the pregnancy and require careful monitoring by a healthcare professional.

Inflammatory bowel disease (IBD) is a prime example where appropriate disease management is important in pregnancy to avoid outcomes such as preterm birth, low birthweight (under 5.5 pounds or 2,500 grams), and Caesarean section (C-section) birth. Studies show that when conception occurs during IBD remission, the mother has about the same risk of experiencing a symptom flare as she had before the pregnancy. But if pregnancy occurs when the IBD is active, unfortunately the majority of women find that the status of their disease remains the same or worsens during pregnancy. (Interestingly, however, the number of IBD flares may be reduced in the years following pregnancy.) Ideally, those with IBD should inform their doctor three to four months before planning to attempt pregnancy. Adjusting certain IBD medications may be necessary.

REMEMBER

Strict adherence to a gluten-free diet is essential in pregnancy for those with celiac disease because uncontrolled disease is linked to a greater risk of miscarriage, preterm labor, low birthweight, and stillbirth. Given these major risks, individuals with a family history of celiac disease may want to explore being tested for the disease before attempting to become pregnant, even if no digestive symptoms are immediately evident.

Being aware of pregnancy-related digestive diseases

Sometimes a new digestive disease emerges during pregnancy. The two main examples are as follows:

» **Hyperemesis gravidarum (HG):** This condition, occurring in 2 to 3 percent of pregnancies (including, most famously, the pregnancies of The Duchess of Cambridge), is a severe form of nausea and vomiting accompanied by weight loss of more than 5 percent of a person's pre-pregnancy weight. Dehydration and electrolyte imbalances may also occur. HG can be life-threatening to the mother and is associated with developmental risks to the fetus. The cause of HG was recently discovered: In individuals who (because of their genes) normally have low levels of the hormone growth differentiation factor 15 (GDF15) before pregnancy, the rapid release of GDF15 by the fetal cells in early pregnancy triggers the debilitating symptoms. Medical management can include intravenous fluids, and other treatments are in development.

» **Gallstones:** Increased hormone levels in pregnancy cause higher cholesterol and delayed emptying of the gallbladder, increasing the risk of gallstone formation. An estimated 8 percent of pregnant women develop new gallstones, but only about 1 percent experience symptoms. Abdominal pain is the most common symptom, and gallstones can be identified safely during pregnancy using abdominal ultrasound.

Eating for trillions plus two

Increasing evidence shows that diet has an important impact on the gut microbes and overall health of a pregnant individual, with implications for the developing fetus. The ideal diet during pregnancy is centered around whole fruits and vegetables, whole grains, lean sources of protein, and monounsaturated fatty acid-rich foods such as olive oil. Yet the majority of U.S. women who are pregnant don't follow a healthy diet pattern before or during pregnancy. After pregnancy occurs, the challenge of healthy eating only tends to increase, when in the first trimester some individuals have a decreased appetite or can no longer stand the sight of some of their favorite nutritious foods.

REMEMBER

The health of the mother depends on having adequate nutrition during pregnancy. Studies show a healthy diet pattern both before and during pregnancy not only controls excessive weight gain and the related complications, but also reduces the risk of several maternal health issues: gestational diabetes mellitus (GDM), pre-eclampsia, and gestational hypertension.

Dietary intake during pregnancy affects fetal health as well. When the mother receives inadequate nutrition, the outcomes may include fetal growth restriction, a baby with low birthweight, or conversely, a fetus that is larger than average or born large for gestational age. A healthy diet is also shown to reduce the chances of preterm birth and the risks it brings to the baby, including longer-term health consequences.

Just as diet affects the gut microbiota in nonpregnant individuals (refer to Chapter 10), it also shapes the gut microbiota of pregnant women. Given the gut microbes' close involvement with the metabolic changes that occur in pregnancy, nutritional intake should be designed to feed the trillions of microbes living in the digestive tract — so a pregnant individual isn't eating for two, but for trillions plus two.

REMEMBER

These microbes crave fiber to support good metabolic health. One study found that a higher intake of dietary fiber (as well as omega-3 fatty acids) in pregnancy shaped the gut microbiota and predicted the newborn's gut microbiota and healthy growth in the first 18 months of life. In addition, studies in mice indicate that dietary fiber has an unmistakable impact on the gut microbial composition of the mother and is responsible for accompanying differences in the offspring's gut microbiome setup and development of its immune system.

As a side benefit, increased fiber in the diet while pregnant has the benefit of preventing or reducing some troublesome digestive symptoms that may emerge, such as constipation. When a pregnant woman is experiencing nausea, vomiting, or multiple food aversions, figuring out how to achieve adequate fiber intake may be challenging, but the payoffs to maternal and fetal health can be significant. A registered dietitian may be able to provide some personalized nutritional strategies for achieving optimal nutritional intake during pregnancy.

Supplementing with biotics

Specific biotic substances — probiotics, prebiotics, synbiotics, and postbiotics (refer to Chapter 10 for more information) — have been studied as ways to enhance the health benefits of a nutritionally balanced diet in pregnancy. Among these, probiotics (which target the gut, even if they don't always change the gut microbiota) demonstrate the greatest potential for benefits.

Overall, both the potential benefits and the potential risks of probiotics during pregnancy highlight their metabolism-modulating effects, as the following research shows:

>> According to one meta-analysis, consumption of probiotics during pregnancy (typically starting in the second or third trimester) improves metabolic parameters such as blood glucose level, lipid profile, inflammation, and oxidative markers, which indicate a lower predisposition of the mother to GDM.

On the other hand, another analysis concluded that probiotics may not lead to an actual reduction in the occurrence of GDM.

>> As for the safety of probiotics in pregnancy, most of the time the reported adverse effects are limited to mild boating or diarrhea.

However, some evidence suggests probiotics increase the risk of preeclampsia or hypertensive disorders during pregnancy and should therefore be used with caution.

More research on specific strains or strain combinations is needed to assess whether some probiotics offer the benefits without the attendant risks.

Studies suggest that probiotics taken in the third trimester of a healthy pregnancy have no adverse effects on the fetus. And in fact, some specific probiotics are shown to reduce the risk of eczema when taken for the last two months of pregnancy and the first two months after birth for breastfed infants. Consult a healthcare professional for guidance on whether a probiotic during pregnancy is advisable for you.

Managing chronic stress

A busy life doesn't usually grind to a halt when someone becomes pregnant — they still experience the same everyday stresses or sources of chronic stress that existed before the pregnancy.

REMEMBER

Chronic stress seems to have particularly negative effects in pregnancy, both for maternal and fetal health. When a mother's stress response is chronically activated, her endocrine and immune systems are on high alert and function abnormally. She may experience high blood pressure, potentially leading to preeclampsia. Severe stress (including trauma) seems to affect birth outcomes the most when it occurs early in pregnancy, and it's associated with preterm birth, lower gestational age at birth, and low birthweight. Prenatal stress may contribute to the following consequences long after birth:

>> Attachment difficulties

>> Hyperresponsiveness to stress

>> Asthma and allergy

>> Mood disorders

Although scientists don't fully understand the underlying causes of these stress-related health consequences, one study showed that maternal general anxiety in late pregnancy was associated with particular gut microbial changes, which could potentially be transmitted to the offspring. Several animal studies have found that maternal stress in pregnancy results in gut microbiome alterations, which cause abnormal behavior in the offspring.

Controlling stress during pregnancy — and particularly in the first trimester — is important for the health of both the mother and the fetus. This goal may feel unachievable in some circumstances, but incorporating stress-reduction techniques such as exercise, yoga, or meditation may help with feelings of calm. Consider consulting a qualified therapist or a healthcare professional on how to manage stress and anxiety during pregnancy. Meanwhile, much more research is needed on stress in pregnancy, including specific understandings of how racial and cultural stress experienced by people of color may increase levels of prenatal stress.

Using antibiotics wisely

Antibiotics may be necessary during pregnancy for treating bacterial infections — and in fact they're prescribed sometime during pregnancy for around one in four

U.S. women. The type of antibiotic is important, however, because some are associated with risks to the fetus, including the following:

>> Streptomycin is associated with congenital deafness if taken in the first trimester.

>> Tetracycline is linked to fetal abnormalities and liver toxicity in the mother.

>> Folate antagonists (also called *antifols*) increase the risk of neural tube and cardiac defects in the fetus.

Yet even the antibiotics that are deemed safe for use during pregnancy may potentially affect the fetus and influence health over a longer term. Studies across large populations show that antibiotics taken during pregnancy, especially during the second and third trimesters, puts the infant at greater risk of metabolic conditions as well as allergic disorders (such as asthma and eczema) in childhood. Some antibiotics have effects on the maternal gut, drastically reducing diversity temporarily, but it's unclear yet whether the long-term effects of the antibiotics have to do with this maternal modulation of the gut microbes, which is somehow passed on to the fetus. When antibiotics must be taken during pregnancy, especially in trimesters two and three, consider a strategy to offset the effects — taking a probiotic that's been proven effective for antibiotic-associated diarrhea (see Chapter 10).

Controlling infections

During pregnancy, individuals become more susceptible to many infections. The placenta is generally constructed to keep microbes out, including potentially infectious microbes that may cause harm to the fetus. However, some viruses such as Zika, rubella, and cytomegalovirus have the skills to cross into the placenta, with potentially tragic consequences that include miscarriage or major birth defects.

Even infectious microorganisms that don't get into the placenta, however, can cause a maternal response that could adversely affect the fetus. Large population studies show that viral infections during pregnancy are associated with preterm birth as well as central nervous system and cardiovascular abnormalities in the fetus. The way these fetal effects happen is still a mystery, but the latest understandings of infection in pregnancy include a maternal immune system (headed up by the GALT in the digestive tract) that responds to the presence of harmful microbes, as well as a separate immunological organ consisting of the placenta and fetus, which aids this maternal response. Thus, the fetus is a participant in a maternal infection. Moreover, the consequences of some infections may last until after birth. Animal studies indicate that even when the mother has a short-term infection with certain microorganisms in pregnancy, the offspring is born with an altered gut immune system, with overactive immunity that lasts into adulthood.

TIP

With these latest findings in mind, you want to prevent infections as much as possible during pregnancy. Here are some of the best practices for preventing infection and thereby avoiding complications for the mother and the fetus:

>> Receive all recommended vaccinations (including the seasonal flu shot and COVID-19 booster) before and during pregnancy.

>> Handwash frequently.

>> If possible, avoid direct care of others who have infections (but if necessary, wear a mask, and wash hands frequently when caring for someone who's sick).

>> Use gloves when gardening.

>> Avoid undercooked meats, sushi, and deli meats (which all carry a higher risk of infectious microbes).

>> Avoid the handling of feline litter boxes (to prevent infection with parasite called *Toxoplasma gondii,* which is shed in cat feces).

Comprehending How Events at Birth Influence the Gut

Despite potential microbial influences on the fetus, labor and birth mark the grand entrance of the baby into a world rich with microorganisms. The moment the water breaks is the beginning of a big transition, microbially speaking. For the first time, the baby experiences continuous exposure to a wide variety of microbes, which will continue for the rest of its life.

Before birth, the fetal large intestine is filled with *meconium,* a sticky substance that precedes the presence of stool. Meconium is considered sterile in utero, whereas it apparently becomes rapidly infused with bacteria after birth. These bacteria likely originate from breastmilk, maternal gut and skin, and other sources in the surrounding environment.

Generally speaking, bifidobacteria are the first microorganisms to establish themselves in the newborn's gut, having been transmitted from the mother's gut and vagina or acquired from the surrounding environment. This group of bacteria remains dominant in the gastrointestinal tract of a breastfed infant for the first several months of life.

Just as scientists lack specific knowledge on what makes a healthy gut microbiome for adults, they don't yet know the specific features of a healthy infant gut microbiome. However, the gut microbiota of a healthy, full-term, vaginally delivered, breastfed infant is generally considered the gold standard for a gut microbiota that supports optimal health in early life. The following factors surrounding birth have the potential to disrupt this ideal pattern, potentially causing health problems.

Considering birth mode

How the infant is delivered — whether by vaginal birth or C-section — is known as the *birth mode*. The procedures for carrying out a C-section safely and with minimal pain and inconvenience are a wonder of modern medicine. This single intervention has made having a baby much less risky, having saved many mothers' lives and reduced newborn complications. But today, not all C-section births are initiated for safety or lifesaving reasons. Instead, the decision to deliver a baby by C-section at times is motivated by convenience or other nonmedical factors.

Looking at how birth mode affects the initial microorganisms

The process of vaginal birth exposes the infant to microbes from all along the birth canal as well as from the maternal gut. Because C-section birth occurs in a sterile operating theatre, these exposures don't occur. Some early microbiome studies found that birth mode had striking effects on the initial microorganisms that established in and on the infant's body, as follows:

>> Vaginally delivered infants show a higher proportion of bacteria from the groups *Bacteroides* and *Bifidobacterium*, as well as lactobacilli, in the first few days of life. The microbiomes on their bodies are dynamic in the following weeks.

>> C-section delivered infants show delayed establishment of bifidobacteria, with less diversity overall and an enrichment of bacteria typically found on maternal skin or hospital surfaces: *Staphylococcus*, *Streptococcus*, and *Clostridium*.

Examining how C-section birth affects health

These findings might be unremarkable were it not for the observation across large populations that infants born by C-section have a higher risk of some health problems later in life, including:

>> Asthma and allergy

>> Attention deficit hyperactivity disorder

>> Autism spectrum disorder

>> Obesity

>> Type 1 and type 2 diabetes

One existing theory is that the increased risk for these conditions among C-section-born infants has to do with the birth mode's disruption of the infant gut microbiota during a window of time that's critical for immune system development. More research is necessary to confirm this mechanism, but some scientists believe it's prudent to take steps to normalize the infant gut microbiota of C-section-born infants.

C-sections and antibiotics tend to occur together, making it somewhat difficult to separate out the health effects of birth mode alone. However, one study that aimed to separate birth mode from the effect of antibiotics (by waiting until the baby was born and the umbilical cord was clamped before administering them to the mother) found that the differences in gut microbiota driven by birth mode are distinct, and they in fact persist through the entire first year of life.

Several studies have explored an approach called *vaginal seeding* or *maternal vaginal microbial transfer* to normalize the infant microbiome after C-section birth. This procedure involves swabbing the infant's body immediately following birth with a gauze that contains microorganisms from the mother's vaginal tract. This procedure results in an infant microbiome that temporarily looks more like that of a vaginally born infant (although not identical). However, no studies have shown whether this attenuates the health risks that accompany C-section birth. Because the risks of the procedure haven't been clearly defined, the procedure isn't recommended except as part of an approved clinical trial.

Lowering the health risks associated with a C-section

Changing the C-section microbiome immediately after birth may not be necessary because other factors may compensate for these different microbial exposures. Promising ways of modifying the infant gut microbiota and possibly reducing the health risks associated with C-section birth include the following:

>> Exclusive breastfeeding for a minimum of six months after C-section birth, which may help infants develop a gut microbiota similar to vaginally born infants

>> Infant consumption of certain probiotics may affect the gut microbiota, but it's unknown at this time which specific strains of bacteria, amount, or duration of probiotic supplementation results in a more favorable gut microbiota profile

Grappling with antibiotics at birth

Antibiotics are frequently administered to women during labor and delivery, most commonly to prevent infection during C-section birth or to prevent a bacterium called group B streptococcus (GBS) from being transmitted from the mother to the infant. Antibiotics disrupt the gut microbiota of the mother — and of the infant too, even if they're administered before the baby is born. Infants exposed to antibiotics in the time surrounding birth show reduced levels of bifidobacteria and increased levels of *Escherichia coli* in their guts, and the effects on gut microbiota may persist up to one year.

Antibiotics administered in the time surrounding birth are associated with an increased risk of infections later on for the infant, but whether the antibiotics themselves are driving this association is unclear. Nevertheless, the following tips may help mitigate the effects of antibiotics at birth:

>> When making a birth plan and preparing for all scenarios, inquire about the possibility of administering antibiotics after the umbilical cord has been clamped, should they become necessary. This may reduce their direct influence on the infant's gut.

>> If antibiotics are required during birth, focus on breastfeeding after birth to help normalize the infant's gut microbiota.

Looking at gestational age and preterm status

Gestational age is the time a fetus has developed since the beginning of pregnancy. *Preterm* infants are those born before 37 weeks' gestation.

REMEMBER

Gestational age at birth is one of the strongest determinants of the gut microbiota composition of the infant. Children born with a higher gestational age have a more diverse gut microbiota than those with a lower gestational age (although the overall diversity of the infant gut microbes isn't especially high) — and remarkably, the traces of gestational age persist in the gut microbiota up to 4 years of age. Preterm infants have a gut microbiota that reflects their earlier stage of gastrointestinal tract maturation, with lower levels of specific bacteria, including those from the *Bifidobacterium* genus, along with higher levels of potential pathogens. Preterm infants often receive more hospital care, including antibiotics, which may further influence their gut microbiota.

A SERIOUS MATTER: GBS INFECTION IN LATE PREGNANCY

Group B streptococcus (GBS) is a bacterium that, when present in a woman's rectum or vagina at the time of birth, is associated with preterm birth and stillbirth. GBS can also be transmitted to the infant, resulting in potentially life-threatening complications such as sepsis or meningitis.

To avoid these serious outcomes, women in many countries are typically tested for the presence of GBS at 35 to 37 weeks of gestation. A positive result means they're given antibiotics during labor to avoid GBS transmission to the infant. Around 25 percent of women carry GBS — which leads to the question, is there any way to keep the infant safe from GBS while still avoiding antibiotics?

The best strategy may be to reduce the chance of testing positive for GBS, eliminating the need for antibiotics. A systematic review in 2022 found that certain probiotics taken in the third trimester (starting at 30 weeks) reduced vaginal GBS colonization and appeared safe. Vaginal probiotic suppositories containing lactobacilli are also under investigation for this purpose.

Preterm infants are susceptible to a serious disease called *necrotizing enterocolitis (NEC)*, in which inflammation and death of intestinal tissue occurs. NEC is associated with a 20 to 30 percent risk of infant death, with serious health problems even among survivors: short gut syndrome, liver disease, and/or neurocognitive delay.

The notion that the gut microbiota are somehow involved in NEC susceptibility is supported by several clues:

>> Preterm infants have an altered gut microbiota that may fail to provide protective, anti-inflammatory functions.

>> Evidence from dozens of studies — collectively involving more than 10,000 infants — shows that probiotics are effective for preventing NEC.

A recent meta-analysis found that probiotics containing multiple strains are the most effective in reducing the risk of NEC and death in preterm infants. Few adverse events were reported across studies, although bacterial infection was observed in very rare cases. Several medical societies have examined the evidence and endorsed probiotics as an intervention for NEC prevention.

REGULATORY HURDLES IN ADMINISTERING PROBIOTICS TO PREVENT NEC

A wealth of research shows that probiotics are effective for preventing NEC in preterm infants, with a low risk of adverse events. But in 2023, an extremely premature infant who received a probiotic product for NEC prevention in the hospital developed a bacterial infection and tragically died. This case prompted the U.S. Food & Drug Administration (FDA) to issue a warning to healthcare professionals about probiotic supplementation in preterm infants.

The FDA subsequently warned several probiotic product manufacturers to stop selling their products as dietary supplements because they aren't subject to the same standards as drug products that specifically address disease. Some doctors caring for preterm infants are dismayed that access to probiotics is reduced for this population and that a lifesaving intervention will no longer be used so frequently.

Despite the convincing science on probiotics for steering preterm infants away from NEC, however, regulatory factors play into the ability of healthcare professionals to administer this lifesaving treatment. See the nearby sidebar for more information.

Developing a Healthy Gut in the First Three Months of Life

The first three months of an infant's life are a time of rapid change and development — in the gut as well as in the rest of the body. During this time, the digestive tract becomes better able to digest and absorb nutrients and fluids. And this window is a time of particularly rapid immune development, with the intestinal barrier and immune system learning to keep a lid on disease-causing microbes while tolerating the infant's normal gut microbial community. Newborns are more susceptible to infections during this three-month developmental window, and alterations in the gut microbiota during this time are associated with the development of immune-linked diseases such as asthma later on (even at five years of age). In parallel with the immune development that occurs during the first three months, brain development also proceeds rapidly, enabled by the brain receiving some timely signals from the gut microbes.

What does the gut microbiota of a healthy infant in the first three months of life look like? Even though it's in a constant state of flux, the gut microbial community is dominated by species and strains of bifidobacteria. Its relatively low diversity gradually increases over time. A disruption in this pattern may set up the immune system differently and predispose the child to immune-linked diseases later in life.

A couple of factors — chief among them the infant's diet — modify the gut microbiota during this critical time, with potential consequences for health. The following sections examine the two main factors.

Supporting the infant gut through diet

Ample research points to breastmilk as the optimal infant food for supporting gut and overall health — so the WHO recommends exclusively breastfeeding infants for the first six months of life and continuing at least partial breastfeeding for two years. The composition of human milk has never been replicated, even by the best-quality infant formula.

REMEMBER

The infant's early diet, whether human milk or formula, is a powerful shaper of gut health and infant gut microbes in the first three months. Compared with infants who are exclusively breastfed, formula-fed infants show a higher abundance of potentially harmful bacteria such as Enterobacterales and *Clostridium* and a higher abundance of antimicrobial resistance genes in their intestines. It's unclear, however, if these differences have any health consequences.

Important beneficial components of human milk are the human milk oligosaccharides (HMOs): complex carbohydrates that are synthesized in the mammary gland. Scientists have discovered more than 200 different types of HMOs, and the breastmilk of each mother contains a slightly different mixture of HMO structures. When ingested by the infant, most HMOs bypass the small intestine to reach the colon, becoming food for specific microbes in the infant gut. The bacteria equipped to digest HMOs are shown to have beneficial effects — supporting the infant's gut, immune system, and brain in different ways. For example, *Bifidobacterium* species that grow on HMOs prompt the release of metabolites that tame the intestinal immune system.

Human milk also contains live microorganisms, which originate in the mammary gland and are ingested by the infant. So far the functions of these microorganisms are somewhat unclear, but they could act as probiotics for the infant gut, conferring specific health benefits that are difficult to gain in other ways.

Overall, breastmilk is the optimal way to support the baby's gut health and development in the first three months. In the real world, however, breastfeeding isn't always easy and often formula feeding is the best way to provide the infant with all of its nutritional needs. In such cases, a parent may choose a formula that not only provides basic nutrition, but also mimics some additional features of human milk. See the nearby sidebar for more details.

Making use of probiotics

Besides potential administration of probiotics through infant formula, probiotics administered separately may provide health benefits to infants in the first three months. A prime example is for colic. Nearly 20 percent of infants are affected by colic — persistent and inconsolable crying, which can cause considerable distress to parents. Certain probiotic strains are shown to effectively treat colic and also may reduce daily crying time in infants without colic. If you decide to go this route, look for evidence on the specific probiotic product you're considering.

WHAT'S THE BEST FORMULA FOR SUPPORTING THE INFANT GUT?

Many options for formula are available on the market today. Some formulas now go beyond the basic nutritional components and add various ingredients to more closely approximate human milk: probiotics or postbiotics to imitate the milk microbiota, and oligosaccharides or synthetic HMOs to imitate the HMO structures in breastmilk. When these substances are present in formula, they're present in stable amounts even though their amount and composition in real human milk is specific to the mother and changes constantly with the development of the infant.

These added substances are generally deemed safe by regulators, but pediatric medical societies say more research needs to be done before recommending routine administration of these substances to healthy, term infants. Deciding whether or not to use them is a parent's choice.

Here's a rundown on some of the components added to infant formula:

- **Probiotics:** These are live microorganisms that confer a health benefit when administered at an adequate dose, with the exact benefits depending on the strain. Most infant formulas that contain probiotics have one or more strains of bifidobacteria or lactobacilli, which have a long history of safe consumption.

- **Postbiotics:** These are nonviable microorganisms, present in some fermented infant formulas that have been commercially available in Europe for several decades. So far, most postbiotics in infant formula are derived from strains of live bifidobacteria or lactobacilli.

- **Oligosaccharides:** These prebiotic fibers are included in some infant formulas because of their stability and safety for infant consumption. Different mixtures of galacto-oligosaccharides (GOS) and fructo-oligosaccharides (FOS) have been studied and are added to formula in an amount comparable to HMOs in human milk, around 8g/L. Health benefits for the infant may include stool softening and a reduced risk of infections.

- **HMOs:** So far two HMOs — 2'-fucosyllactose (2'FL) and lacto-N-neotetraose (LNnT) — have been produced synthetically and are sometimes added to infant formula to promote the growth of bifidobacteria in the infant gut.

Chapter **18**

Fostering Good Gut Health in Children and Teens

From infancy through childhood to adolescence, normal growth and development can't happen without a well-functioning digestive system. Not only does the digestive tract break down and absorb what the body needs according to its developmental stage and level of physical activity, but also the microbes living in the gut engage in continual dialog with the developing immune system.

On a daily basis, busy parents may not have their children's gut health at the top of their priority list. But gut health in childhood may help explain some important observations about disease that have puzzled researchers for years:

» Children with many older siblings have a lower risk for asthma and hay fever later in life.

» Children who grow up on traditional farms (especially ones with cowsheds and cow's milk) have half the risk for asthma and allergies.

» Children living with a dog in the household also have a lower risk of asthma and allergies as well as eczema.

The theme of these observations is that children in certain environments are less likely to have a group of diseases characterized by overactive immune systems. Is there something about siblings, farms, and dogs that can help tame the immune system at an early age? The answer is yes. All three put a child in contact with a much wider array of microbes compared with children who don't encounter them. Scientists are gathering evidence for the idea that exposure to diverse microbes early in life provides the developing immune system (both in the gut and the respiratory tract) with inputs that it scans and learns to tolerate. This learned tolerance pays off later when the immune system doesn't overreact to outside substances that frequently cause allergic reactions, such as peanuts or pollen. Underlining the gut's role in this phenomenon is the fact that these three protective factors leave traces on gut microbiota composition, in the form of a more diverse gut microbiota or enrichment in certain health-associated bacteria.

This area of research supports the notion that gut health in childhood helps set the stage for adult health, so it's important for caregivers to have an idea of how the gut develops and what science says about protecting it. Not every child can have older siblings or live with a pet dog or grow up on a farm. Nevertheless, it may be a revelation to parents and other caregivers that, in addition to their efforts to keep children away from disease-causing microbes through good hygiene, seeking out exposure to diverse, harmless microbes is also important for health.

This chapter covers three phases in human development — the first year of life, the remainder of childhood, and adolescence — and specifies the scientifically supported actions for gut health, with special attention paid to microbial exposures. I explain, throughout these phases, how caregivers can skillfully walk the tightrope of giving children exposure to lots of diverse microbes while avoiding the small minority of disease-causing microbes.

Cultivating Good Gut Health through the First Year of Life

Chapter 17 covers the critical first three months of life and the factors affecting the baby's gut health. The period that follows, from 3 to 12 months, is also important because the digestive tract matures in ways that allow it to process solid foods: The teeth start to erupt, salivary secretions change to become suitable for breaking down a variety of solids, and stomach capacity increases.

The gut microbes, too, continue a rapid pace of change during the first year of life. By 4 months old, the child's gut microbiota has an increased capacity to produce amino acids and vitamins. The gut microbial ecosystem gradually shifts over time (a process called *ecological succession*) and becomes more diverse. By one year, any traces of birth mode (vaginal delivery versus C-section) have disappeared from the gut microbiota, and infants and mothers living together share some of the exact same microbial strains.

REMEMBER

During the first year, a child's digestive system is still underdeveloped and sensitive to new substances that are ingested, so transient digestive symptoms such as vomiting, regurgitation, stomach pain, diarrhea, and constipation are common. The following symptoms, however, may signal more serious issues and should prompt you to visit your doctor:

>> Spitting up most or all of a meal (whether milk or solids)

>> Vomiting greenish bile or blood

>> Difficulty breathing during or after feedings

>> Regularly choking on food (not to be confused with usually-harmless gagging)

>> Experiencing watery diarrhea or blood in the stool

For generally healthy children in the first year of life, three actionable factors have an outsized influence on gut health: the transition to solid foods, ingestion of antibiotics, and exposure to diverse (outdoor) microbes.

Making a healthy transition to solid foods

Babies younger than 3 months old subsist only on milk or formula. But between 4 and 6 months, the baby's digestive system becomes ready to handle solid foods as well. This dietary transition marks a turning point in gut health, with a dramatic shift occurring in the gut microbes: The number of bacteria in the baby's gut sharply increase, and the diversity of the microbial community increases as well. Over the first year, the gut microbiota becomes equipped to break down many types of complex sugars and starches, with short-chain fatty acid production ramping up.

Continuing breastfeeding if possible (even occasionally) does a lot to ease the baby's transition to solid foods because the biggest gut microbiota shift of all happens when complete weaning takes place. At weaning, the baby's gut sees an increase in a group of microbes called Proteobacteria, which are normally associated with inflammation, but in healthy babies may change the chemical environment of the gut in a way that encourages establishment of a more mature microbiota (that is, one with fewer oxygen-tolerating species).

The timing of solid food introduction can have consequences on health later in the child's life. Although human milk provides all of an infant's nutritional requirements through to 6 months of age, professional recommendations generally specify introduction of solid foods no earlier than 4 months of age and no later than 6 months. Introducing solid foods too early is linked with nutritional problems and diarrhea in the infant, as well as later eczema, obesity, and adult-onset celiac disease.

Research is mixed on whether the timing of an infant's introduction to foods such as eggs and peanuts has an effect on allergy development later in life. The data currently support purposeful introduction of peanuts and eggs (as well as other possible allergens) around 6 months, but not before 4 months. If anything, a solids diet consisting of high-fat and high-sugar foods (including fried and highly processed foods) may be associated with the development of food allergies later on.

TIP

Here are some potential ways to support a healthy gut through diet in the first year of life:

>> Continue to provide the baby with breastmilk throughout the entire first year or beyond, even when solids are the main meals.

>> Introduce new foods one at a time, waiting 3 to 5 days before introducing another new food.

>> On a daily basis, offer a variety of foods that are high in fiber, including appropriate whole grains and a variety of fruits and vegetables (for example, rye bread, banana, melon, and cooked sweet potato or broccoli).

>> For infants at risk of allergy, introduce allergenic foods around 6 months. After a food has been introduced, offer it several times per week to maintain tolerance. Between 4 and 7 months is also the ideal time to introduce wheat to children who are susceptible to celiac disease.

Managing antibiotics in year one

A little more than a century ago, around 16 percent of all children born in the United States didn't survive to see their first birthday, and all the leading causes of fatality were different types of infections. Children born today have much better odds of survival because two incredibly effective interventions — vaccines and antibiotics — make them much less susceptible to fatal infections.

So let it be acknowledged that antibiotics are lifesaving treatments for many infants around the world. Yet today, antibiotics are used far more often than necessary; for example, they're often prescribed when infants display general symptoms of illness because of the possibility of developing a serious bacterial infection, even if bacterial infection hasn't been proven in a lab test.

REMEMBER

Awareness is growing about the potential downsides of antibiotics, however, especially before 12 months. Antibiotics in the first year of life are associated with negative health consequences — not just antibiotic-associated diarrhea and anti-microbial resistance in the short term, but also a higher risk of chronic conditions in the long term, such as inflammatory bowel disease (IBD), asthma, celiac disease, and increased weight in childhood or adulthood. One study also found that children who received antibiotics in their first year were more likely to have behavioral challenges, lower scores on executive function tasks, and a decreased vocabulary.

Some of the health consequences of antibiotics in the first year of life may be attributable to how they disturb the rapidly developing gut microbiome. Antibiotics have been shown to interrupt gut microbiome development during this time in a child's life, altering composition as well as function. The interruption may shape immune system development to increase susceptibility to certain immune-related diseases later in life.

TIP

Here are some ways to try reducing antibiotic use in the first year of life:

>> Prevent infections in the first place by reducing exposure to sick individuals and by washing hands frequently.

>> Take advantage of lab testing (or rapid testing) if possible to confirm a suspected bacterial infection that would necessitate the use of antibiotics.

>> Never specifically ask your doctor for antibiotics, and instead ask if close monitoring (also known as *watchful waiting*) is appropriate given your child's symptoms.

Getting exposure to safe diverse microbes

As I explain in this chapter's introduction, siblings, a farm environment, and a household dog in the first year of life all provide lifelong health benefits, likely because they provide exposure to a variety of diverse microorganisms. Early exposure seems to be crucial for these benefits to occur. Even though specific microbes that are potentially responsible for the health benefits haven't yet been identified, scientists hypothesize that beneficial microbes may either come from outside of the home (for example, from a barn) or from a natural outdoor environment.

Houses on traditional farms tend to have house dust that contains microorganisms not found in urban homes or industrialized farms. These same microorganisms are linked with less airway inflammation in mice. The evidence points to the idea that increased outdoor time may provide valuable microbial exposures that could benefit health. Also, diverse microbial exposures may be provided by either cats or dogs, because both types of pets are shown to change the gut microbiota composition of people who live in the same household.

TIP

Here are some ideas for increasing a child's exposure to diverse microbes, preferably from the outdoors, during the first year of life:

>> Have outdoor playdates with other children — not just at the playground, but in safe natural environments such as the beach or wooded areas.

>> If you have a pet dog or cat that gets along well with the baby, let the child touch it and cuddle with it.

>> If your child plays in an outdoor space such as a yard or patio, bring materials — rocks, sticks, pinecones, leaves, and other items — from the natural environment into the space if appropriate.

Nurturing Gut Health in Childhood

The gastrointestinal tract continues to grow and change throughout childhood, from the ages of 1 to 12. A complete set of baby teeth is generally acquired around age 2, equipping the child to consume a variety of differently textured foods, including tough or crunchy foods.

TECHNICAL
STUFF

Rapid change characterizes the gut microbiota during childhood, and particularly from ages 1 to 3. *Bifidobacterium* gradually lose their dominance in the child's gut during this time. One large study followed more than 900 children from four countries (Germany, Finland, Sweden, and the United States) for the first three years of life and found their gut microbiota to develop in three phases, based on the most abundant groups of bacteria:

>> **Up to 14 months:** Developmental phase, with rapid changes in composition and diversity

>> **15 to 30 months:** Transitional phase, in which some groups of bacteria stabilize, while diversity continues to fluctuate

>> **Above 30 months:** Stable phase, in which levels of most bacterial groups are sustained and diversity levels off

This analysis supports the idea that the gut microbiota becomes mostly adult-like by the third year, although other studies confirm that after age 3, the gut microbiota continues to increase in diversity and stability — both of which indicate a health-associated gut microbiota, as Chapter 3 covers.

Throughout childhood, household members also have a marked influence on the gut microbiota. In contrast with infancy, when a child primarily shares gut microbes with their mother or primary caregiver, an older child is likely to share microbial groups with all others who live under the same roof, whether they're genetically related or not.

In the following sections I focus on what a normal gut microbiota looks like in children. Furthermore, I examine several factors that support gut health in childhood: good dietary habits, outdoor microbe exposure, and reduced adverse experiences.

Knowing what constitutes normal gut development

Because the gut microbiota is a moving target in childhood, scientists have devised ways to figure out if a child's gut microbiota development is progressing as expected. For specific groups of children in research studies, scientists have developed metrics to score the maturity of the gut microbiota compared with healthy children of a similar age from the same area. These tools are useful in research but aren't yet suitable for clinical practice.

Some early research indicates that the gut microbiota of children may be more sensitive to external factors than the gut microbiota of adults. For example, a daily serving of almonds was found to produce a greater shift in the gut microbiota of children compared to adults. Another interesting study examined how adults and children fared when they visited a rainforest village far from home and consumed the local diet; the researchers found the gut microbiota response was more pronounced in the children than the adults.

Digestive symptoms such as mild abdominal pain, gas, vomiting, heartburn, diarrhea, and constipation are fairly common in healthy children and usually resolve on their own. Allergic reactions to foods can also occur throughout childhood, but they can sometimes be difficult to identify, with a wide range of symptoms (from a rash to a runny nose to difficulty breathing) that can occur from minutes to hours after ingestion of the food. The majority of allergic reactions aren't serious, but if the child has difficulty breathing or swallowing, you should seek medical attention right away.

Some digestive diseases are frequently diagnosed in childhood, too. Celiac disease may be detected, and its symptoms tend to be more obvious than in adults with celiac disease. IBD (either ulcerative colitis or Crohn's disease) can slow growth or delay puberty if present in children.

TIP

As a parent, trust your gut about your child's gut; if you observe a change or a symptom you're worried about, see a doctor. Here are some definite reasons to seek medical attention:

>> Blood is visible in your child's stool.

>> Your child has pain or difficulty passing stool on a regular basis.

>> Your child's stool appears greasy, runny, and particularly smelly.

>> Your child vomits persistently or has vomit that is green or bloody.

Establishing good dietary habits for life

On the one hand, many caregivers in industrialized countries are well aware of messages about healthy eating for children and the need for lots of fruits and vegetables. But on the other hand, the readily available foods that are deemed kid-friendly in grocery stores and restaurants — from sugary breakfast cereals to mac 'n cheese and chicken fingers — aren't nutritionally ideal. In addition, many kids who are accustomed to consuming sweet and high-fat foods sulk when faced with high-fiber foods such as lentils or broccoli. These circumstances can make healthy eating for kids an uphill battle.

REMEMBER

Aside from overall nutritional needs for supporting healthy growth, however, a child particularly needs a diverse range of fiber-rich foods to support the development of the gut microbiota and overall gut health. Just as increased intake of fiber is a gut-friendly diet principle for adults (as Chapter 10 explains), it also can be a guiding principle for healthy eating in kids. While a Western-style dietary pattern (high in both sugar and fat and low in fiber) has detrimental effects on children's health, increasing fiber makes all the difference and mitigates these negative effects.

A focus on fiber may help set children up for better eating habits that will last throughout their lives. With my two children, I talk a lot about fiber in a relaxed way — which foods have lots of it and which foods lack it. Sometimes we read labels together, and sometimes we do a quick online search. The goal is to be aware of fiber in the foods we consume and try to make sure we include it regularly (even though we don't necessarily try to consume a set amount per day). When one of my kids asks for a cookie after school, I ask, "What fiber have you had?" If he hasn't consumed any fiber recently, I first provide him with something higher in fiber (for example, a banana or some carrot sticks) and afterward give him the cookie he really wants. And even though I did try to restrict sugar consumption during the first two years, now that my kids are school-aged, I don't ban cookies in the house — because they're going to encounter cookies their entire lives and I want to empower them to make responsible decisions about how to balance their diets, while fully aware that fiber is the key to many health benefits.

REMEMBER

A registered dietitian specializing in children's nutrition can offer personalized advice for encouraging children to eat their fruits and veggies. These tips support gut health in childhood through adequate nutritional intake and increased fiber:

>> Start every day with a higher-fiber food, such as sliced fruit.

>> Get in the habit of presenting a high-fiber food before giving your child a sweet or salty food.

>> Slow down to eat and enjoy meals together so your child can observe your own balanced meal.

>> In a developmentally appropriate way, explain that good bugs (microbes) live in your child's tummy and that it's their job to take care of the bugs by feeding them fiber. Several great kids' books are available for introducing this topic.

Enjoying some good ol' fashioned dirt

Exposure to diverse microbes, preferably from outdoor sources, is important not just in the first year (when it can pay extra dividends for health) but all throughout childhood. This area of research is relatively new, but one intervention study tested children between the ages of 3 and 5 after playing with a regular sandbox and one that was enriched in biodiverse microbes. They found that the biodiverse sandbox changed the microbes on the children's skin and led to positive differences in their immune system activity. Another study of children in a ten-week nature play program found their gut microbiota was changed after the program, and the children also showed a reduction in stress and anger. These findings reinforce the idea that diverse microbial exposure through a little dirt is a good thing.

Not all dirt is equal, so it's important to make educated guesses about where disease-causing microbes may be lurking. The trick is to maintain good hygiene while allowing your child to have close contact with natural environments. The good hygiene part comes more easily to many parents: washing the child's hands and face, preventing the child from eating food that has fallen to the floor, or encouraging the use of a tissue to wipe their nose. But contact with natural environments can be encouraged, too: taking children outside often, inviting contact with woodchips, sand, and soil, or seeking kids' help with gardening tasks.

TIP

Here are some ideas for increasing outdoor microbial exposures while reducing infection in childhood:

>> For outdoor time, dress kids in clothes that are okay to get dirty and don't stop them from playing in the mud or dirt (within reason).

>> When outside, encourage children to touch natural materials (except animal waste).

>> Never drink untreated water from a stream or lake.

>> Wash children's hands with soap after touching animals, before eating, and after using the toilet but avoid antibacterial soaps. Handwashing is critical after kids who are playing outside may have come into contact with raccoon feces, as they harbor roundworms (*Baylisascaris*), which can cause life-threatening brain infection especially in young children.

>> Scrub children's toys only after a sick child has played with them or when visibly dirty.

>> Eat home-grown vegetables straight out of the garden but wash store-bought fruits and vegetables with plain water before consuming them.

Mitigating childhood adversity

Certainly the ideal environment for a child to grow up in is calm and stress-free. Nevertheless, many children unfortunately have stressful or adverse experiences in their early years.

TECHNICAL
STUFF

Scientists have different ways of measuring the stress experienced by children:

>> Going through a list of adverse experiences and counting how many have occurred in a child's early years with the assumption that the consequences of stress are due to repeated exposure, regardless of the type of stress.

>> Listing the specific types of stressors, under the premise that different categories of experiences have different effects on the developing brain.

>> Considering each stressor and the child's reaction to it individually because a given adverse event such as neglect has different effects on different children.

But no matter how adverse events are measured, they make a child more vulnerable to mental and physical disorders later in life.

SHOULD HEALTHY CHILDREN TAKE PROBIOTICS?

Some probiotic products are aimed specifically at children, raising the question of whether generally healthy children should take a probiotic on a daily basis. Probiotics may be a little pricey — not to mention that pills and supplements may not go over so well with children (although probiotics in gummy format may be more palatable).

On the plus side, many available probiotics for kids are shown to be very safe from birth to adolescence. Some probiotic strains are well-studied and have been shown to provide a range of benefits to children, from reducing chronic constipation to improving gut motility and shortening the duration of diarrhea. Other probiotics may reduce the occurrence of upper respiratory tract infections — in other words, the common cold. So although probiotics have the potential to confer benefits on healthy children, this ability depends on the strain(s) used. Make sure you do your homework on the product (see Chapter 12).

Research in animals shows gut microbes may be involved in how adverse experiences have ripple effects on health through the rest of life. Mice separated from their mothers in early life experience long-term changes in gut microbiota as well as long-term exaggerated stress responses. In humans too, the gut microbiota of mothers and children have distinct features that occur under circumstances of social disadvantage and psychosocial stressors. These observations raise the intriguing possibility that one day scientists could find interventions that normalize the adversity-associated microbiota, thereby attenuating the ways that early trauma persists in the body.

Protecting a child from these experiences whenever possible — or providing physical and emotional support if they do happen — may bring the child invaluable benefits for health later in life.

Encouraging Good Gut Health in Teens

Adolescence, from puberty to around the age of 18 years, is a time of skeletal maturation in the body as well as continued maturation of the digestive tract. The gut microbiome doesn't yet look exactly like that of an adult, but it does show differences in some key bacterial groups compared to early childhood.

REMEMBER

Digestion may change around puberty, with new gastrointestinal symptoms emerging. The most common gut symptoms during this time are as follows:

» Abdominal pain

» Constipation

» Symptoms of lactose intolerance (vomiting in particular, but also abdominal pain/cramps, bloating, gas, or diarrhea)

In this age group, IBD is the major chronic digestive disease that may emerge, with around 25 percent of people with IBD being diagnosed before the age of 20. Teens also sometimes receive a diagnosis of gallstones or pancreatitis.

According to the latest research, diet and outdoor time are the main ways to support gut health in the phase of adolescence.

Supporting teens to make good diet choices

During adolescence, individuals tend to gain around 40 percent of their adult weight and 15 percent of their adult height. Dietary choices are important for supporting this major bodily transition.

As a teenager's priorities shift toward social connections and independent activities, a balanced diet may not always be the top priority. However, the consequences of a poor diet during this time of life are potentially long-lasting, especially with regard to mental health. One large study found in adolescents aged 11 to 18 that poorer diet scores (high-fat, high-sugar intake) correlated with lower mental health scores. This association is seen in multiple studies, and dietary effects on the gut microbiota — with subsequent effects on the brain through the gut-brain axis — is a leading hypothesis for why this occurs.

TIP

Some ideas for supporting gut health through diet in teens are as follows:

» When hungry, teens may tend to eat the first thing that's readily available, so leave nutritious, high-fiber foods — vegetable sticks or trail mix, for example — where they're easily seen and grabbed.

» Model balanced eating. At this highly impressionable time, if caregivers don't eat a variety of high-fiber foods that nourish their gut health, teens may not see the point in doing it themselves.

>> Introduce fermented foods if your teen doesn't already consume them. Teens may seek out novelty, and fermented foods offer a wide variety of new flavors and textures to try.

>> Prompt teens with language related to intuitive eating — that is, knowing when to eat by relying on physiological signals such as hunger, rather than emotional or situational cues. For example, rather than commenting on how much or how little your teen is eating at a meal, provide reassurance that you trust them to know how much food their body needs. (The exception is for teens who have a diagnosed eating disorder; in that case, follow the suggestions of your doctor or dietitian.)

Getting a dose of nature

Adolescents today spend a lot of time indoors, especially with screens that facilitate social connections without having to set foot outside. Yet exposure to natural environments is shown to replenish the cognitive, social, and behavioral resources they need for physical and mental wellness in everyday life.

One study found that more time spent in a woodland environment was associated with higher cognitive scores and a lower risk of emotional and behavioral problems for adolescents. More time outdoors appears to benefit teens in multiple, complex ways, and one of the mechanisms may occur through the microbial exposures they get from it.

TIP

Adolescence is known as a time when individuals form habits that will last into adulthood. Here are some suggestions for helping teens get in the habit of spending time outside:

>> Don't just send your teen outside — join them! Go for a walk together or visit the park to sit and read books.

>> Ask your teen to invite one of their friends for an outdoor family activity such as a hike.

>> On holidays, deliberately plan some outdoor activities (for example, a picnic or an afternoon at the beach).

>> Leave your teen's favorite sports equipment (for example, a basketball or a baseball and gloves) in a handy spot such as a vehicle trunk so you're equipped to play if you come across an appropriate outdoor area.

>> Encourage your teen to try something new — kayaking, zip-lining, snowboarding, or another outdoor activity.

Chapter **19**

Maintaining Gut Health in Older Age

O ccasionally in the media, a self-professed biohacker claims to have reduced biological age by 5 or even 25 years through a special lifestyle regimen that includes ice baths, chia seed smoothies, strength training, or early bedtime. In truth, no one has ever really been able to turn back the clock on their age, yet it's clear that not everyone experiences the same physical and cognitive deterioration as the years advance. For some individuals, aging means day-to-day activities become more challenging as physical and cognitive functions slowly ebb and age-related diseases take their toll. For other individuals, age is just a number that advances as they stay sharp and active with an overall sense of well-being. The individuals with greater well-being are said to have a longer *health span* — defined as "the period of life spent in good health, free from the chronic diseases and disabilities of aging."

What makes the difference between those who remain fit and robust past the age of 65 and those who start to experience *frailty* (that is, physiological decline and vulnerability to poor health)? Given that healthy aging tends to run in families, genes certainly contribute to the length of one's health span. But lifestyle factors are also powerful tools for shaping what happens with advancing age.

REMEMBER

Gut health and gut microbes are emerging as cornerstones of healthy aging. This status is rooted in their close connections with overall health (as Chapters 3 and 5 describe) and bolstered by emerging evidence that shows the heightened importance of gut-related lifestyle factors at age 65 and higher. While in younger adulthood the gut microbiota may buffer the effects of some lifestyle choices that could be detrimental to health, in older adulthood the gut microbiota becomes more vulnerable and loses resilience, making healthy lifestyle choices even more important.

Some of the positive lifestyle choices that are likely to increase your health span may exert their biological effects through the gut microbiota. This chapter covers the primary ways you can protect your gut health in older age (65 to 99) and what researchers have learned about longevity from people who reach their 100th birthdays.

Finding Out How to Maintain a Healthy Gut in Older Age

During the normal aging process, some of the changes that occur in the digestive system are as follows:

>> Missing/broken teeth or dental pain, affecting what one eats

>> Reduced digestive enzyme secretion

>> Slower motility in the colon

>> Decreased immune function in the intestine and other mucosal sites of the body

These physical changes may be associated with more frequent digestive symptoms — primarily an increase in constipation, but also swallowing difficulties, loss of appetite, abdominal discomfort, or sometimes fecal incontinence.

Aging is also associated with an increased risk of some digestive diseases. A growing number of individuals with inflammatory bowel disease are diagnosed after age 65, and diagnoses of celiac disease are increasing in this population as well. The risk of colon cancer also increases with age.

The following sections examine the changes that occur in the gut microbiota as you age and delves into some ways to support your gut health in older adulthood, which may pay dividends for overall health.

Identifying what causes changes in the gut microbiota as you age

Changes occur in the gut microbiota as you age. In older age, the gut microbes show less similarity to other people, with fewer of the microbial species that are common among younger adults. Scientists have figured out two overlapping and interacting drivers of these gut microbiota shifts:

>> **Normal aging-related changes:** These changes in the gut microbiota are characterized by a reduction in bacterial groups that are dominant in younger people, and a marked loss of bifidobacteria (which are normally associated with health) and anti-inflammatory bacteria. Diversity decreases, and the gut may see an increase in *Akkermansia* and in potentially disease-causing bacteria.

Gut microbiota may also interact with the immune system to influence the general process of *inflammaging*, which is a chronic low-grade inflammation that occurs in older adults. Inflammaging may kick off a cycle of gut microbial changes — primarily an increase in oxygen-tolerating species — that, in turn, reinforce inflammation in the intestines.

>> **Age-linked diseases and frailty:** These diseases also cause particular shifts in the gut microbiota that are distinct from the effects of aging per se (see Chapter 5 for more details). Studies show the individuals with greatest frailty tend to have certain gut microbes in common, and it appears that gut microbes may hasten the transition to a frail state.

The good news is that scientists are actively studying how lifestyle factors such as dietary intake and medications may be able to delay the effects of aging and disease on the gut microbiota, potentially modifying age-related physical and cognitive impairments. In fact, particularly healthy older people, who have fulfilling and active lives, show a less pronounced loss of microbes that produce the short-chain fatty acid (SCFA) butyrate, and as such their intestinal microbial communities look similar to younger individuals.

Living environment and geography seem to leave their marks on the gut particularly in older age. Studies on older individuals in South Korea, China, Japan, Italy, and other countries show distinct differences in gut microbiota composition based on the geographical area. In addition, individuals who move from a community setting into a residential care facility see a marked change in gut microbiota that continues to change over a period of one year before leveling off. Although some studies find these gut microbial changes are associated with health status, cause and effect aren't yet clear.

Paying attention to diet

Older adults don't require as many calories in their daily diet even though they have the same nutrient needs as a younger person, which means a high-quality diet is necessary for optimal health. Toast and tea, unfortunately, doesn't cut it. Neither do some of the meals offered at residential care homes, which sometimes favor palatable and easy-to-eat foods such as gelatin and mashed potatoes over the nutrient-dense foods that older individuals really need.

A lower-quality diet in older age markedly impoverishes the gut microbiota. One initial study in the field found major differences in gut microbiota structure and lower diversity in older people who lived in residential care homes compared to people of the same age who lived in the community. The community-dwellers' gut microbiota looked like healthy younger adults. The main lifestyle factor accounting for the gut microbiota differences was diet: The community-dwellers consumed much more fiber than most of the individuals in residential facilities; sure enough, the pattern of a low-fiber diet and distinctive gut microbiota was also associated with poorer health overall and greater frailty. A separate study also backed up dietary intake as an important factor for gut microbiota and healthy aging: Poor appetite and reduced food intake in older adults led to a less diverse gut microbiota, changes in its composition, and reduced muscle strength.

REMEMBER

On the positive side, fiber-rich diets are correlated with enhanced markers of health as well as health-associated microbes in the gut. One important study found that people over age 65 who adhered to a Mediterranean-like dietary pattern for one year showed distinct differences in their gut microbiota, with more SCFA–producing bacteria and metabolites associated with health. Compared to a control group, the Mediterranean diet group also had lower markers of inflammation, better cognitive function and less frailty, and less incidence of chronic diseases. The study provided compelling evidence that diet can affect gut health in a way that staves off normal aging-linked physiological decline.

Worthy gut-related aims for dietary interventions in older age are to increase the abundances of lactobacilli and bifidobacteria as well as other butyrate-producing bacteria, thereby extending or improving health. Certain dietary supplements may be particularly helpful for achieving these ends. Biotic substances have the advantage of delivering health benefits in this age group with very little preparation or effort.

Here are some examples of biotic supplements that may be able to complement foods in the diet to improve health in older age (see Chapter 10 for more information on biotics):

>> **Prebiotics:** Certain prebiotics increase bifidobacteria while improving parameters of immune function or metabolic health. Polyphenols may also act as prebiotic substrates; in fact, some polyphenol supplements and polyphenol-rich foods are shown to be more effective in older adults (especially those with frailty as well as obesity and insulin resistance) than in younger adults. Resistant starch powder, another type of prebiotic, is generally palatable when added to cold drinks and is effective at increasing bifidobacteria and potentially improving metabolic health.

>> **Probiotics:** Some probiotic strains (or groups of strains) are effective for increasing bifidobacteria and lactobacilli while improving measures of immune activity. Newer formulations leveraging gut-brain axis mechanisms are also shown to improve stress and benefit mood, anxiety, and/or sleep quality.

>> **Synbiotics:** Specific combinations of bacterial strains with prebiotic substrates are shown to bolster either bifidobacteria or lactobacilli in the gut, with health effects that range from improved immune function to better metabolic function.

REMEMBER

The effects of these interventions may depend on a person's baseline gut microbiome composition; so, if an older individual lacks a certain group of bacteria, for example, the intervention may not have the intended effect. This factor highlights the importance of maintaining a high-quality diet from earlier in adulthood so that important bacterial groups are retained with age.

Managing medications

Polypharmacy — the use of multiple drugs that address disease — is more common in older adults than younger adults. And even though each prescribed drug has a specific use, polypharmacy itself is associated with negative outcomes such as adverse drug reactions as well as a higher risk for hip fractures. Polypharmacy is also associated with gut microbiota differences, with increased or decreased abundance of 15 bacterial groups. Consider these medications:

>> **Antibiotics:** They're known for their impacts on gut health and gut microbiota composition — and their effects may be particularly pronounced in older individuals. Antibiotic-induced gut microbiota changes are associated with diminished markers of immunity and poorer cognitive function in older people. A mouse study found the gut microbiota in older mice took longer to recover after a ten-day antibiotic treatment.

>> **Proton pump inhibitors (PPIs):** These drugs address symptoms of gastro-esophageal reflux disease, and their use tends to increase with age. One large study in Spain found more than half of those older than 65 were prescribed a PPI. These drugs have pronounced effects on the gut microbiota at any age with compositional shifts and decreased diversity.

>> **Nonsteroidal anti-inflammatory drugs (NSAIDs):** They're a common pain-relief medication available without a prescription. Even though they're effective for relieving pain temporarily, their long-term use can cause damage to the upper digestive tract. Aging increases the risk of gastric ulcers or other complications from NSAID use. Additional drugs reducing acid in the stomach, such as PPIs, can help prevent the digestive tract damage from NSAIDs, but these may have negative effects on the gut microbiota.

TIP

Judiciously using medications, especially antibiotics, in older age is important. Where possible, older adults should leverage lifestyle factors for improving gut health and overall health, to avoid the consequences of both individual drugs and polypharmacy.

Discovering the Secrets of Gut Health and Longevity

Certain areas of the world, known as longevity blue zones, have an abnormally high proportion of people who live past 100. These areas include Okinawa (Japan), Nicoya Peninsula (Costa Rica), the island of Ikaria (Greece), Sardinia (Italy), and Loma Linda in California.

Scientists studying these remarkable populations have determined that about one-third of longevity is accounted for by genes, and the remainder is attributed to personal and lifestyle factors. Here are factors associated with living past 100:

>> Strong family connections

>> Close social ties

>> A sense of meaning in life

>> Continuous, low-level physical activity

>> Stress management

>> Moderate amounts of alcohol consumption

>> Belief in a higher power

When tallying all the effects of normal aging as well as disease and lifestyle factors on gut health, can the gut actually support greater longevity? The connection between gut health and longevity has been a topic of speculation for many years. Famously in 1908, the Russian scientist Elie Metchnikoff studied long-lived individuals in rural Bulgaria and proposed that the fermented milk they drank was the secret to their longevity. He surmised that aging was attributable to pathogenic microorganisms poisoning the large intestine and that the microbes in the fermented milk were able to offset this process.

Unfortunately, subsequent work has found that humans need more than a little yogurt or kefir to live a long, healthy life. It's true that in some animal models, manipulating the gut microbiota can delay age-related impairments and sometimes actually prolong lifespan. In humans the gut isn't the silver bullet for longevity, but it may indeed be a worthwhile target for increasing lifespan as well as health span.

The gut microbiota of healthy centenarians retains some of the features of normal aging (such as a lower abundance of health-associated bacteria) but also has distinct features — high diversity in composition and an increased proportion of butyrate-producing bacteria — which are found in individuals older than 100 living in very different geographic areas. An intriguing study of very healthy centenarians from Jiangsu, China, found these individuals' gut microbiota looked similar to that of middle-aged adults, reinforcing the notion that the gut is an engine of healthy aging.

Overall, centenarians reinforce the notion that the gut microbiota can be a target for healthy aging — even though scientists need to do much more work to find out what specific interventions can increase longevity. However, the top potential areas for interventions are related to dietary intake and psychosocial factors.

Diminishing calories

Diet seems to be a highly important lifestyle factor that contributes to longevity. Analyses of centenarians find that they usually avoid overeating, and many have a diet lower in calories than other individuals or follow a fasting regimen. These behaviors amount to *caloric restriction* (CR), which is a lower intake of calories without malnutrition. Across both animal and human studies, evidence shows that CR contributes to longevity.

CR also affects the gut microbiome's composition and function, increasing butyrate-producing microbes and decreasing groups of proinflammatory bacteria. The gut microbiota may be responsible for some beneficial metabolic effects of CR, as demonstrated in mouse studies. Further research is needed to determine the mechanisms of CR's effects and any gut bacterial groups that could be responsible for effects on health and longevity; in the meantime, some form of CR is advisable in older age as a lifestyle change to promote longevity. Consult with a doctor or registered dietitian for guidance on how to implement a form of CR that works for you.

Attending to psychosocial factors

Recent research on the microbiota gut-brain axis (see Chapter 3) raises the possibility that psychosocial attributes of long-lived individuals could help maintain health through the gut. At least four psychosocial domains warrant more study in people of extreme age:

>> Life events and personal history

>> Personality

>> Cognition

>> Socioeconomic resources and support systems

So far researchers don't know if people with happy childhoods and laid-back personalities, for example, are predisposed to having a longer life. These factors could plausibly leave their marks on gut health, thereby contributing to health or longevity, but more research is needed to determine any specific interventions that could be applied in the psychosocial domain for a longer health span.

6
The Part of Tens

Discover the top gut-friendly foods to include in your diet.

Clarify common misunderstandings about gut health.

Chapter **20**

Ten Foods for Better Gut Health

The name of the game for gut health is diversity of (plant) foods; research shows that consumption of at least 30 types of plants per week leads to the most diverse gut microbiota. So the idea of focusing on a small number of superfoods actually runs counter to the ethos of gut-friendly diets. But on the other hand, picking out some foods that are high achievers in the realm of substances that contribute to gut health is possible. These foods either have high amounts of prebiotic fibers or high numbers of diverse live cultures — both of which are associated with gut health as well as overall health.

TIP

What follows are ten of the best foods to incorporate into your diet for gut health. To be clear, don't consume them excessively (lest they actually reduce the diversity in your diet); rather eat moderate portions of these foods regularly to round out a diverse diet.

The first five foods in this chapter — onions, garlic, leeks, Jerusalem artichokes, and dandelion greens — are high in *prebiotics,* substances that alter your gut microbes in a way that benefits your health. Although many different vegetables and fruits contain prebiotics, researchers from San José State University who analyzed the prebiotics contained in 8,690 foods in the Food and Nutrient Database for Dietary Studies singled out the ones in this chapter. These five foods contain between 100 and 240 milligrams of prebiotics per gram of food.

The proof for prebiotic benefits is in the science: When researchers in Belgium studied what happened when they gave individuals a diet high in prebiotic-rich vegetables (preparing dishes such as Jerusalem artichoke soup and globe artichoke salad), not only did the participants' gut microbes re-configure (with more health-associated bifidobacteria), but also they felt more satisfied after their meals and their cravings for sweet, salty, and fatty foods notably decreased. Note that the dose (or amount) of prebiotic foods is important for the health benefits you receive. By eating the prebiotic-rich foods suggested in this chapter the dose may vary so you aren't guaranteed to have a specific health benefit such as reduced cravings. However, these foods are ideal for giving you more general health benefits and boosting the levels of health-associated bacteria in your gut.

The final five foods in this chapter give you a hearty dose of live microorganisms. Of the rich variety of fermented foods that exist in the world, the ones in this chapter are relatively common to find in grocery stores and/or easy to make yourself, and they typically contain a diverse mix of live cultures when you consume them raw. The live cultures in these foods don't generally meet the criteria to be considered probiotics, but nevertheless, higher quantities of these live dietary microbes (no matter the type, as long as they're safe for consumption) are associated with health benefits that include better blood pressure and blood sugar control, lower inflammation, and a lower weight.

TIP

If some of the foods in this chapter are new to you, start with small steps: First try a tiny amount, then gradually increase the portion over time. But if your home is already stocked with some of these foods on a regular basis, you can try a new way of eating the food or increase how frequently you consume it. The ultimate goal is to consume a minimum of one or two of the foods in this chapter every day.

Onions

The onion, with its many layers and papery skin (yellow, white, or red) is a common staple in kitchens around the world. But don't let its humble appearance fool you — this vegetable has an esteemed history. In ancient Greece, athletes ate copious amounts of onions with the belief that they'd gain exceptional strength. And onions were considered sacred in ancient Egypt because their concentric circles symbolized eternal life.

Onions are an important flavor in many recipes and can be used as a main vegetable, a condiment, or both. The smell of cooking onions is often the first sign that something good is going on in your kitchen — mouthwatering for certain, but also eye watering when you cut them. (*Tip:* Chill onions for 30 minutes in the fridge before slicing them to cut down on the tear factor.)

TIP

Onions are high in a prebiotic fiber called *fructo-oligosaccharides* (FOS). Try consuming more onions by putting into action these ideas:

>> Slow cook onions to make a French onion soup.

>> Remove the skin and inner layers and then stuff the onions and bake them.

>> Sauté onions in a mixture of butter and olive oil and use as a topping for burgers or meats.

Garlic

Garlic, a bulbous herb made up of a cluster of tightly packed cloves, has been cultivated by humans for more than 5,000 years. Today, many varieties of garlic exist, falling into two categories:

>> **Softneck:** Many smaller cloves in each bulb, with a more papery skin

>> **Hardneck:** Bulbs made up of fewer, larger cloves that have a thicker skin; a rigid stalk in the center

Garlic releases its flavor when cut, crushed, or chopped. You can use it either raw or cooked, but its strong, lingering flavor and smell means it's typically used sparingly when raw.

Garlic was traditionally used for alleviating digestive symptoms, and today scientists know it does indeed have gut benefits because it's high in prebiotics (FOS). Even though many people already use small amounts of garlic in cooking, it's better for your gut microbes if you think beyond just the flavoring that garlic has to offer and look for ways to consume a higher amount — several cloves at a time.

TIP

To incorporate more garlic into your diet, buy fresh, whole bulbs rather than preminced garlic because they're more versatile. This list has some ways to eat more garlic — and the garlic breath part is optional, depending how you choose to consume it:

>> Cut the whole bulb in half horizontally and slow roast it in the oven; the cloves become buttery soft and make a delicious spread for bread or crackers.

>> Make aioli by crushing together minced garlic, egg yolks, olive oil, lemon juice, salt, and pepper.

>> Add a few whole cloves of garlic into a soup without crushing them and let them simmer for a gentle garlic flavor. You can eat the cloves in the soup after they're well cooked.

>> Make garlic bread by mixing together crushed garlic and butter (with herbs if desired) and then spreading over crusty bread and broiling in the oven.

Leeks

Leeks are members of the onion and garlic family — and with their white flesh and dark green leafy tops, they look like a giant version of scallions. Leeks have a milder flavor than some closely related plants, making them versatile veggies for eating raw or cooked.

Leeks are generally high in fiber (with around 1.6 grams per cup) and are an excellent source of prebiotics — no wonder they were traditionally used to improve digestion and sometimes alleviate constipation.

TIP

Here are some ways to consume more leeks in your diet:

>> Make *vichyssoise,* a soup made with pureed potatoes and leeks and typically served cold.

>> Use finely chopped raw leek instead of raw onion in salads if you prefer a milder flavor.

>> Chop and sauté leeks, and then drizzle them with a vinaigrette or cream sauce for an easy side dish.

Jerusalem Artichokes

Jerusalem artichokes are root vegetables that somewhat resemble knobby brown potatoes. The plant is a variety of sunflower that originated in North America and was later brought to Europe and beyond.

These vegetables aren't really artichokes, nor do they come from Jerusalem. Their name may have originated from a mispronunciation of the Italian *girasole articiocco,* meaning "sunflower artichoke" — a name that came from knowledge of the plant type plus the fact that, when eaten raw, the vegetable's nutty, crunchy flavor is reminiscent of genuine artichokes (that is, the thistle-shaped globe artichokes with green leaves that can be pulled apart). Sometimes Jerusalem artichokes are also called *sunchokes* or *earth pears.*

TIP

Jerusalem artichokes are abundant in a prebiotic called inulin. They can be boiled, roasted, or eaten raw. Here are some more delicious ways to enjoy Jerusalem artichokes:

>> Make a pureed soup of them.

>> Roast and serve them with aioli.

>> Make a Jerusalem artichoke and potato *au gratin.*

>> Shred some raw Jerusalem artichoke over a salad.

WARNING

Take it slow if you're not used to eating Jerusalem artichokes because large doses can cause uncomfortable gas and bloating. Start with a small portion and increase your consumption over time.

Dandelion Greens

When you see dandelions on the lawn, eating them may not be top of mind. But make no mistake, the entire dandelion, apart from the stem, is delicious to eat. Dandelion greens are the leaves of the dandelion plant. Rather than harvesting the leaves from random dandelions, however, you can grow the plants in a pot or garden and trim off the flowers as soon as they appear, encouraging the leaves to grow larger. You can then eat these leaves as nutritious greens.

TIP

Dandelion greens are high in the prebiotic fiber inulin, and their spicy, bitter taste slightly resembles arugula. Dandelion greens can be eaten raw or cooked — and when cooked they can be prepared like spinach or kale. To reduce bitterness, blanch the greens in boiling water for one to two minutes before cooking. Here are some ways to try dandelion greens:

>> Add them to soups that have spinach or kale, adding brightness to the green vegetable flavors.

>> Sauté and then blend them with garlic, pine nuts, salt, and Parmesan cheese to make a flavorful pesto.

>> Create a salad of dandelion greens and other greens dressed with strong flavored oils and vinegars (for example, wine vinegar or raspberry vinegar).

>> Sauté them with small pieces of bacon.

>> Make a salad from dandelion greens, bacon, warm vinaigrette, and garlic croutons.

Yogurt

Yogurt — the most common microbe-rich food to be found in the average supermarket — is made when milk is fermented with two bacterial species, *Streptococcus thermophilus* and *Lactobacillus bulgaricus*. During the first part of the fermentation the *Streptococcus* do the work, but after the milk mixture starts to turn sour, the lactobacilli dominate the fermentation. Overall, the process of making yogurt makes milk more digestible.

Meanwhile, Greek yogurt is made when regular yogurt is strained, removing some of the liquid (called *whey*), to create a thicker product that's higher in protein and calories per serving.

SCIENTIST SAYS

Bob Hutkins, Professor of Food Microbiology at University of Nebraska in Lincoln, Nebraska, says if you're a newbie to fermented foods, trying different brands of yogurt is a good first step. He says, "Yogurt is the most accessible fermented food in the grocery store. Its health benefits are well established." He adds that plain yogurt is the best option because some sweetened versions can contain as much sugar as a can of soda. For gut health you don't need to choose low-fat or fat-free yogurt unless you prefer the taste. (Chapter 10 discusses how fats affect gut health.)

Yogurt is a great source of live cultures, but only some commercial yogurts contain microorganisms that qualify as probiotics. If a product has probiotics added after fermentation, you should find the probiotic strain or strains listed on the label.

TIP

Yogurt is easy to eat by itself and is normally available as many different types of convenient products. Here are some ideas for eating more yogurt:

>> Make a yogurt parfait in a tall glass by layering plain yogurt, granola, and fruit or jam.

>> Add a dab of plain yogurt on top of a curry, soup, or stew.

>> Stir yogurt into oatmeal in place of milk.

>> Blend herbs and salt into yogurt for a green goddess dressing to eat with salad or rice dishes.

Kefir

Describing kefir as yogurt's thinner, sourer cousin doesn't do it justice — it's a tangy dairy drink that's made by simply combining milk with *kefir grains* (which are gelatinous granules resembling tapioca pearls, made up of yeasts and bacteria). Yeasts transform the lactose in the milk into carbon dioxide and alcohol, so trace amounts of alcohol may be present in the final product. Commercial kefir is typically found in the dairy section of the grocery store, next to the yogurt.

Besides yogurt, kefir, which is an excellent source of live cultures, is one of the most studied types of fermented foods. Research demonstrates that, unlike other fermented foods, kefir consumption results in detectable changes to the gut microbiota. For example, experiments show that daily consumption of kefir leads to a reconfigured gut microbial community, with once-rare species growing in abundance.

TIP

Try these ways to consume more kefir:

>> Create a mango lassi with kefir and mango, adding honey to sweeten according to your preference.

>> Put a few pieces of frozen fruit in a bowl with kefir and let it sit on the counter to thaw for about one hour before consuming.

>> Use kefir as a base for a creamy salad dressing.

Kimchi

One of the oldest known examples of lacto-fermented vegetables, kimchi is a spicy fermented cabbage that appeared to originate between 2,500 and 3,000 years ago in Korea. Kimchi is a $2 billion industry in Korea today, which is not to mention the kimchi produced in people's homes. Its popularity has spread all around the globe with many different variations being produced using radishes, cucumbers, and other vegetables.

Kimchi (unless it's cooked) is rich in live cultures. Studies across populations associate kimchi with various health benefits such as a lower incidence of metabolic dysfunction and asthma. Some lactic acid bacteria isolated from kimchi seem to have anti-inflammation and anti-obesity effects when tested in animals.

TIP

Here are some ideas for eating kimchi:

>> Add it to any egg dish (perhaps in place of Tabasco sauce).

>> Top ramen noodles or a rice bowl with a few spoonfuls of kimchi.

>> Chop it finely and add it to a hot dog or hamburger.

>> Sauté greens and then remove them from the heat and stir in kimchi for instant flavor.

Sauerkraut

Sauerkraut is pleasantly sour cabbage that's made with two simple ingredients: fresh cabbage and salt. Although today sauerkraut is associated with eastern Europe, its history goes back to ancient China as well as ancient Greece and Rome.

The fermentation process for sauerkraut involves a succession of different microorganisms growing in the fermentation vessel. To start, species of *Leuconostoc* tend to bloom, but they're soon replaced by acid-producing lactobacilli. After it's properly fermented, sauerkraut should contain at least 1.5 percent acid (that is, lactic acid produced by the bacteria).

TIP

Raw fermented sauerkraut is a good source of live dietary microbes. When sauerkraut is cooked, you don't get live microbes, but you still get fiber and other nutrients. Here are some ideas for eating sauerkraut:

>> Enjoy a classic sauerkraut-topped hot dog.

>> Use it instead of plain shredded cabbage in fish tacos.

>> Add zip to avocado toast by topping it with some sauerkraut.

>> Chop it finely and add it to potato salad.

Fermented Pickles

Several ways exist to preserve cucumbers, but if you ask me, fermenting them creates the best pickles, hands down. Fermented pickles are a completely different food from the shelf-stable vinegar brine pickles you see on grocery store shelves. Fermented pickles are made with cucumbers and salt brine, with a slightly higher salt concentration than in sauerkraut, creating a slightly less diverse community of microorganisms in the fermentation.

TIP

Fermented pickles are another good source of live dietary microbes, and here's how you can incorporate more of them into your diet:

>> Create a dill pickle dip for vegetables using sour cream, dill, salt, and chopped fermented pickles with a few spoonfuls of brine.

>> Add chopped fermented pickles to egg or chicken salad.

>> Finely chop fermented pickles and use them as a relish to serve with meat, especially rich, fatty types of meat.

Chapter **21**

Ten Myths about Gut Health Debunked

A huge amount of online content exists on the topic of gut health, but beware because you can find misinformation everywhere. When the same information is repeated over and over again online, it takes on the appearance of truth despite experts' efforts to debunk it. And the top search results for gut health topics aren't necessarily written by gut health experts or verified for accuracy. The task of sifting through and finding what's true can be daunting.

Some of the content in this chapter may surprise you because you may not have realized some of the basic information you've read (even on supposedly reputable websites) is false or incomplete. But after you discover these myths and correct the record, you'll be savvier about gut health than the vast majority of individuals.

Many of the common gut health myths have to do with probiotics because they're the most well-known gut-targeting intervention. Here are ten prevalent myths related to gut health along with an explanation of the facts on each one.

All Beneficial Microorganisms Are Probiotics

By far the most frequently touted myth you may encounter in the world at large pertains to something incredibly basic: What is a probiotic? Countless media articles, blog posts, and company websites get the answer to this question wrong. In fact, if you enter this question into your search engine of choice right now, chances are the correct answer won't be among the top results for your search.

REMEMBER

Probiotics are live microorganisms that, when administered in adequate amounts, confer a health benefit on the host. They must be microorganisms whose name and quantity are known, and they must be deliberately ingested. Chapter 10 discusses probiotics in greater detail.

Here are some false definitions of probiotics that you may encounter and why they are incorrect:

>> **Probiotics are a mixture of live bacteria and/or yeasts that live in your body.** Probiotics can be any live microorganisms, not just bacteria or yeasts. And the microorganisms that normally live in your digestive tract or elsewhere in your body — as beneficial as they may be — don't qualify as probiotics because they aren't ingested to give you health benefits.

>> **Probiotics are good bacteria that help keep your gut healthy.** Calling any group of bacteria inherently good is misleading because even so-called good bacteria may be harmful in certain contexts (for example, when the dose is too high or when the immune system that keeps them in check is dysfunctional). For this reason, it's essential to specify the exact bacteria and dose that give you a health benefit. Furthermore, even though many probiotics are ingested via the gut and successfully provide gut health benefits, the probiotic category includes live microorganisms that benefit body sites outside of the gut too, such as the respiratory tract or the vaginal tract.

>> **Probiotics are live microorganisms that are intended to have health benefits when consumed or applied to the body.** If you're taking a scientific approach to finding out if something really works, intention isn't good enough. Either you have proof something works, or you lack proof. Therefore, if a group of live microorganisms is to qualify as probiotics, they need to be tested and shown to give a certain health benefit, not merely seen as having potential or intended to have an effect.

>> **Probiotics are live, active microorganisms ingested to alter the gastrointestinal flora for health benefits.** This incorrect definition implies that the health benefits of probiotics are attributable to the way they alter the

gastrointestinal microbiota. However, probiotic scientists have shown, in most cases, probiotics that successfully provide a health benefit can't be detected in the colon after ingestion so altering the gut microbiota isn't how they manage to achieve their health benefits.

REMEMBER

Remember, any uncharacterized (or unnamed) live microorganisms you can safely consume in foods that don't meet the criteria for being probiotics fall under the catch-all category of live cultures or live dietary microbes. Research on this larger category of live microbes has shown the potential for modest, general health benefits when you consume live cultures in higher numbers in your diet — mainly through fermented foods (see Chapter 20 for some options) or fresh fruits and vegetables.

Fermented Foods Are Good Sources of Probiotics

Many online sources of information misinform you that you can obtain probiotics from a dish of fermented kimchi, a glass of home-fermented kefir, or other fermented foods that contain live microorganisms. This assertion is misleading for two reasons:

>> Even though live cultures are required to create fermented foods, they may not be present by the time the food is consumed because of processing steps such as pasteurization, baking, or filtering. (For example, the microorganisms in sourdough bread are killed when the bread is baked.)

>> If the fermented food does in fact contain live cultures when you consume it, these microorganisms aren't likely to qualify as probiotics because they haven't been tested and shown to give any specific health benefits (which is, by definition, what a probiotic must do). Indeed, testing the microbes in many fermented foods would be more challenging than herding cats — the microbes may not be the same from one batch to the next, making it difficult to know even what the microbes are and their amounts, let alone whether they provide any consistent health benefits.

Don't get me wrong: Fermented foods are a great addition to your diet to promote gut health. But even though fermented foods may be healthy and sometimes provide a source of live cultures in your diet, they don't provide probiotics unless bona fide probiotics (with known types and amounts) are added after the fermentation process is complete. These added probiotics may be present in some commercial versions of fermented foods such as yogurt or kombucha, with the strain or strains specified on the label.

Probiotics Add Healthy Bacteria to Your Gut Microbiome

Over the past two decades, gut microbiome research has yielded some truly exciting results and has given scientists many insights into the mechanics of how diet and other factors affect your health. So I don't blame the probiotics companies for jumping on the gut microbiome bandwagon and trying to make a connection to their products. In fact, I'd argue that probiotic companies, through their marketing efforts, have managed to greatly increase awareness of the gut microbiome among members of the general public.

Yet the claims that probiotics "balance the friendly bacteria in your gut" or "add healthy bacteria to your microbiome" aren't supported scientifically. Some companies' entire schtick is to promise to give you a healthy microbiome — never mind that scientists haven't yet defined a healthy microbiome.

REMEMBER

A probiotic must confer a tangible health benefit of some kind. For many (maybe even the majority of) probiotic products on the shelves, no proof exists that they give any health benefits. But say a certain probiotic does have a study showing it gives you a benefit — for example, alleviating antibiotic-associated diarrhea. Provided it reliably gives this benefit, any effects it has on your gut microbiome along the way (such as balancing or adding bacteria) are less important.

In fact, saying probiotics change your gut microbiome in some beneficial way is almost the opposite of the scientific truth because many scientific studies show that probiotics typically pass right through the digestive tract without leaving a trace. They rarely alter the gut microbiota composition, in other words. Taking all of the science on probiotics together, it's clear that even when probiotics successfully give you a health benefit, they rarely do so by taking up residence in your gut microbiome. They have many possible mechanisms of action — interacting with immune cells or directly affecting gut cells, for example — but changing your gut microbial community isn't a common one. Thus, probiotics aren't a reliable strategy for balancing or adding so-called healthy bacteria to your gut microbiome over the long term.

Different Probiotics Are Interchangeable

This myth is common in the probiotics world. For example, a study on one probiotic *formulation* (that is, a specific form of a product) shows it doesn't reduce the risk of *Clostridioides difficile* infection in hospitalized individuals after they take antibiotics. In the media coverage of this study, the headline typically reads something like "Probiotics ineffective for stopping hospital infections," implying that the entire category of probiotics is no good for this purpose. Yet another probiotic formulation in another study may be shown to provide benefits in this same medical situation. Those who see the media coverage may dismiss the entire probiotic category because one type of probiotic is ineffective for a specific purpose.

Imagine the same logic applied with medicines. A study is released, for example, saying the anti-inflammatory medication adalimumab (which is effective for some autoimmune conditions) doesn't help diabetes. The headline reads "Medications prove ineffective for diabetes." But clearly that's false because many effective diabetes drugs exist and only this one drug is shown to be ineffective in the study.

This example shows why it's important not to paint all probiotics with the same brush. Each probiotic strain has slightly different abilities, and each strain or group of strains is tested for specific health effects. When talking about how effective probiotics are, you should be as precise as possible and talk about the specific strain or formulation in question.

TIP

Normally every strain or formulation must be specifically tested for its safety and efficacy, even if a closely related strain is already shown to work. If you're choosing a probiotic for a certain health issue, find out which exact strain or formulation is shown to give the benefit you're looking for.

The fact that different strains of microorganisms can have different characteristics and activities is exactly why probiotic science is so exciting. The complex jungle of bacteria that exists inside your body is a rich source of strains that haven't all been studied yet. As scientists discover what these microorganisms are capable of and how they interact with the human body, they'll likely discover some that can be administered as new types of probiotics for novel benefits to human health.

Multiple Strains Are More Effective Than Single Strains

Diversity in the gut microbiome is shown to support health, so isn't it better to add a diversity of strains to the gut microbiome when you take probiotics? This logic would seem to support multi-strain products over single-strain products.

But probiotic products with more strains don't necessarily provide greater health benefits than those with single strains — it all depends on what the relevant scientific studies have shown. If your goal is simply to add a greater quantity of live cultures to your diet without seeking a specific health benefit, a multi-strain product may indeed be desirable. But if you want a certain benefit, some single-strain products may be tested and shown to be better for helping you achieve that benefit. Because different probiotic microbes work in different ways according to their characteristics, some may work better alone and others when they're paired with additional microbes.

Note that the same microorganisms may act differently when they're by themselves than when they're members of a complex probiotic mixture, so the benefits of each single strain can't be assumed to be maintained when the strains are part of a group.

You Shouldn't Take Probiotics While Taking Antibiotics

You may have heard that taking probiotics and antibiotics at the same time is a waste of money and effort.

As Chapter 3 explains, living things are too complex to be assigned simple labels of good or bad. This is an example of where the good versus bad narrative falls flat: If you're thinking about probiotics as good bacteria and antibiotics as bacteria-killing agents, logic would seem to dictate that sending good bacteria into your gut while the killing agents are on the loose is a complete waste. But the scientific reality shows otherwise. Certain strains of bacteria, when ingested at the same time as the antibiotics, do in fact produce better health outcomes compared to not taking them. So whatever bacterial warfare is happening in the gut, it ends up being beneficial for your health.

An important caveat, however, is that not all probiotics are beneficial in the context of an antibiotic onslaught. One well publicized study in 2018 showed that a specific probiotic mixture inhibited the recovery of the gut microbiota after antibiotics. The health benefits weren't tracked in this study, however, so it's not certain whether the individuals noticed any changes in health that accompanied their disrupted gut microbiota recovery.

Probiotics Aren't Regulated

You can thank your lucky stars you live in a time when the food and drug supply in most countries is well regulated. Otherwise, what would stop a company from putting a bottle of glue paste on the shelf and calling it peanut butter? You wouldn't know which products you could trust. But currently when you enter a grocery store in most regions you know with reasonable certainty that the products are safe and that they contain what they say they contain.

A common myth is that probiotics aren't regulated, but they're regulated just like any other item for human consumption. Frameworks exist to make sure probiotics are safe, efficacious, and appropriately labeled. Each country regulates probiotics slightly differently, but in general the regulatory framework that applies to probiotics when they are offered for sale to the public generally depends on their intended use: either to maintain health in a healthy person or to treat a certain medical condition.

REMEMBER

Here are some of the common categories that probiotics may fall under in a regulatory sense:

>> Dietary supplement

>> Natural health product

>> Food for special medical purposes

>> Drug

The category determines the applicable regulations — for example, the standards used to judge the effectiveness and safety of the probiotic and also the manufacturing standards.

If a company wants to sell a probiotic product, it must generally go through the required testing, followed by marketing and selling it to customers. Depending on the category as well as the specific country, the timing may differ for when a regulatory authority intervenes or requires notification. Here are some examples of the timing for exercising oversight:

>> The authority must review and approve the data on the product before it is offered for sale.

>> The authority must simply be notified before the product is offered for sale.

>> A company must meet certain conditions and then directly offer the product for sale, with the authority monitoring compliance after it's on the market.

The regulatory oversight isn't necessarily lax in situations where companies can directly offer a probiotic for sale. In these situations, the authorities may exert more control after products are on the market. Such post-marketing surveillance is one way the U.S. Food and Drug Administration (FDA), for example, tries to prevent misleading information and claims about probiotics. Companies are also expected to inform paid social media influencers about what can and can't be said about their products.

With this said, not all companies are equally conscientious. Some companies take the regulatory frameworks very seriously and develop scientific and marketing strategies that take all the nuances into consideration whereas others seemingly flout the regulations to try to give their products an edge. One example of regulatory boundary-pushing occurred during the COVID-19 pandemic: Several companies claimed that their probiotics boosted immunity and therefore were potentially protective against the novel pathogen SARS-CoV-2. Yet they had no actual proof that their product was protective against COVID-19. The FDA sent warning letters to the companies asking them to stop making these claims.

Prebiotics and Fiber Are the Same

A common myth about prebiotics is that they're the same thing as dietary fiber.

Both fiber and prebiotics are items in your diet, undigestible by your body, which promote health in certain ways. But whereas fiber is broad, prebiotics are a much more restricted category.

REMEMBER

Run-of-the-mill fiber may or may not alter the gut microbiome to achieve its health benefits. But for common prebiotic fibers such as inulin, fructo-oligossacharides, and galacto-oligosaccharides, proof exists that they alter the gut microbiome, and this alteration is how they achieve their health benefits. Furthermore, when prebiotics are ingested, most of the microbes in the gut microbiota aren't affected but certain key microbes thrive.

What's important to remember about prebiotics is that their end goal isn't just to help beneficial bacteria grow. When they do help these bacteria grow, they're doing so in service of a health benefit.

Postbiotics Are Metabolites Produced by Bacteria in Your Gut

Be alert when you hear the term postbiotics: Is it referring to molecules produced by bacteria in the gut, such as short-chain fatty acids? Or is it referring to a preparation of killed microbes that provides a health benefit?

TECHNICAL STUFF

The biotics scientific community is still somewhat divided on this postbiotics semantic issue, but by now, most agree with the official scientific definition of postbiotics: a preparation of inanimate microorganisms and/or their components that confers a health benefit on the host. After all, no special name is really needed for the metabolites in your body that are produced by bacteria, because you can simply call them by their chemical names without highlighting their relationship to microbes in the gut. But inanimate/killed/inactivated microorganisms deserve a special category to themselves to mark them as distinct from their live microbial counterparts (that is, probiotics). Notably, the live originator microbe for a postbiotic doesn't have to be an official probiotic.

Despite the growing scientific and regulatory agreement on the term postbiotic, the most common definition you may still find online from nonscientific sources is the one relating to metabolites. The scientific community is working to raise awareness of this term more widely so that regulators, consumers, and other groups are on the same page.

Gut Microbiome Tests Can Give You Information to Shape Your Diet

The promises made by microbiome testing companies can be attractive: Simply test your gut microbes and reveal a personalized diet plan and/or probiotic regimen that benefits your health and gets rid of all your gut troubles.

REMEMBER

The problem is that the science isn't advanced enough to make these kinds of recommendations from knowledge about gut microbes alone. Yes, you can feel free to spend your money and receive an analysis of what groups of microorganisms are living in your gut. This part of the gut microbiome testing service is likely accurate. But the difficulty comes with knowing how to use these results. The largest and most sophisticated research studies in the world haven't managed to find out how manipulating the gut microbiome through diet leads to guaranteed health benefits for an individual person, so no company can truly do this either. Furthermore, most of the diet recommendations from microbiome tests aren't given with overall nutritional balance in mind and may have the inadvertent consequence of narrowing the diversity and nutritional completeness of your diet.

In the future, when the science is solid enough, these gut microbiome analyses will pass the criteria to qualify as medical tests and medical doctors will use them to provide useful clinical information. But currently the tests are offered directly to consumers without verified clinical usefulness.

REMEMBER

The upshot is that you shouldn't rely on the diet advice you get from a gut microbiome test; instead, consult with a registered dietitian who can help you balance and personalize your diet for optimal health.

Index

A

AAD (antibiotic-associated diarrhea), 58

abdominal pain/discomfort, as a digestive symptom, 104–105

abdominal ultrasound, 119

acquired immune deficiency syndrome (AIDS), gut connection with, 91

active cultures, 190

active fluorescent units (AFU), 190

acupuncture, as an intervention for digestive disorders, 132, 139

AD (Alzheimer's disease), gut connection with, 82–83

adaptive immunity, 44

additives, 181–183

adolescence. *See* children and teenagers

adversity, childhood, 312–313

AFU (active fluorescent units), 190

aging. *See* older age

AI (artificial intelligence), 221

AIDS (acquired immune deficiency syndrome), gut connection with, 91

Aidy, Sahar El (professor), 46

Akkermansia, 61, 62, 319

Akkermansia muciniphila, 42, 88, 94

al dente, 248

alcohol
  impact on gut health of, 65
  sleep and, 205

Alidina, Shamash (author)
  Mindfulness For Dummies, 211

allergies, gut connection with, 82

almonds, in Mediterranean Tomato Almond Chicken, 254

ALS (amyotrophic lateral sclerosis), gut connection with, 83

Alzheimer's disease (AD), gut connection with, 82–83

The American Gut Project, 171

The American Journal of Clinical Nutrition (journal), 77

amino acid, 45

AMR (antimicrobial resistance), 60

amyotrophic lateral sclerosis (ALS), gut connection with, 83

anecdotes, 225–226

ankylosing spondylitis (AS), gut connection with, 84

anorexia nervosa (AN), gut connection with, 83–84

antacids, 142

antibiotic-associated diarrhea (AAD), 58

antibiotics
  at birth, 296
  during first year, 306–307
  history and overuse of, 57–58
  influence on gut of, 57–60
  myths about, 342
  during older age, 321
  during pregnancy, 291–292
  probiotics and, 188

antimicrobial resistance (AMR), 60

anus, 26–27

anxiety, gut connection with, 84

apples, 279

applesauce
  Banana Oat Muffins, 271
  Pumpkin Spice Baked Apples, 279

apps, specialized, 154

archaea, 35

arthritis, gut connection with, 84–85

artificial intelligence (AI), 221

artificial sweeteners, impact on gut health of, 65

AS (ankylosing spondylitis), gut connection with, 84

ascending colon, 26

asparagus, in Buckwheat Noodle Miso Soup, 238

asthma, gut connection with, 85

atopic dermatitis, gut connection with, 85–86

autism spectrum disorder (ASD), gut connection with, 86–87

Avocado Dressing recipe, 242

avocados
  about, 183
  Avocado Dressing, 242
  Mexican Lentil Salad, 242

axis, 74

B

Bacillus anthracis, 35

bacon, in Rustic Noodles and Cabbage, 256

bacteria, 34, 35, 340

balanced diet, 176

balancing fats, 179–181

Balsamic Glazed Mushrooms recipe, 259

Banana Oat Muffins recipe, 271

bananas
  Banana Oat Muffins, 271
  Peanut Butter Oat Cookies, 278

barium swallow, 121

barley, in Chicken Barley Soup, 236

basil, in Roasted Vegetable Ratatouille, 247

bathing outdoors, 215

bathroom finding apps, 154

Beanie Brownies with Chocolate Kefir Icing recipe, 277

beer, as a fermented food, 173

behavioral bedtime delay, 204

bell peppers
  Fantastic Veggie Frittata, 249
  Greek Quinoa Salad, 243
  Kale Sausage Soup, 237
  Mediterranean Tomato Almond Chicken, 254
  Quick 'n Tasty Veggie Curry, 250
  Roasted Vegetable Ratatouille, 247

Berman, Rachel (author)
  Mediterranean Diet For Dummies, 66

best before date, on product labels, 226

beverages, 183

Bifidobacterium genus, 38, 77, 296, 299, 308

The Biggest Loser (TV show), 93

Bioessays (journal), 77

bioinformatics, 36

biotics
  about, 131, 184
  confusion around, 184–185
  implementing, 139–140
  postbiotics, 194–196, 301
  prebiotics, 190–193, 196, 321, 344
  during pregnancy, 290
  probiotics, 175, 186–190, 195, 290, 298, 300–301, 313, 321, 338–345
  synbiotics, 193–194, 196, 321

birth
  gut health during, 16–17, 283–284, 293–298
  microbes at, 49–50

birth mode, 294

black beans
  Beanie Brownies with Chocolate Kefir Icing, 277
  Kale Sausage Soup, 237
  Mexican Lentil Salad, 242

Blaser, Martin (author)
  Missing Microbes: How the Overuse of Antibiotics Is Fueling Our Modern Plagues, 80

bloating
  as a digestive symptom, 105
  implementing dietary interventions for, 141
  wardrobe changes for, 142

blood-brain barrier, 48

blue poop challenge, 29

Bodian, Stephan (author)
  Meditation For Dummies, 211

body position, implementing, 140

brain, influence on gut health of, 67–68

breastfeeding, 50, 300

breathing, deep, 212

Bristol Stool Scale, 29, 30

broccoli
  Buckwheat Noodle Miso Soup, 238
  Fantastic Veggie Frittata, 249
  Quick 'n Tasty Veggie Curry, 250
  Savory Miso Noodle Bowls, 252

Buckwheat Noodle Miso Soup recipe, 238

burping, as a digestive symptom, 107–108

Orange Kefir Cake, 272

Peanut Butter Oat Cookies, 278

Pumpkin Spice Baked Apples, 279

Rhubarb Cake, 273

detoxifying, 31

development, guiding, 47–48

diabetes, gut connection with, 89–90

diagnoses

of digestive disorders, 116–121

embracing, 125–126

not having, 135–144

recognizing possible, 15

researching, 126

diarrhea

as a digestive symptom, 106–107

implementing dietary interventions for, 141

infectious, 70

as a symptom of antibiotics, 58

Dicke, William (pediatrician), 122

diet

establishing good habits, 310–311

implementing interventions, 140–141

importance of, 10–11

myths about, 345–346

for newborns, 50

during older age, 320–321

during pregnancy, 289–290

for teenagers, 314–315

diet and exercise apps, 154

dietary changes

about, 216–217

as an intervention for digestive disorders, 128–131

making, 15–16

dietary pattern, 65–66

digestive disorders

about, 115

diagnosing, 116–121

embracing diagnoses, 125–126

major, 122–125

types of interventions for, 127–133

digestive function, as a parameter for assessing gut health, 11

digestive health, 10

digestive symptoms

abdominal pain/discomfort, 104–105

about, 101–102

bloating, 105, 141, 142

burping, 107–108

clarifying, 103–112

constipation, 106, 132, 140

diarrhea, 58, 70, 106–107, 141

distension, 105, 142

gas, 107–108, 141, 142

gastrointestinal (GI) bleeding, 108–109

heartburn, 109, 141, 142

incontinence, 110

managing during pregnancy, 287–288

nausea, 110

regurgitation, 110

small intestinal bacterial overgrowth (SIBO), 111

swallowing difficulties, 111

as a symptom of antibiotics, 59

vomiting, 112

who gets, 102–103

digestive system

about, 19–20

anus, 26–27

esophagus, 24–25

glucagon-like peptide 1 (GLP-1), 31

gut barrier, 20–21

gut chemistry, 30

gut function essentials, 28–31

gut motility, 28–30

gut's nervous system, 28

immune system interactions, 31

large intestine, 26–27

mouth, 24

oropharynx, 24

parts of digestive tract, 22–27

small intestine, 25–26

stomach, 25

G

gallbladder disease, 123–124

gallstones, 288

GALT (gut-associated lymphoid tissue), 31, 43, 284

gamma-aminobutyric acid (GABA), 77

Gandhi, Anusha (patient advocate), 149, 150, 157

garden work, 215–216

garlic
  about, 329–330
  Balsamic Glazed Mushrooms, 259
  Cannellini and Parsley Dip, 266
  Classic Creamed Spinach, 260
  Italian White Bean Soup, 235
  Quick 'n Tasty Veggie Curry, 250
  Savory Miso Noodle Bowls, 252

gas
  as a digestive symptom, 107–108
  implementing dietary interventions for, 141
  wardrobe changes for, 142

gastric emptying study, 120

gastroesophageal reflux disease (GERD), 109, 124, 132, 287

gastrointestinal (GI) bleeding, as a digestive symptom, 108–109

gastroparesis, 124

GBS (group B streptococcus), 297

gene sequencing, 36

genes, microbes and, 51

geography, as a factor influencing gut health, 71

GERD (gastroesophageal reflux disease), 109, 124, 132, 287

germ-free mice, 42

germophobes, 35

gestational age, 296–298

GI (gastrointestinal) bleeding, as a digestive symptom, 108–109

Gibson, Glenn (professor), 190–191

ginger
  Buckwheat Noodle Miso Soup, 238
  Savory Miso Noodle Bowls, 252

glucagon-like peptide 1 (GLP-1), 31, 47

gluten, 87–88

gluten-free diet, 129–130, 168

gluten-testing devices, 155

The Gospel of Wellness (Raphael), 219–220

graft-*versus*-host disease (GvHD), gut connection with, 90–91

Greathouse, K. Leigh (dietitian), 168

Greek Quinoa Salad recipe, 243

group B streptococcus (GBS), 297

guiding development, 47–48

gut
  how it works, 13
  linking to specific diseases, 81–95
  microbes, 13–14
  relationship with physical/mental health, 14
  research on, 78–81

gut barrier, 20–21, 41–43

gut chemistry, 30

gut function, essentials of, 28–31

gut health
  about, 9–10
  components of, 11–12
  conditions and, 112–114
  diagnoses, 15
  dietary/lifestyle changes, 15–16
  identifying symptoms, 14
  importance of, 12
  influences on, 55–72
  managing, 14–17
  meaning of, 10–11
  relationship with overall health, 73–97
  staying proactive, 16–17
  talking about, 143

gut microbiome
  about, 34
  bacteria, 35
  composition, 36–39
  culturing, 35
  diversity and resilience of, 51–53
  gene sequencing, 36
  microbes in, 35–36
  microbes in digestive tract, 39–40
  microorganisms in, 34–35

myths about, 340

role of, 41–48

roles of microorganisms, 40–41

uniqueness of, 48–51

gut microbiome testing, implementing, 141

gut microbiota characteristics, as a parameter for assessing gut health, 11

gut motility, 28–30

Gut: The Inside Story of Our Body's Most Underrated Organ (Enders), 26

gut transit time, 29

gut-associated lymphoid tissue (GALT), 31, 43, 284

gut-brain axis function, 11, 75–77

gut-friendly diets, principles of, 169–184

gut-kidney axis, 78

gut-liver axis, 77–78

gut-lung axis, 75

gut-skin axis, 74–75

GvHD (graft-*versus*-host disease), gut connection with, 90–91

H

Haas, Sidney (doctor), 122

halibut, in Crispy-Topped Halibut, 255

Haskey, Natasha (dietitian), 180

health, progressing toward, 136–142

health-associated microbiome, 52, 73–97

heartburn

as a digestive symptom, 109

implementing dietary interventions for, 141

wardrobe changes for, 142

Helicobacter pylori (H. pylori), 51, 70–71

hemorrhoids, 106

herbal therapies, implementing, 141

HG (hyperemesis gravidarum), 288

HIV infection, gut connection with, 91

HMOs (human milk oligosaccharides), 192, 299, 301

home

as a factor influencing gut health, 72

managing symptoms at, 147

managing symptoms in other people's, 149

honey

Miso Snack Mix, 265

Peanut Butter Oat Cookies, 278

hope, maintaining, 143–144

hormones

about, 31

producing, 77

relationship with the gut, 74

Hudson, Kate (actress), 219

human immunodeficiency virus (HIV), gut connection with, 91

human milk oligosaccharides (HMOs), 192, 299, 301

hydrolysis, 30

hygiene hypothesis, 80

hype, 219, 223

hyperemesis gravidarum (HG), 288

hypnotherapy, implementing, 141–142

I

IBD (inflammatory bowel disease)

about, 75

exercise and, 132

gut connection with, 91–92

managing during pregnancy, 288

IBS (irritable bowel syndrome)

about, 57, 124

exercise and, 132

gut connection with, 92

Ice Bucket Challenge, 83

ice cream, 183

icing sugar

Beanie Brownies with Chocolate Kefir Icing, 277

Chocolate Kefir Icing, 277

icons, explained, 4

identifying symptoms, 14

ileum, 26

immune cells

in gut barrier, 43

modulating, 77

immune system, 43–44, 74

immunosuppressive drugs, as an intervention for digestive disorders, 127

implementing interventions, 139–142

incontinence, as a digestive symptom, 110

indole, 47

infancy, gut health during, 283–284, 298–301

infections
  avoiding, 217–218
  controlling during pregnancy, 292–293
  influence on gut health of, 69–71
  as a symptom of antibiotics, 59

infectious diarrhea, 70

inflammaging, 319

inflammatory bowel disease (IBD)
  about, 75
  exercise and, 132
  gut connection with, 91–92
  managing during pregnancy, 288

insomnia, 69

insulin resistance, 47

interventions
  for digestive disorders, 127–133
  implementing, 139–142

intestinal gas, 29

intestinal permeability test, 120

intestine
  large, 26–27, 40
  small, 25–26, 40

intimacy, managing symptoms during, 152–153

iodine, 165

iron, 164

irritable bowel syndrome (IBS)
  about, 57, 124
  exercise and, 132
  gut connection with, 92

Ishiguro, Ed (professor), 44

Italian White Bean Soup recipe, 235

J

jejunum, 25

Jerusalem artichokes, 330–331

jet lag, influence on gut health of, 69

jicama
  about, 263
  Tangy Jicama Sticks, 263

Johne's disease, 123

journaling, 144, 214

K

kalamata olives, in Greek Quinoa Salad, 243

kale
  Italian White Bean Soup, 235
  Kale Sausage Soup, 237

Kale Sausage Soup recipe, 237

kefir
  about, 333
  Avocado Dressing, 242
  Beanie Brownies with Chocolate Kefir Icing, 277
  Butternut Cheesy Mac, 248
  Chocolate Kefir Icing, 277
  Cranberry Breakfast Cake, 274
  as a fermented food, 173
  Mexican Lentil Salad, 242
  Orange Kefir Cake, 272
  Pumpkin Spice Baked Apples, 279
  Rhubarb Cake, 273

kimchi
  about, 333–334
  Buckwheat Noodle Miso Soup, 238
  as a fermented food, 173
  Kimchi Pancakes, 267
  Savory Miso Noodle Bowls, 252

Kimchi Pancakes recipe, 267

kitchen, equipping and organizing, 198

Koch, Robert (scientist), 35

kombucha, as a fermented food, 173

L

L. johnsonii, 77

labeling, 185, 226–227

Lactobacillus, 38

lactose intolerance, 124–125

lactulose, 120

lactulose breath test, 120
large intestine
  about, 26–27
  microbes in, 40
leaky gut syndrome, 21, 114
leeks
  about, 330
  Double Pea Soup, 239
  Italian White Bean Soup, 235
lemons
  Cannellini and Parsley Dip, 266
  Cardamom Oat Cookies, 276
  Cranberry Breakfast Cake, 274
  Mediterranean Baked Rice, 262
  Quick 'n Tasty Veggie Curry, 250
  Spiced Chickpeas, 268
lentils, in Mexican Lentil Salad, 242
lifestyle changes
  about, 201–202
  avoiding infection, 217–218
  diet, 216–217
  improving sleep habits, 202–207
  making, 15–16
  medical interventions, 218
  outdoors, 214–216
  regular exercise, 207–210
  stress management, 210–214
light, for sleep quality, 205
light exercise, 208
limes
  Avocado Dressing, 242
  Mexican Lentil Salad, 242
  Tangy Jicama Sticks, 263
Linnaeus, Carolus (botanist), 36–37
liquids, for sleep quality, 205
Listeria monocytogenes, 70
live cultures, 190
live microorganisms, 177–178
Living Gluten-Free For Dummies (Van Noy), 130
loperamide, 142
Lotito, Michel, 24
lower esophageal sphincter, 25

low-FODMAP diet, as an intervention for digestive disorders, 130
low-grade inflammation, 47
lumen, 20
lupus, gut connection with, 95

M

macronutrients, 64, 162
macrophages, 43
magnetic resonance cholangiopancreatography (MRCP), 120
main courses
  about, 245–246
  Butternut Cheesy Mac, 248
  Crispy-Topped Halibut, 255
  Easy Chickpea Feta Bake, 251
  Fantastic Veggie Frittata, 249
  Mediterranean Tomato Almond Chicken, 254
  Quick 'n Tasty Veggie Curry, 250
  Roasted Vegetable Ratatouille, 247
  Rustic Noodles and Cabbage, 256
  Savory Miso Noodle Bowls, 252
maintenance diet, as a phase in elimination diets, 129
managing
  gut health, 14–17
  metabolism, 46–47
  stress, 210–214
  symptoms, 137–139, 146–153
mannitol, 120
MAP (*Mycobacterium avium paratuberculosis*), 123
maternal vaginal microbial transfer, 295
meat, 253. *See also specific types*
meconium, 293
medical doctors, 229
medical history, 117
medical interventions, impact of, 218
medications
  as an intervention for digestive disorders, 127–128
  influence on gut of, 57–63
  modifying, 46
  during older age, 321–322

N

NAFLD (non-alcoholic fatty liver disease), 90

nature, as a factor influencing gut health, 72

nausea, as a digestive symptom, 110

necrotizing enterocolitis (NEC), 93, 297–298

neurons, 77

neurotransmitters, producing, 77

news, science, 223

n-of-1 studies, 138–139

noise, for sleep quality, 206

non-alcoholic fatty liver disease (NAFLD), 90

noncaloric sweeteners, as additives, 182–183

noncommunicable diseases. *See* chronic diseases

nonsteroidal anti-inflammatory drugs (NSAIDs)

  influence on gut of, 61–62

  during older age, 322

norepinephrine, 209

NOVA food classification, 184

nutrition, basics of, 162–165

nutritional yeast, in Classic Creamed Spinach, 260

nuts

  Banana Oat Muffins, 271

  Miso Snack Mix, 265

O

oat milk, in Butternut Cheesy Mac, 248

oats

  Banana Oat Muffins, 271

  Cardamom Oat Cookies, 276

  Cranberry Breakfast Cake, 274

obesity, gut connection with, 93–94

old friends hypothesis, 80

older age

  about, 317–318

  changes in microbiota, 319

  diet, 320–321

  maintaining healthy gut in, 318–322

  medications, 321–322

  microbes and, 51

  protecting gut health during, 17

  tips for, 322–324

oligosaccharides, in formula, 301

Oliver, John (talk show host), 222

olives

  Greek Quinoa Salad, 243

  Mediterranean Baked Rice, 262

omega-3/6 fats, 180

165 rRNA gene sequencing, 36

onions

  about, 328–329

  Chicken Barley Soup, 236

  Double Pea Soup, 239

  Easy Chickpea Feta Bake, 251

  Fantastic Veggie Frittata, 249

  Greek Quinoa Salad, 243

  Kale Sausage Soup, 237

  Quick 'n Tasty Veggie Curry, 250

  Roasted Vegetable Ratatouille, 247

  Rustic Noodles and Cabbage, 256

  Zucchini with Parmesan, 261

online information, evaluating, 220–221

oral cavity. *See* mouth (oral cavity)

Orange Kefir Cake recipe, 272

oranges

  Cranberry Breakfast Cake, 274

  Orange Kefir Cake, 272

organ systems, relationship with the gut, 74–78

oropharynx, 24

outdoors, 214–216, 315

over-the-counter medications, implementing, 142

P

Paltrow, Gwyneth (actress), 219

PAMP (pathogen-associated molecular patterns), 78

pancetta, in Rustic Noodles and Cabbage, 256

panko breadcrumbs

  Butternut Cheesy Mac, 248

  Crispy-Topped Halibut, 255

Parkinson's disease (PD), gut connection with, 94

R

RA (rheumatoid arthritis), 85

radiation therapy, influence on gut of, 60–61

randomized controlled trial, 222

Raphael, Rina (author), 228

  The Gospel of Wellness, 219–220

raw foods, 253

rectum, 27

red miso, in Buckwheat Noodle Miso Soup, 238

regulation, myths about, 343–344

regurgitation, as a digestive symptom, 110

relaxation, sleep and, 204

Remember icon, 4

research

  on diagnoses, 126

  on gut, 78–81

resilience, 51–53, 210, 214

resistant starch, 192

restrictive diets, 168

rheumatoid arthritis (RA), gut connection with, 85

Rhubarb Cake recipe, 273

rice, in Mediterranean Baked Rice, 262

Roasted Vegetable Ratatouille recipe, 247

Roberfroid, Marcel (author), 190–191

Rook, Graham, 80, 214

Roseburia intestinalis, 41

rotini pasta, in Butternut Cheesy Mac, 248

Rustic Noodles and Cabbage recipe, 256

S

saccharin, 182–183

salads and soups

  about, 233–234, 240

  Avocado Dressing, 242

  Buckwheat Noodle Miso Soup, 238

  Chicken Barley Soup, 236

  Dijon Dressing, 241

  Double Pea Soup, 239

  Greek Quinoa Salad, 243

  Italian White Bean Soup, 235

  Kale Sausage Soup, 237

  Mexican Lentil Salad, 242

  Summer Watermelon Salad, 243

  Tangy Tuna and White Bean Salad, 241

Salmonella species, 70

SAM (severe acute malnutrition), gut connection with, 94–95

satiety hormone, 31

saturated fats, 179

sauerkraut, 334

Savory Miso Noodle Bowls recipe, 252

scallions

  Kimchi Pancakes, 267

  Summer Watermelon Salad, 243

  Tangy Tuna and White Bean Salad, 241

SCD (specific carbohydrate diet), as an intervention for digestive disorders, 131

SCFAs (short-chain fatty acids), 40–41, 45, 47, 61, 75, 90, 163, 168, 171, 207–208, 319

science

  about, 219–220

  artificial intelligence (AI), 221

  evaluating online information, 220–221

  news, 223

  products and tests, 224–230

  studying, 222

science-washing, 219–220

Scientist Says icon, 4

screens, sleep and, 204

seafood. *See* fish and seafood

Selye, Hans (physician), 210

serotonin, turning tryptophan into, 45

serving size, on product labels, 226

sesame seeds, in Miso Snack Mix, 265

severe acute malnutrition (SAM), gut connection with, 94–95

Shigella, 82

short-chain fatty acids (SCFAs), 40–41, 45, 47, 61, 75, 90, 163, 168, 171, 207–208, 319

SIBO (small intestine bacteria overgrowth), as a digestive symptom, 111

sides and snacks

  about, 257–258, 264

  Balsamic Glazed Mushrooms, 259

  Cannellini and Parsley Dip, 266

vegetable broth
  Buckwheat Noodle Miso Soup, 238
  Chicken Barley Soup, 236
  Double Pea Soup, 239
  Italian White Bean Soup, 235
  Kale Sausage Soup, 237
  Savory Miso Noodle Bowls, 252
vegetables. *See also specific types*
  Fantastic Veggie Frittata, 249
  Quick 'n Tasty Veggie Curry, 250
  raw, 178
video swallow, 121
vigorous exercise, 209
viruses, 35
vitamin A, 164–165
vitamin D, 164, 165
vitamins, 44, 164–165
vomiting, as a digestive symptom, 112

W

walnuts, in Pumpkin Spice Baked Apples, 279
wardrobe changes, implementing, 142
Warning icon, 4
watermelon, in Summer Watermelon Salad, 243
websites
  Cheat Sheet, 5
  Clinical Guide to Probiotic Products Available in Canada, 225
  Clinical Guide to Probiotic Products Available in USA, 225
  U.S. Probiotic Guide, 188
wellness gap, 137
Western diet, 65, 176
white flour
  Banana Oat Muffins, 271
  Cardamom Oat Cookies, 276
  Cranberry Breakfast Cake, 274
  Rhubarb Cake, 273
white miso
  Buckwheat Noodle Miso Soup, 238
  Miso Snack Mix, 265

whole wheat flour
  Banana Oat Muffins, 271
  Cranberry Breakfast Cake, 274
  Rhubarb Cake, 273
whole-fruit challenge, 178
whole-genome sequencing, 36
wine, as a fermented food, 173
work travel, managing symptoms during, 150
workplace, managing symptoms in, 152
World Health Organization (WHO)
  on antimicrobial resistance (AMR), 60
  on chronic diseases, 12
  on noncaloric sweeteners, 182

X

xenobiotic metabolism, 46
X-ray tests, 121

Y

yeasts. *See* fungi/yeasts
Yoga For Dummies (Payne, Feuerstein, and Feuerstein), 211
yogurt
  about, 332
  Beanie Brownies with Chocolate Kefir Icing, 277
  Cranberry Breakfast Cake, 274
  as a fermented food, 173

Z

zinc, 164
zucchini
  Fantastic Veggie Frittata, 249
  Quick 'n Tasty Veggie Curry, 250
  Roasted Vegetable Ratatouille, 247
  Zucchini with Parmesan, 261
Zucchini with Parmesan recipe, 261

About the Author

Kristina Campbell M.Sc., a science and medical writer from Victoria, Canada, has spent the past decade covering gut health and microbiome science for online and print media throughout Europe and North America. She has written hundreds of articles and is coauthor of the textbook *Gut Microbiota: Interactive Effects on Nutrition and Health*, first and second editions (Academic Press) with Drs. Edward Ishiguro and Natasha Haskey. She's also the author of the Amazon bestselling *Well-Fed Microbiome Cookbook* (Rockridge Press). She holds degrees from the University of Toronto and the University of British Columbia.

Kristina is passionate about making science fun and accessible for everyone and building scientific and health literacy. You can find her on X and Instagram at @bykriscampbell and on Mastodon at @bykriscampbell@sciencemastodon.com.

Dedication

Twelve years ago, I was a blogger with an insatiable curiosity about the gut microbiome who wanted to learn as much as possible. This book is dedicated to those amazing scientists (most memorably, Stanley Falkow) who first picked up the phone, answered my emails, or jumped on video calls — you helped me create a foundation of knowledge in this field that serves me well to this day.

And to Danielle and Françoise, you offered me my first important opportunity as a gut health writer, and a front row seat to your incredible skill and strategic thinking. I'll always be grateful.

Author's Acknowledgments

Thank you to Callum, my partner and biggest supporter, who understands what writing takes and always picks up the slack. And Clara and Lewis, your zest for life brings me joy and makes every day an adventure.

Sincere appreciation goes to my wonderful and supportive agent Matt Wagner, who gave this project wings. I also appreciate the team at Wiley — especially Tracy — who managed the project so cheerfully and efficiently. Developmental editor Chad Sievers was a joy to work with and made my words so much better. And I am honored to have worked with Christine Lee, MD as technical editor — she's full of wisdom both as a physician and an academic.

By far the best part of my job is meeting and speaking with all the amazing scientists and other professionals who work in this field. It's a thrill to have some of the people whose work I admire most quoted in this book: Lawrence David, Sahar El Aidy, Natasha Haskey, Bob Hutkins, Ed Ishiguro, Anusha Gandhi, Glenn Gibson, Leigh Greathouse, and Rina Raphael.

Publisher's Acknowledgments

Senior Acquisitions Editor: Tracy Boggier
Project Editor and Copy Editor: Chad R. Sievers
Technical Editor: Christine Lee, MD

Production Editor: Tamilmani Varadharaj
Cover Image: © Atlas/Adobe Stock Photos